AF621518

THE BUTCHER'S BOY FROM CLUN

THE BUTCHER'S BOY FROM CLUN

MY LIFE AS A HEART SURGEON

Francis Wells MA, MS, FRCS FRCPI FEACTS

FONTHILL

First published in Great Britain in 2026 by
Fonthill
An imprint of
Pen & Sword Books Ltd
Yorkshire – Philadelphia

Copyright © Francis Wells 2026

ISBN 978-1-03615-673-2

The right of Francis Wells to be identified as Author of this work has been asserted by him in accordance with the Copyright, Designs and Patents Act 1988.

A CIP catalogue record for this book is available from the British Library.

All rights reserved. No part of this book may be reproduced, transmitted, downloaded, decompiled or reverse engineered in any form or by any means, electronic or mechanical including photocopying, recording or by any information storage and retrieval system, without permission from the Publisher in writing. NO AI TRAINING: Without in any way limiting the Author's and Publisher's exclusive rights under copyright, any use of this publication to "train" generative artificial intelligence (AI) technologies to generate text is expressly prohibited. The Author and Publisher reserve all rights to license uses of this work for generative AI training and development of machine learning language models.

Typeset by Simon and Sons ITES Services Pvt. Ltd., Chennai, India.
Printed and bound in the UK by CPI Group (UK) Ltd, Croydon, CR0 4YY

MIX
Paper | Supporting responsible forestry
FSC www.fsc.org FSC® C013604

The Publisher's authorised representative in the EU for product safety is Authorised Rep Compliance Ltd., Ground Floor, 71 Lower Baggot Street, Dublin D02 P593, Ireland.
www.arccompliance.com

For a complete list of Pen & Sword titles please contact

PEN & SWORD BOOKS LIMITED
47 Church Street, Barnsley, South Yorkshire, S70 2AS, England
E-mail: enquiries@pen-and-sword.co.uk
Website: www.pen-and-sword.co.uk
or
PEN AND SWORD BOOKS
1950 Lawrence Road, Havertown, PA 19083, USA
E-mail: uspen-and-sword@casematepublishers.com
Website: www.penandswordbooks.com

To my parents and grandparents, without whom none of this would have been possible and Joanna, Nicholas, Olivia, Emily, Archie, Florence, Wilfred, Arthur and to Claudia, who are all important in my life.

Learn to preserve your health and in this you will better succeed as you shun physicians, because their drugs are a kind of alchemy about which there are no fewer books than there are medicines.

Leonardo da Vinci. Windsor 19009r.

Preface

If I can stop one heart from breaking,
I shall not live in vain;
If I can ease one life the aching,
Or cool one pain,
Or help one lonely person
Into happiness again
I shall not have lived in vain.

Emily Dickinson, 1890

You may well ask, 'Why did you write this book?' The reasons are several. The first driving force was something of an apologia to my children for the little they saw of me when growing up. I wanted to leave an explanation and description of the reasons that contributed to that. Also, to honour and to highlight the superhuman efforts of my parents to drive me and my two sisters onwards to a better life, despite a difficult family setting. My mother developed severe and progressive multiple sclerosis at a time when the diagnosis was poorly recognised and was entirely by exclusion, with no treatment of any kind available, including supportive care in the home. What she and my father endured can only be imagined. All whilst running a physically demanding business. Watching her suffer and experiencing the humility of our family in a quiet English backwater, treating everyone as an equal prepared me for a life in service to others in a profound way that continues to influence me and my medical practice to this day. Nothing was too much trouble for my father, who gave of himself completely every single day, both in support of my mother and in providing the best service that he could to his customers.

Then I would like to leave some kind of picture of life in the countryside, a world that is disappearing all too rapidly. In a world devoid of mobile phones, online gaming and other addictive distractions, it truly was the last of the idyl of play outside and a real appreciation of nature.

Overcoming the struggle that I faced in getting a place in medical school, coming from a non-medical background, and as the first child to enter university from our valley, I hope may encourage others always to follow their dream and not to be put off by naysayers. To describe the intense and often hellish training that we, the generation of young doctors, experienced having to endure the expected demands of working in excess of 100 hours a week in our aspiration to become professional surgeons in an era of intense competition. The advent of the working time directive has changed all of that, but the profession of medicine remains a hard task master. There are new challenges of overreaching management control and the heightened risk of litigation as a result of often unrealistic expectations raised by the media and cash hungry lawyers.

The two most important mentors in my life were my father and grandfather. Both always had a wise word for any situation and one of my greatest regrets is not really appreciating the profundity of their experience of life, which they gently tried to pass on to me. In my career at Papworth my mentor was Ben Milstein (1918–2013). Ben had graciously stayed on as consultant surgeon at Papworth to allow me to carry out my research year in Alabama. Prior to taking over his job as consultant cardiothoracic and vascular surgeon at Papworth, I had asked him for some sage advice. He replied along the following lines. First, just as does the juggler, keep all your balls in the air. In other words, don't focus on too small an area too soon as you cannot foretell future developments and thus retain a degree of totipotency, to use an embryological term. Second, start preparing for your retirement now.

This first piece of advice led me to a fascinating career in general thoracic, oesophageal, vascular and cardiac surgery along with cardio-pulmonary transplantation. By the second piece of advice, he meant that you should develop interests outside of surgery at an early age and pursue them in such a way that on retirement you can move easily from one world into the next. Ben loved his garden and discussing plants by their Latin names with other expert gardeners. He was a very competent watercolourist, but his greatest love was making stringed instruments. At his retirement event, students from the music department at the university, played for him on a violin, viola and cello, all made with his own hands. That piece of advice was what led me to continue my own love of the arts, art history and the piano. He is sorely missed.

Finally, despite training and working through probably the most exciting period of intrathoracic surgery, it is important for me to say that this is not intended to be an exhaustive review of life as a heart surgeon in the later twentieth and early twenty-first century. Rather it is intended as an overview of my life as a whole, which for me has been as much to do with things outside that world as within it. I hope it may inspire, to some small degree, younger surgeons starting out, to look outside of the world of surgery and find additional ways of enriching their lives.

Francis Wells
November 2025

Acknowledgements

The stars of the show are the patients who have put their trust in me over the decades of my career. The courage and humanity of all of them, along with their relatives, has been truly moving. It is an immeasurable privilege to take a fellow human being into your hands and to reconstruct their heart and lungs, or to remove a diseased portion safely in an attempt to return them to a heathy and normal life. The kindness and gratitude that so many of them show has moved me to frequent tears. The occasions when we fail to restore them to health are devastating and the emotions that are evoked by such failure is difficult for those who are not surgeons to understand. But even in those darkest of moments I have been lifted in spirits by the bravery and generosity of some truly remarkable families. Many continue to stay in touch, still decades later, and their cards and letters always lift one's spirits even on the darkest of days.

There are several people to whom I owe a great debt of gratitude. First and foremost, my parents and grandparents without whom this career would not have been possible. Their total commitment to ensuring that all three of us, their children/grandchildren, had the opportunity to make a successful life for ourselves, was made on the back of severely restricted lives for themselves. Claudia is a rock of stability, and her loving support has been immensely helpful in the resetting and refinement of my life and also in the development of this project.

Helen, mother of Joanna and Nicholas bore the brunt of their development, and her efforts are manifest in two beautiful adults with model children of their own. Thereza gave to me Olivia, who is developing into an admirable young woman. All of my children and grandchildren give me a deep pleasure and it is enormously satisfying to observe them as they grow in life.

The headmasters of respective primary and secondary schools, Mr Guppy and Rev. Jeff Roberts, both played significant parts in helping me along by seemingly believing in me despite my initial scholastic mediocrity. Once through the starting gate for medicine Professors Hamilton, Glenister, Sir Tiny Maini and Arthur Makey were bulwarks in my training. Dr J T Scott, Professor Hugh de Wardener and John Pendower were inspirational for me.

Once graduated Christopher Lincoln, Matthias Paneth, Peter Goldstraw, Professor Sir Roy Calne and Jim Mousley propelled me onwards through the ranks of surgical training. Latterly Ben Milstein, Sir Terence English, Dr Jim Kirklin, Professor John Wallwork, Drs Craig Miller, Tyrone David, Randy Chitwood and Professor Alain Carpentier played significant parts in my development as a cardiac surgeon.

Colleagues at Papworth Hospital were always, and remain, supportive and encouraging, even in the most difficult of times. Special mention must be made of Stephen Large, direct contemporary of mine with the most robust and obtuse sense of humour I have ever encountered. Even after turning his Volvo car upside down after ramming a hospital tug whilst exhausted from untold hours in the operating room, he staggered from the wreckage with a huge smile on his face. Len Shapiro, consultant cardiologist, with whom I almost grew up in the specialty, holds a special place. Implacable in the direst situations and always honourable, his skills in the catheter laboratory were second to none.

In chest medicine Dr Robert Rintoul is one of the smartest physicians I know and has carried forward the lung cancer centre that I started with energy and commitment to a research-based approach that is respected throughout the world. In earlier years the support from Drs John Shneerson and John Stark for me as a young enthusiast enabled me to achieve a great deal in reshaping the respiratory service.

Throughout my time at Papworth I could not have completed the work that I have without excellent secretarial support. Jackie Manson was the first and helped me set up my practice when I was even more disorganised than usual. Annette followed her and was extremely efficient and admired by our patients. Julie Mazzone took over and was with me for over twenty years and managed my several faux pas, such as leaving vital radiographs in the overhead bin on an Air France jet on a trip to Paris for an international meeting, finding a way to retrieve them and to get them to me just before I had to speak. Finally Joanna Aveling, my ever patient and hard-working current secretary, who is greatly loved by the patients and for whom nothing is too much trouble. Her calming voice and cheerful demeanour is quoted to me almost every day by patients that she has dealt with. The role of these wonderful people has never been properly recognised by the management who have physically divorced them from us by placing them in an office 14 miles away.

In management there are fewer memorable faces, but head and shoulders above them all is Stephen Bridge, the most empathic and supportive manager of them all. Most Friday evenings he would make his rounds to enquire how his consultants were getting on and offer his support; something not seen since his departure.

None of what we do is possible without anaesthetic, perfusion and nursing support. There are too many to list all by name but Dr Amo Oduro, with whom I tackled some of the most remarkable lists on a Friday, Don Bethune and John Kneeshaw and Ray Lattimer stand out. Amo, always with a ready smile even as things were turning for the worst, Don with his steady and sound skills and John, one of the swiftest anaesthetists I have worked with. All have bailed me out of difficult situations, and I am ever grateful to them. There are myriad nurses, but standing out more than most was lovely Pam Blomiley. Aunty Pam was always there to support patients and doctors alike, with a gentle voice and a heartwarming laugh. She is greatly missed.

Pathologists Martin Goddard, Susan Stewart and Peter Stovin provided expert support, and all worked beyond the hours that they should have done. In earlier years, bacteriologist Bill Newsom encouraged me in useful research and was not slow to challenge management in the improvement of facilities where he saw it necessary.

These people, and many more are the ones who have made Papworth what it became. Their skill, knowledge and sheer hard work gave that small tuberculosis hospital, founded out in the countryside, the worldwide reputation that it gained steadily over the years. Sadly, the new generation of managers have no sense of historical perspective and the importance of the real champions of our progress is not celebrated by them at all. Indeed, it seems that the consultants are to be reduced to just another employee to be controlled and demonised if necessary, to allow control of the dedicated professionals with really intelligent minds, by those of real mediocrity.

Contents

Introduction

Shouts of 'Look out, jump, quickly, get out', rang loudly around the ring. I was swept off my feet high into the air and passed from one pair of strong hands to another with men leaping over the five barred fence around the sales ring. As I turned to look back at where I had been ejected, I could see a long horn steer charging across the ring from the weighing scales. A few remaining men of every shape, size and age, desperately trying to get out of its path. But then, pinned between the horns of the raging animal, I could see a large, elderly farmer going down under the force of the animal's charge. Then in my peripheral vision a shape flashed over the bars and into danger. Without hesitation, the raging animal was wrestled to the ground by its horns, freeing the hapless downed farmer. Eager hands reached in to grab and drag the winded man to safety. Once the injured farmer had been secured on the safe side of the rails, the hero in the ring released the horns of the steer and leaped to safety, to tumultuous cheers from everyone present. The hero… my father Frank Wells, the butcher from Clun. That day at the auction was unlike any other, but for Dad, the business of buying livestock had to continue as usual.

We were in the process of buying animals for the forthcoming week for our shop in that beautiful, unspoiled village, in south-west Shropshire. Each Monday, alternating, between Craven Arms and Ludlow, there was a market for the sale of sheep, pigs and cattle between farmers and butchers. Dad would arrive at the auction yard mid-morning in either Craven Arms or Ludlow, having spent the early part of the day cleaning the slaughterhouse with Charlie (my great uncle) and Grandad, so that it was spotless. On arrival he would go around all of the animals in their pens to pick out which ones he would bid on.

They were arranged in groups of animals from each of the farmers, all of whom Dad would know personally. At the opening of the sale the animals would have been inspected by the auctioneers, usually Jackson and

McCartney's, along with professional meat inspectors. The sale progressed quickly with each bidder having their own private way of signalling, almost imperceptibly, to the auctioneer. The sheep and pigs were sold in their pens, but the cattle were brought into the parade ring, having entered over a large weighing scale. The auctioneer was elevated above the bidders on a wooden dais. He called the rapidly rising bids in staccato fashion, bringing down the hammer at the final price. It was all very exciting for a young boy accompanying his father into the big world of business on the hoof, literally speaking. Prizes were awarded for the best animals in their class. Indeed, Dad prided himself on buying the best. The rosettes indicating those animals, were prominently displayed in the shop along with the well-hung meat. On market days in the interwar years, elaborate exhibitions of the meat adorning the outside of the shop were a common site. We grew up in a world where moderate exposure to 'dirt' was perceived as a good thing for our immune development. Not so with the advent of heavy-handed health and safety regulations in the modern world.

It was well-known that the Wells's sold only the finest quality meat, personally chosen, bought on the hoof, and prepared on site in our own slaughterhouse in Clun. It was not bought generically from an abattoir, where quality could not be controlled to the same degree. In later years, as the word spread, customers travelled from as far afield as Shrewsbury and Birmingham for their meat, especially for important occasions. On market day, following the sale, we would go to the cashier's office at a pre-arranged time to pay for the animals that we had bought. The farmers that we had bought from would also be there. Then a rather archaic practice of exchanging 'luck money' would take place. After paying the auctioneers, Dad, the buyer, would secretively palm money in notes to the farmer from whom the animals had been bought. The practice was expected, and, as far as I am aware, is still in use, especially in the Welsh border market Towns. It seemed like a quaint form of bribery to me, but it didn't alter the animals that Dad wanted to buy, which were chosen on the grounds of quality.

Butchery was a business that I hated but was the source of our livelihood. Much later in life my father confided in me that he had hated it as well, especially the slaughter of those poor animals. After his retirement, thinking he would appreciate it, I gave him a large painting of the heads of cattle. We both found them quite beautiful animals. To my surprise, on my next visit I found that the picture had been relocated to wall space that was not readily visible and on questioning him, he declared that he was sorry, but it reminded him of all the animals that he had slaughtered over the years, and that now he was removed from it, he found it disturbing. This brought home to me just how difficult life must have been for him, unable to remove himself from an occupation that he had found so distasteful.

Dad was born in an apartment in the walls of Ludlow Castle on 28 May 1927. He became the only child of Gertrude (née Brookes) and Charles Edgar Wells, my grandfather. His sister Dorothy sadly died before reaching the end of her first year of life. She was spoken about only very rarely and I know no more of her.

My grandfather had served throughout the terrible ordeal of the First World War. During that catastrophic conflict, he had volunteered for the Royal Engineers. He had been in charge of some of the trains that moved the massive guns to the front, the so-called, Big Berthas. His story was a fascinating one, signing up immediately to fight for his country at the commencement of the war, but more of his experiences later.

On returning from France, Grandad had worked with relatives on his wife's side of the family, the Brookes and Babbages, in a shop in Ludlow prior to buying the business in Clun. However, I know little of his choice to set up his own butchery business. Shortly before Dad was born in 1926, Grandad took over the butcher's shop in the main square in Clun and began the family business.

My father was just too young for the Second World War, but became snarled up in the now almost occult war of partition in the middle east; a messy conflict whose legacy, conflated with the divisive Balfour declaration of 1917 and the Sykes/Picot agreement of 1918, continues to this day with murder and mayhem on a massive scale. Uncountable lives have been lost and lives ruined.

He was a very tall and athletic figure, with angular good looks. He was kept fit by the arduous work in the butchery business. I would see him, with a complete side of beef on each shoulder, running from the slaughterhouse to the shop to minimise wasted time. He always had a ready, broad and warm smile in almost any circumstance and effused an aura of safety and kindness. Nothing was too much trouble for his customers. He was frequently to be heard advising the young farmers' wives on the preparation and cooking of all cuts of meat and knew the differences between French and traditional English cuts. He was interested in everything around him and despite a limited education was very well informed and remarkably knowledgeable. Both he and my grandfather were extremely hard working, and I cannot ever remember either of them complaining about anything, but always having a determination to get things done and in as pleasant a way as possible for all concerned. Their commitment to working until the job was completed infected my own attitude towards work which had consequences for a life in medicine, as there is never an end to what needs to be done. They both had an exceedingly good sense of humour and always saw things through the eye of reasoned optimism. Both loved music and were given to bursting into song, my grandfather with renderings of the old First World War and music hall ditties and my father with his version of the American classics of Bing Crosby with a very similar voice. They both loved people and were well loved in return by the folk in the town. Wherever we went they had a smile and warm greeting for everyone they met, friend or stranger alike. I am tempted to add, 'regardless of colour, creed or persuasion', but it really is redundant to speak of them in that way as they were blind to perceivable differences and treated all with the same respect, so that my sisters and I were really unaware of racial, social or religious bias until we left the confines of the Clun valley.

My mother was equally as hard working and respectful of others. Mother and father had quite different qualities. Mum was much stricter and something of a disciplinarian, suffering fools less gladly than my father. Although she didn't really have the opportunity to develop her intellect in a demonstrable way, it was clear to see a sharp mind with a speed of computation of maths and English that was clearly above the average. She had trained as a primary school teacher and taught in Clun School, which is probably how she had met my father, although the details of that story are not known to me. I remember reports from villagers of how much she had been liked as a teacher and how grateful they had been to her for her patience and help. This latter appreciation was interesting, as we seemed not to receive a lot of those qualities in the home; towards us, her own children, there seemed to be quite a lesser degree of tolerance. This, of course, is seen from the perspective of us as children, who were not always able to understand how our presence and behaviour impacted upon her as a parent. What is clear is the fact that she fiercely fought our corner in all situations and almost certainly was the one who, in the most determined way, drove us on to achieve important things in our lives.

The utterly disabling impact of severe progressive multiple sclerosis from her early forties had an impact on all of us, but of course maximally upon her. The strength of mind that she exemplified was remarkable and its power only becomes more and more clear to me and my siblings as we progress through life. It was the void that multiple sclerosis produced that our grandparents filled. Both acted in loco parentis, and our grandmother in particular maintained the daily running of the house, both before and after the appearance of multiple sclerosis. Prior to its development, Mum was very active in running the business in all of its phases, from serving in the shop to delivering the meat from the delivery vans, to completing the necessary book work.

Prior to commencing work in the business, my father's ambition was to be an engineer, a subject that he showed significant talent for whilst serving in the R.E.M.E. (Royal Electrical and Mechanical Engineers). His notebooks remind me of the Renaissance notebooks of Alberti and Leonardo, a wonderful combination of beautifully legible writing and technical drawings. His ambition was thwarted by the premature death of my grandmother Gertrude Wells at the age of fifty-nine of a myocardial infarction one month before my birth in February 1950. Being an only child, he was forced, out of loyalty to my grandfather, to enter the family business. His ambitions dashed, and with only the school certificate from the local secondary modern school in Bishop's Castle (the only local secondary school for many miles around), my father was pushed into a life in the world of butchery. I am certain that he could have escaped from it, if given different circumstances, and the opportunities that he and our mother were to give to me and my two sisters Rosamond and Charmian. However, it was a family business and with the premature death of his mother, he felt the duty to support my grandfather Charlie Wells (1895-1974). Had not my father (28 May 1928–16 May 2019) and my mother, Violet (17 December 1920–20 January 2003) stepped in to share in the running of the business it would probably have been too much for my grandfather alone, especially having also to bear the grief of losing his wife at such a relatively young age. Theirs was a particularly close and loving relationship.

They were redoubtably assisted by Charlie Griffiths, who turned out to be my great uncle on my mother's side of the family. Surprisingly, I was not to know this for many years. Charlie had also survived the First World War, spending most of the time as a runner, as depicted in the recent movie *1917*. That he survived at all is little short of a miracle as the great majority of those men were killed running to and from the front under intense sniper fire and heavy bombardment. Perhaps his short stature, standing little more than 5 feet tall in his stockinged feet helped make him a more difficult mobile target, but still his survival was almost miraculous.

Charlie's sister, my maternal grandmother Minnie Mold (1894–1994) was the lynchpin of the family. Granny was essential to keeping everything running behind the scenes, cooking, cleaning and really acting in loco parentis to us children as mother and father were in the shop from dawn to dusk, Monday to Saturday.

Sunday mornings were taken up by 'doing the books'. This was an energy sapping exercise because of my mother's meticulous approach to detail. Dad would have been happy to complete it in half the time. Gifted with a mathematical brain which undoubtedly would have allowed her to complete a degree in mathematics, Mum could add long lists of numbers in her head, which were always checked with an early calculator only to find that she was consistently, and infuriatingly, correct.

Voluble arguments were common, and I came to hate these mornings and usually escaped to my paternal grandfather's house for peace and quiet, returning for the Sunday lunch together. This was always a roast with all the trimmings and a pudding, often a steaming suet pudding with lashings of Lyle's golden syrup and homemade custard, a glorious atherosclerotic enhancing diet from which we all seemed to prosper in fine health, fortunately living quite long lives. This was the setting in which my sisters and I grew up.

It all seems such a very long time ago now and so far away from the life I moved on to. Now a heart surgeon with more than forty years practice behind me and experience of a lot of the world, my move from local butcher's boy to senior heart surgeon in Cambridge seems almost mythical. It could not and would not have been achieved without all the effort, commitment, unstinting support, and massive compromises that our parents and grandparents made for us. Both of my sisters achieved great things also, one a lawyer, the other a person of significance in the regulatory affairs in the pharma business.

In recent times, Clun produced one notable person of modest fame: Simon Kirk. Simon and I sat next to each other at the back of the class in St George's Primary School. Simon's brother Miles was murdered by the IRA on a tour of duty in Northern Ireland. A shocking event which brought home to us the depth of the tragedy that was then euphemistically named 'The Troubles'. The shock was felt throughout the community. Simon and I used to pretend to play the drums together on our wooden desktops with a pair of twelve-inch rulers, maddening the teacher in the room. Simon went on to become the drummer in the highly successful rock band The Free. Many years later, on a trip to New York with my son Nicholas, we managed to get tickets to see Ringo Star and his All-Star band at the famous Radio City Music Hall in the centre of Manhattan. Towards the end of the show, Ringo was calling onto stage several rock friends to play with the band and to my astonishment he called on Simon, whom he then told to take over the drums as he regarded him as a better drummer than himself. At the end of the show I said to Nicholas, 'Let's go round to the stage door and see if I can reconnect with Simon.' We rushed around and were in the first row behind a cordon of police and a low barrier. Eventually our patience paid off as out he came with Ringo and other members of the band. I called across to him, 'Hey Simon, do you remember me?' He turned and after a short, but intense gaze he called out, 'Yes of course, it's the butcher's boy from Clun.'

My journey from a small country town to the hot bed of heart surgery has not been easy and I have often been told that I don't have the characteristics of a typical heart surgeon, not brash or arrogant, and far too sensitive, but I always had the desire to do something practical with my hands and the romanticism to envisage working on the human heart as the ultimate human endeavour. I have been lucky to have been able to follow that path, even though it has generated a lot of trauma in my life.

This, then is my story: from butcher's boy to heart surgeon, from slaughterhouse to operating theatre. The paradox, as will become clear, is that I am a surgeon whose heart truly lies in the world of the arts. Whether that could ever have led to success as measured by any of the usual means is conjectural and, as I hope to show, a life in surgery has been and continues to be immensely rewarding.

1

Life in a Sleepy English Village

> Clunton, Clunbury, Clungunford and Clun, Are the quietest places under the sun.[1]

My childhood in Clun was truly a special time. The town lies at the junction of three valleys amongst beautiful rolling hills on the Welsh border. Nine miles away, on the main Shrewsbury to Ludlow Road, is Craven Arms which, as the name implies, is an unattractive town. Turning off this highway you take the road towards Clun. Very quickly a wide, flat-bottomed, post-glacial valley opens up in front of you. The fairly steep bordering hillsides are covered with pine forests and meandering along the floor of the valley is the River Clun. The fields are verdant and the hamlets of Clunton and Clunbury that you pass through are centuries old. You truly feel as though you are stepping back in time.

The town of Clun sits in the northern region of the Welsh Marches. The term is used in the Domesday Book and refers to that area of south Shropshire and its environs using the term, the Marche of Wales. Interestingly, the population of Clun recorded in The Domesday Book is 650, which is almost identical to that recorded in the 2011 census of 680. Thus emphasising its importance as a centre for trade in those early days, as a crossing point of the river for drovers taking their flocks from central Wales to markets within England. The meaning of the word marche is 'a border area' and is derived from the old French word *marche* [walk].

The Clun valley has a history from the dawn of known civilisation with early stone tools from the Neolithic period discovered there, and evidence of lake dwellings on stilts from that period. In the 780s, Offa, King of Mercia (747–796), commanded the building of a defensive dyke to keep out the Welsh as part of his plan to quell their frequent incursions. The earth wall and ditch, Offa's Dyke can be seen running across the Clun valley, very close to our home, and indeed visible from my father's retirement house.

In latter times, there were heroic stands against the Romans led by Caractacus, a first century British chieftain and early guerilla leader, with several hit and run victories over the Romans. He was only finally defeated by Publius Ostorius Scapula when, as myth has it, he took on the Romans in open battle. Caer Caradoc (Fort Caradoc), an early earthworks fortress in the hills between Knighton and Clun is said to be one of his strongholds, although much of the works may pre-date that period. The outline can still be seen in the hills on the road between Clun and Knighton. Between the two hills there is a romantic gulley with a stream running through it, where Caractacus was supposed to have wooed a beautiful local peasant girl and made her is wife. Old drovers' tracks, now mostly single-track roads, wind all around and over the hills with solitary farmhouses scattered along their path, the inhabitants all known to my parents and to whom their regular deliveries of meat were made.

There are elements of Clun church that are Saxon. The entrance and tower are from the tenth century. On the west door, which is medieval, are a lot of rusty nails. The story goes that miscreants had their ears cut off and pinned to the door as a deterrent to others. The nave has the classical dog-toothed decorative Norman arches. There has been heavy restoration over the years and clear distinction between restored parts and authentic original work is difficult to decipher. It is, however, a beautiful and serene old church where, as children, we spent most Sunday mornings in Sunday school.

With evidence of continuous human settlement going as far back as 5,000 years, it was impossible not to feel immersed in history, growing up in this beautiful countryside. It was quite common for us children to find stone-age flint tools as we wandered around on the tops of the hills. Amongst them would be flint arrow heads and knives. The romance of holding a flint knife so beautifully chosen and knapped to fit the palm of the hand never lost its excitement for me. Those that we found we gave to the museum and many of them still exist in that collection today.

My grandfather used to regale me with mythical stories of these sacred places as we drove between the towns in our delivery van. The stories were made more memorable by the somewhat uncomfortable fact that the van was filled with suffocating smoke from Grandad's strong cigarettes, a habit inculcated in most of the soldiers in the First World War to still their nerves in the face of the onslaught of battle.

Following his invasion of England in 1066, William, Duke of Normandy, the conqueror of Harold, who was head of the Anglo-Saxon forces, had persistent struggles to retain his hold on the English. He established the

Marcher Barons to control the marauding Welsh. Roger de Montgomery had been given twenty-seven manors by William after defeating Eadric the Wild, whose forces had been harassing those of William in the area. Roger was then created Earl of Shrewsbury, and gifted Clun to Robert Fitz Picot de Say who was an early arrival with William and his forces. For loyal services rendered during the conquest, William also granted Robert the estates at Stokesay, a nearby estate on the outskirts of what is now Craven Arms, and styled him Lord of Clun. Robert ordered the construction of Clun Castle which, to this day, is an impressive building of the classical motte and bailey style. Its purpose was to defend the border from marauding Welsh tribes who regularly plundered across the region. During much of this time Clun was considered a part of Wales rather than Shropshire, hence the border was a virtual one and was challenged regularly. As a result of this proximity to Wales the south Shropshire accent has a significant Welsh influence, which can be heard clearly in the singing voice of the locals.

The family name of Say, is derived from the village of Sai in Orne, eastern France. Domesday records that Robert held twenty-six other manors. His wife Isabel outlived him and went on to have two further marriages. The last, to William FitzAlan around 1155, brought the barony and lordship of Clun to the FitzAlan family. Just away from the centre of the town is a large house that I always found quite foreboding as a child, named FitzAlan house, reprising the distant influence of that family.

By 1319, the earl of Arundel administered the law in that 'hundred' and it has remained in the barony of the Duke of Norfolk Lord Arundel, who remains the baron of Clun to this day. The hundreds were small areas of land capable of supplying 100 men to fight when required. Clun was granted an early town charter in the fourteenth century.

Stokesay castle also played its part some two centuries later in memorable history as a place that the two princes Edward V and Richard of Shrewsbury, Duke of York, spent some time. It was owned by Richard, Duke of Gloucester, who later became King Richard III. How long the young princes stayed there is not known, but it is believed that it was a temporary residence for them as children. Myth has it that it was from there that they were taken to the Tower of London, from whence they disappeared.

The region was popularised in the late nineteenth century by the romantic novelist Mary Webb and an English cleric Francis Kilvert in his diaries.

During that period in the middle of the last century, contact with the outside world seemed remote and was achieved mainly through the radio. Television was a late feature, made even less relevant to daily life because of the terrible local reception. To visit any other village or town, meant a drive through exquisite country in every direction. The rolling hills of the

Clun Forest, extend into the sparsely inhabited Welsh hills. This was our playground, where we were allowed to roam from dawn to dusk. We still had very distinct seasons. Winter brought snow and ice, and the summers, seemingly endless sunshine. The winter of 1964 saw twenty-foot drifts on the hills around Clun, through which we had to battle our way to deliver the meat to hill farms.

Still today the campaign for the protection of rural England has suggested that Clun is one of the most tranquil locations in the country. Relatively unspoilt, it is still a true representation of the words of A. E. Houseman in his celebrated poetry collection, *A Shropshire Lad*, whose poem continues:

> In valleys of springs or rivers, By Ony, Teme and Clun, The country for easy livers, The quietist under the sun.[1]

Clun remains a little known, quiet idyllic place, barely discovered other than by a few hardened hill walkers and the Green Man followers, who descend upon the town in their hordes on a Monday in early May, bringing welcome income into the town. Smothered in green velvet, Phrygian caps, and other mock medieval garb they approach the centuries old bridge in the centre of the town for the fight between the Ice Queen and the Green Man. Ominously, a myth suggests that should the Ice Queen win, there will be no summer. I don't think that this has been put to statistical test.

That fourteenth century bridge at the nadir of the town, gave rise to the saying that, 'whoever crosses Clun bridge returns sharper than when went'. Having to cross it in both directions every day to go to school, it seemed that I was exempt from this myth.

Although Clun is a very small town, it was quite self-contained in the shops and utilities that were available. Butchers, bakers, grocers, clothes shops, sweet shops, haberdashery and ironmongers and even a tailor were all there. I was reliably informed that for the approximately 600 inhabitants in the town and environs there were no less than thirteen public houses of various sizes and scale, from someone's front room with the beer brewed in the outhouse on Church street, to large establishments like the Buffalo's Head, opposite our butcher's shop, where Sir Walter Scott is said to have stayed and written part of his novel, *The Betrothed*. My grandfather bought the post office across the square from our shop and turned into a sweet shop; joy of joys for us as children, although not so good for the teeth. Visits to the dentist in Knighton, 7 miles away, were anxious times. He seemed to be very short of local anaesthetic and only to have blunt dental drills. I can still hear the shrill sound of the drill and the sudden bursts of pain as drilling ensued. One memory that stands out in my mind is of my sister Rosamond returning with Dad in our white car, with her head out of the window and blood smeared along the side of it, swept there with the passing wind. Knowing that it was my turn the following week caused a degree of anxiety.

Early in his development of the business, one of my grandfather's innovations was to rent out the front room of our house to a travelling dentist. He used to visit on a Tuesday afternoon to service pre-arranged appointments. A service for the town but also a small money spinner for the family. Despite this practice ending before my memory becomes reliable, there remained a brass plaque on the wall outside our front door advertising it.

Being something of a shy child my world only extended beyond the market square with the walk to school. It was the central focus of the town and buzzed with activity on market days. Strangely, being sent on an errand to the newsagent or hardware store at the far end of the town always instilled a slight sense of foreboding in me.

The coming of the supermarkets has caused a gradual change in the town, bringing about the closure and forced adaptation of some of the shops. Also, there has been a slow migration from Birmingham and other major cities to the country, buying properties often occupied by the same families for many generations. Other than farming and related trades, occupation for the younger folk is limited, driving many to leave for more varied professional opportunities, my sisters and I being among them.

Before the advent of the tractor and other heavy farm machinery, life in this farming community relied heavily on real horsepower. To service the horses there were two blacksmith forges. They were only fifty yards apart, close to the old bridge. One had closed before my memory begins but the remaining functioning one was at the foot of Bridge Street. On our way back from school, it was a treat for us children to stand at the entrance of the forge and watch the blacksmith super heating the fire with hand or foot pumped bellows; the coals glowing white hot and the metal horseshoes yellow with the heat. The smell of the burning keratin of the horse's shoe when the hot metal was fixed to the hooves remains in the memory. There were several Shire horses, used to pull the heavily laden drays, still in regular use. Those magnificent beasts were favourites of mine. They exude power and grace. In the Middle Ages, they were bred as war horses capable of carrying knights in full armour. As that tragic purpose declined, they were transitioned into farm horses, doing everything that a modern tractor went on to do. For heavier jobs they were aided by yet another common sight at that time: steam traction engines. These were used to pull the very heavy machinery. My grandfather, a steam train driver himself before and during the great war, used to revel in the sight and sound of these enormous beasts of steam and steel. He used to take me to an annual steam engine rally in Bishop's Castle, a nearby town. The sight of these majestic machines being driven by steam power, the drivers' faces usually caked with coal soot from feeding the boiler which generated the steam, was mesmerising to a young child.

At that time the railway ran through a village close to us, Aston-on-Clun, and we would go and watch the trains pass by through the countryside with a long trail of steam and smoke streaming from the smokestack and an accompanying whistle to warn of their approach to the station. The unmistakable loud chuffing of the steam driving the wheels lives long in the memory. Those lines all disappeared under the leadership of Dr Richard Beeching, who closed over 2,000 stations and 4,500 miles of track in the early 1960s. It was in response to the conservative government's desire to reduce the costs of running the railways. Very short-sightedly, Harold Macmillan, the then prime minister, enthusiastically backed the plan, thereby isolating many of the poorer citizens of the countryside. Famous for his saying that Britons had 'never had it so good', this act singly reduced the quality of living for many. 67,000 railway workers lost their jobs. It emasculated the railways and the results are felt more than ever today, cutting off those unable to run a car, destroying the ease of travel into the towns and cities from their rural homes. Buses were substituted but had none of the charm and rarely ran on time.

Following heavy rain in the hills above the town, the Clun River overflowed regularly. As a result, the forge and nearby houses were flooded. There was a permanent water mark on their walls, registering the level to which the river rose. Further down the river was a ford which cars were able to drive through when the water was at a normal level. As a child it was always an excitement to cross at that point, not knowing if we might get stuck in the middle of the river.

When we were growing up, the major event of the year was the Clun Carnival and Show. The big day is always a Saturday in early August. The format of this centuries old, daylong celebration begins with a parade through the town of a column of drays (large trailers for moving hay, barrels, and other farming goods) decorated in a variety of themes. Following the drays, children, and adults of all ages, dressed as fictional or political characters, stroll along in procession. They were led by a visiting Welsh mining town band along with the local Clun band, usually led by my grandfather, proudly manipulating his drum major's mace. I always felt my chest swell with pride as he marched by with his head held high and his back as straight as a ramrod, receiving the cheers of the crowd. As little 'Johnny or Jane', in fancy dress passed by, family groups and friends cheered their encouragement. Bringing up the rear on her royal dray was the carnival queen seated, somewhat precariously, on her throne, surrounded by her attendants. The queen and her entourage were chosen at a dance in the memorial hall the week before, where a beauty parade would take place. It is a role highly prized by many of the girls in the town. I don't think that as yet there has been a Carnival King, but it could be a fun idea to explore. Once the parade has completed its tour of the town, the queen's dray is moved to the centre of the main square, near our shop front. After a short speech by a dignitary of some form, she is officially crowned Queen for the following year. In 2016, my father had been honoured with the task but was struck down with a stroke and I was asked to take his place. Although used to public speaking in far flung places, I was surprisingly nervous addressing the home crowd.

During the preceding week, frantic activity could be detected behind closed and locked doors of barns around the valley, as secret preparations were made. The chosen themes for the decorations were a highly guarded secret. Their great unveiling on the Saturday morning as they made their way to the assembly point at the top of the town, always drew a large crowd. Before the parade began, all were judged in varying categories and prizes awarded. The sight of the winning children proudly sporting their rosettes was always moving.

On the Bailey of the old castle grounds, several marquees were erected during the days preceding the carnival. A broad range of arts, crafts, culinary and horticultural produce are put on show within them the night before and, yes, there are prizes for the largest marrow and other horticultural clichés. Judges comprised of local dignitaries, choose the prize winners during the morning. Dad frequently caused quite a stir by beating the ladies of the town with his Victoria sponge cakes and Mum's flower arrangements were rarely topped. We were encouraged to enter artwork or woodwork objects. Competition was fierce. There was tremendous excitement amongst us as we raced up to see the results and whether we had been lucky enough to win anything. Wearied by the excitement of the day we would eventually return home with our spoils. In the evening a dance in the memorial hall threw out music into the night, accompanied by the drunken singing of the younger inhabitants, whose voices had been given volume and the gift of singing out of unison and very much off key, by copious amounts of locally brewed alcohol. A good time was had by all. The following day small groups of us children would be up early to scour the grass around the marquees in the old castle grounds for dropped money. We were always rewarded with plenty of small change. A highlight for me was finding a ten-shilling note, riches indeed.

The river divides the town into two parts, each rising on a hill on either side of the river. Our shop was situated on the north side of the river at the northwest apex of the market square. It nestles into the White Horse pub; one of their guest rooms is directly above the shop. Our house was very narrow and consisted of a small kitchen-dining area with a rarely used sitting room fronting onto the Square. It was kept for special occasions such as Christmas or a birthday. On the floor above were three small bedrooms and a bathroom. Revisiting now it seems so small but to us growing up the size was never a factor. Standing on the corner of the square, the right-angled corner of the house frequently caught out the drivers of large lorries, which used to clip the side of the house, taking out large chunks of plaster. Those with loads of timber from the forests of the Forestry Commission, in the hills above the town, were the worst culprits.

All three of us children attended St George's primary school, which stands at the top of the hill to the south of the village. It sits on the same elevation as the parish church. Our mother taught at this school before marrying Dad and for a while afterwards. She recounted stories of children walking for miles from the farms in the hills in all weathers to attend, some with no proper shoes. It was a very homely little school with a disciplined but caring couple in charge. Mr and Mrs Guppy were their names. Mr Guppy was a tall, quite elegant pipe smoking man with a voice that was clear and carried a long way without shouting. I don't ever remember either of them becoming angry with us.

As I have travelled through life, I have experienced several uncanny associations that have origins in my childhood. One of the earliest arose from an extraordinary association between our village and Ethiopia. A small but interesting museum is situated at the lower side of the Square, twenty-five yards from our shop and house. It was built by Lord Clive of India who had a large early Georgian-style house 6 miles from Clun in a nearby village, Aston-on-Clun. Built from stone plundered from the old castle (as was our house), the lower floor was initially a prison and the upper floor a courtroom. Lord Clive purchased the estate of Aston Hall in Aston-on-Clun in 1762. The modern continuation of the Clive family was friendly with Ethiopia's last emperor Haile Selassie, so much so that he stayed with them several times. On one occasion the family brought him to Clun, and he went into our shop and met my father and grandfather. Years later I would make several visits to Ethiopia with the charity Chain of Hope to carry out surgery on children with heart defects. When sent to boarding school in Newport in north-eastern Shropshire, some of my home sickness was allayed by the fact that our first boarding house was also called Aston Hall and indeed was a similar Georgian-style residence and it brought to my mind the local hall that Clive had built.

Another association is that the preceding Duke of Norfolk and Baron of Clun was Thomas Howard who, on behalf of Charles I, acquired many pieces of art, as well as sculptural and literary artefacts. Among them were the notes and drawings of Leonardo da Vinci, now in the royal collection in Windsor. Those notebooks of Leonardo include all but two of his manuscript sheets on anatomy and what we would now call physiology. As we shall see later, these were to become an important parallel life for me apart from my medical endeavours. Howard gathered around him many men of letters and amongst them was the physician William Harvey, whom Arundel nicknamed 'perpetual motion' on account of his boundless energy.

Yet another coincidence involves the Astronomer Royal. One of the most regular deliveries of meat that we made was to a rather unique private boarding school approximately 9 miles away called Bedstone. Bedstone School is a rare Victorian Calendar house built in 1881 as the country seat of the Ripley family. The family had made its money in the dye industry in Bradford and Henry Ripley was knighted, taking the style of Sir Henry Ripley of Rawdon in the West Riding of Yorkshire and Bedstone in Shropshire. Calendar houses were distinguished by having a chimney for every month, a window for every day, seven entrances and fifty-two rooms. It is said that these facts should never be checked as destitution will visit the perpetrator, a rather convenient guard against criticism of the claim. The school was founded by a Mr and Mrs Rees in 1948, whilst the Ripley family still owned the house. From its inception, my grandfather won the contract to supply meat for the school. In the later 1950s I visited the school regularly with my grandfather. At 7.00 a.m. every day except Sundays, we drove to the school to deliver the meat for the day for the boarding pupils, all boys at the time. From those times I remember meeting the Rees's son Martin, now Lord Rees of Ludlow, currently the Astronomer Royal. On one visit with my grandfather, we were introduced by his father Mr Rees. Coincidently, Lord Rees of Ludlow as he is now styled, was relatively recently introduced as an Honorary Fellow of Clare Hall in the University of Cambridge at the same time as me. Yet another circle of time that has played out in my life.

We were so fortunate to grow up in a village where daily life was idyllic compared with many environments for children in modern times. Everyone was known to each other and I remember few if any internecine hostilities. The open fields were within a few hundred yards of our house and the farms around the hillsides were owned by family friends and acquaintances of our parents. In the school holidays it was usual to spend all day wandering the countryside with friends, playing outside in the fresh air. A strong memory for me was the farm owned by a lovely family, the Breretons. Nestling in a hollow between beautiful rolling hills and surrounded by wooded areas we were free to roam wherever we wished. As the sun reached its zenith in the sky (our clock) we would race back to the farmhouse, Max and I, to find a fresh jug of homemade lemonade with delicious sandwiches standing in the open window of the farmhouse kitchen. Innocently we played cowboys and Indians, armed with bows and arrows made from sticks found in the forest, with faces painted in mud, or pretending to be pirates on the open seas with wellingtons and eye patches; we played for hours splashing around in the Clun River. Ablutions and number twos were achieved in woodland clearings with Dock leaves as universal toilet paper. The days never seemed to end. As night fell, lovely Mrs Brereton would drop me off at the square for bedtime. It was a feral life but utterly absorbing and real.

Television was not really a feature in our lives. Although Dad purchased a black and white set relatively early, much of what was visible was the hiss and crazy haze from what we now know arises from the remnants of the Big Bang microwave background from the early universe; exciting for astrophysicists in the current age, but not of much use to impatient youngsters of the 1950s. When a focussed image could be obtained, much of what was on offer was *Andy Pandy* and later *Blue Peter* and Richard Attenborough's launch platform, *Zoo Quest*. The closest transmitter was in Sutton Coldfield 80 miles distant with several hills in the way, so it was not surprising that the signal and its reception was vague in the extreme. Much later, a relay transmitter was erected on the top of the Brown Clee Hill, around 25 miles away, which continues to be the source of a much-improved signal, eventually allowing the reception of the early colour programmes. Broadcasts began around 5.00 p.m. in the afternoon and close down was around 11.00 p.m., with children's content over by 6.00 p.m. Later, Robin Hood (Richard Greene) and the Lone Ranger (Clayton Moore) became favourites, with Flash Gordon (Buster Crabbe) added for a degree of fear and excitement. Not only was choice very limited but viewing time was strictly controlled by Mum, who was determined that we would read and learn an instrument.

In the absence of social media, we had to be more creative with our leisure time. Drawing and painting, making models and music were mainstays. I can remember making a balsa wood spitfire whilst listening to Cassius Clay (as he was then) fighting Henry Cooper. Cooper should have won that bout, having knocked Clay out in the fifth round, but he was saved by the bell.

Clay, who later after this bout changed his name to Muhammad Ali, as good as admitted this years later. His ring second Angelo Dundee had rubbed salt onto Clay's gloves and loosened the laces on them to cause injury to Cooper's weak eyebrows, which bled easily. Dad and I were outraged as the commentator, Harry Carpenter, described the events, equally outraged himself. The BBC impartiality fell away with his passion. Dear Harry went on to become a friend of Ali, having passed first through a period of hostility towards him rather like the television presenter Michael (Parky) Parkinson. The meetings between the two are still available to see on modern media. It was a great thrill to me to almost walk into 'our 'Enry', as Cooper was affectionately known by his British fans, in Covent Garden when there in my first year as a medical student.

The radio played a large part in life then. On Sundays, around lunchtime, we would listen to Round the Horn, a programme full of gay double entendres, lost on us, followed by the Navy Lark.

In 1963 Mum began to show signs of a serious neurological disease which took years to diagnose. We eventually discovered that it was multiple sclerosis. In the afternoons, for Mum to get a break from the chair in which she was forced to spend most of her days, Dad would take the family out for a drive. The hills around Clun are very beautiful and Dad knew all of the side roads and we would go up on to the tops of the hills with spectacular views in every direction. We would listen to the Semprini serenade on the BBC light programme. Alberto Semprini was born to Italian parents in Bath. He graduated from the Verdi Conservatory in Milan in 1928. He was a concert pianist and cellist and conductor. His opening line was always, 'old ones, new ones, loved ones, neglected ones'. Even now hearing the opening bars immediately transports me back to those Sunday afternoons in the car with the family and our little dog Katie, a west highland terrier-dachshund cross. If I was lucky, part of a Formula 1 Grand Prix would be broadcast after Semprini. I can still remember one very gripping race in which Graham Hill won the Monaco Grand Prix. I longed to attend it one day. A still unrealised dream.

In later years, *Top of the Pops* became a favourite with disc jockeys Derek Jacobs and then Alan Freeman or 'Fluff' as he became known behind the microphone. 'Hi there, Pop Pickers', were his opening words and we knew excitement would follow. The passion for pop music was not shared by Dad, a huge fan of Glen Miller and Bing Crosby. I remember going to the dentist in Knighton with him in the earliest car that I can remember, a Ford Consul, when Elvis Presley came on the radio. Dad's comment that I never let him forget was, 'This pop music is rubbish. It will never catch on'.

Similarly, when at boarding school where there was no access to television, the highlight of the week was crowding round an old, valved radio at 5.00 p.m. on a Sunday in anticipation of the top ten. The lucky ones with some pocket money would queue to buy the number one single from the local record shop in the high-street. I still have a number of those old vinyl forty-five rpm records.

When I was five, my parents arranged for me to start piano lessons with a Mr Bastick in Bishop's Castle. We had a Challen upright piano which both our parents played. Dad was a good extemporiser and could play easily by ear. Vamping, the art of repetitive chordal leaps, was his speciality. With a good tenor voice, he would accompany himself to the American classics popularised by the great crooner, Bing Crosby, whom he could mimic extremely well. Mum was more restrained and stuck to sight reading the classics; her favourite piece was Henry Litolff's scherzo from Concerto Symphonique No 4 in D minor. It was her desire that I should play this piece for her. It would be many years before I could even approach this complicated work.

The first record that Dad bought for me, was a recording of Rachmaninov's second piano concerto played by the relatively well-known concert pianist Joyce Hatto. On the disc was a recording of the Prelude in C sharp minor that I was learning at the time. I suspect it was to encourage me in my efforts. Joyce Hatto and the exploits of her husband William Barrington-Coupe came to play a direct part in my life much later. I had been referred a patient with severe coronary artery disease for surgery. During the consultation the fact that his wife was a concert pianist came up: Joyce Hatto, the pianist on my first LP record. My excitement was obvious, and I was invited to say hello as she was seated outside. I was quite thrilled to meet her and breathlessly told her of the impact that she had had on my life, as I used to play that record over and over. Indeed, whilst learning the C sharp minor prelude, I tried to style my playing on hers. They generously offered to send me some of her CD recordings. Over the ensuing years, all of Joyce's new recordings arrived through the post. Joyce appeared to be accompanied by some of the greatest orchestras in the world, under the baton of conductors at the top of their profession. Then one day I happened to be listening to a news programme when I heard that a huge scam had been uncovered involving the couple. I knew that her husband had a recording studio of sorts at the bottom of their garden, which he told me he used for mixing the final recordings. The bizarre story unfolded and centred upon a New York financial trader, Brian Ventura, who loved classical music and played several of her CDs. Then he noticed one day that the details of the recording listed on his small digital player stated that the orchestra was not the one on the cover of the CD. He had a friend in the recording business and took the CD to him. To their shock and horror, they discovered that Joyce Hatto's piano solo had been dubbed on top of another recording from orchestras that had been copied from other recordings. The whole thing was a massive fraud. They were revealed as such and utterly discredited by the music world. This was a dreadful end to what had begun as a great career for Joyce as she was a very accomplished pianist. In her later years she had struggled to continue through ill-health and her devoted husband had attempted to keep her career alive with this fraudulent behaviour. Eventually the inevitable television documentary about the whole dark business was made, hammering the final nail into their professional coffin. A truly sad story.

My music teacher, a Mr Bastick, lived in Bishop's Castle, a small market border town 6 miles north of Clun with a very long and steep hill, Colstey, in between. It was simply 3 miles up and 3 miles down in both directions. Initially my grandfather would drive me to and from the lesson in one of our two delivery vans, chain smoking and singing all the way there and back, it was an interesting journey. The songs were usually those of the P.B.I. (Poor Bloody Infantry) from the First World War; 'Pack up Your Troubles in Your Old Kit Bag', 'Keep the Home Fires Burning' and 'The Roses of Picardy'. He was a wonderful man, eternally cheerful and profoundly generous. Eventually it was suggested that I should cycle to my lessons. In response Grandad bought me a 'sturdy' bicycle. In my imagination I was looking forward with great excitement to a dropped handlebar racing bike with derailleur gears. My despair, which out of respect towards Grandad was heavily disguised, can only be imagined when a truly 'sturdy' heavy Raleigh bicycle, complete with solid metal chain guard and mudguards was revealed. It was at least three times my own weight. Nevertheless, I was expected to make the journey on the 'new' bike whatever the weather. In the summer I would arrive for the lesson bathed in sweat. In the wintertime my hands would be blue and stiff from the cold air flowing over my hands as I gripped the handlebars tightly with the effort to get the leviathan over Colstey hill and up the steep incline in Bishop's Castle. This final insult, being a one-in-three hill climb to the summit of the town where Mr Bastick lived. I remember entering endless competitions on Cornflake packets and others for a sleek bicycle, but all my attempts failed.

Mr Bastick being a continuous pipe smoker, the small darkened front room in which the piano sat, was filled with heavy tobacco smoke and the musty smell of old leather armchairs. There was a small desk with the upright piano at the far end of the room. There was a large window that occupied much of the wall out onto the street. Through this, the shafts of sunlight could be seen like searchlights on a dark night as they shone through the smoke hanging in the air. The piano sat in the gloom. Occasionally plied with a glass of water and a biscuit I sat at the piano and prepared to play. I was not the most committed student in my practice. Mistakes were rewarded with a nasty wrap on the knuckles with the sharp edge of a twelve-inch ruler with an in-laid metal strip for extra bite. This was supposed to sharpen you up and to create greater focus, or was it just a touch of sadism? A tendency that manifested itself a few years later when it turned into mild abuse with a beating on the bare bottom across an old wooden chair. It never progressed beyond this, but it was quite traumatic. Having lessons at the same time was a delightful girl the same age as me, Kathleen, on whom I had quite a crush between the ages of seven and ten. When I heard that she was receiving the same treatment I reported it to my mother and father who were outraged. The next time my hapless piano teacher appeared in our village driving slowly past the shop Dad set off after him with a carving knife and a meat cleaver. Lessons with Bastick ceased. Perhaps satisfactory justice for a minor offender and a lesson learned by him.

As I mentioned earlier, as with many children I found practice, especially in preparation for the Associated Board of the Royal School of Music exams, quite painful. There is no doubt that my continuation to the higher grades and a lifelong enjoyment of the piano was down to dear Grandad. In the school holidays, when the family had gathered for lunch together (always a meat and two veg feast prepared by Granny, assisted by Dad running in and out of the shop between customers), Grandad would sit next to me at the piano and ask me to play for him. He would tell me how wonderful pieces that I was struggling with sounded (the majority), and plead with me to play them again, and again and again, seeming to rejoice in the disharmony and crashed cords. Without his unstinting support I feel sure that I would have given up before the age of ten. However, success in the Royal College of Music exams followed and that set me up for a life of pleasure with all things to do with that king of instruments. Now in possession of a Steinway grand, my pleasure in the sight and sound of that instrument is undimmed and, if anything, greater than ever. Dear Grandad, I am still playing for you, torturing your otherwise peaceful sojourn in paradise where you surely must be.

I have had only one recurring nightmare in my life and that has the piano as the centrepiece. The dream begins with me entering our main assembly hall at Adams' School. It is the original building from 1666 and a grand affair with a high raised wooden podium on one long wall, with a door leading onto it from a beautiful old library; wooden steps descended into the hall itself.

The headmaster used to appear through that library door for morning assembly with all the pupils lined up by year and form in front of and below him. At the far end of the room is a full concert grand piano. On the wall next to the podium measuring approximately 20 feet long by 10 feet wide, written in large Olde English is the last will and testament of the school founder, William Adams. The text contained the letter 's' written as an 'f', and many words with an 'e' at the end of them. Set into the opposite wall are several very high and large windows. The dream begins with me playing the piano. The door in the main entrance at the far end of the hall opens slowly and a large ghostly black figure enters the room and glides over to me to stand by the side of the piano, overlooking me and glaring at me through red ghostly eyes. The face is largely hidden by a black hood, but enough of it can be made out to reveal one from a horror movie. Light is streaming through the large window behind him onto my hands like a searchlight. As I continue to play, now with increasing apprehension, the ghoul directs his gaze down towards my hands with an intense stare. I look down to see that they are smashed and broken, but without pain. At that moment the headmaster appears through the library door onto the podium, and I look up, appealingly to him. At this point, and always then, I wake in a sweat. Initially the dream came to me at about the age of seventeen. It recurred for practically every night for more than a week and then disappeared. It was at the time that I was wrestling with what to do with my life and mounting fears of failure. Just a few weeks ago it came again for several nights. This was at a time that I have been suffering considerable stress from a horrible senior management team in the hospital. Undoubtedly my hands have been central to my life in surgery and the arts, so perhaps this dream is nothing more than the recognition of their importance and the fear of what would happen if I lost the use of them. The resurgence now can be explained by the turmoil and dilemma I face over how to deal with the current circumstances and when to retire, a question that has been taxing me for some time.

Although our house in Clun was tiny, it seemed adequate as we were growing up, but returning years later, it did appear to be very small, and I wonder how we all functioned within it. We really did live above and around the shop which dominated our lives. Our parents slept above the shop and our front room was next to it. There was a small opening from the back of the shop into the front room, rarely used to prevent the accumulation of animal fat from work shoes onto the paraquet floor. We were only allowed to spend time in that room on very special occasions of which there were precious few. Christmas day was one of them. As O and A level examinations approached, I was allowed to work quietly there. The house was a drawn-out rectangle, one room deep measuring about 15 feet wide. There was a very narrow pavement alongside and people walking past could look straight into the room, something my mother in particular hated. As the sun set and the lights in the room were switched, on we were loudly commanded to draw the curtains as 'the room is now illuminated like a stage set'. Words that I can still hear so clearly. The other side of the room abutted the next-door pub. This was occupied and run by a widowed Austrian lady and her aggressive Alsatian dog. That dog terrified me and frequently chased me down the street, on one occasion succeeding in nipping me on the behind. The anticipation of this attack always deterred me from leaving the house by the back door. The bedrooms were strung out on the floor above with a third-floor attic that could only be accessed through a retractable ladder. This was a treasure trove of memorabilia, and the site of my ever-growing train set courtesy of my Grandfather. We had built it up over several years and it was mounted on a large hardboard base which we painted green to simulate grass. Trees, cars, people and houses were steadily added making it, to my mind, a thing of beauty and endless entertainment.

There was a small communal back yard to the house with the entrance to the slaughterhouse and sheds shared with our next-door neighbour. Beyond that was a small path that led behind the row of small houses between the White Horse Inn and a baker's shop owned by Mr Owen. His son was an older and a somewhat difficult friend, prone to bullying behaviour. On one occasion being provoked to an extreme I am informed that I hit him on the head with a small hammer drawing blood and an end to the bullying. Perhaps the mild cerebral trauma wrought a change in behaviour, as after that we rubbed along together pretty well most of the time.

In the early years, my sister Rosamond and I shared the end bedroom. This room opened on to an extension that Dad had built over the single car garage into which we moved our piano, the record player, a desk and our record collection. Out of sight and sound of the grown-ups, this became our safe space. I would spend hours there in the holidays playing records or drawing. There was a large oak tree overlooking my room which was home to a family of barn owls. Their unforgettable call into the dark hours of the night, the only sounds other than the wind in the trees.

For reasons that I never understood, other than a love of music in all its guises, Grandad had a large collection of instruments: guitars, a drum-kit, violin, and a double bass amongst them. These he kept in the front room of his terraced house on Castle Street. In later years he simply gave some of them away to youngsters in the village who expressed an interest. I have managed to keep a guitar, a violin, and a beautiful lute but the rest have all gone, hopefully to appreciative homes. For many years he acted as master of ceremonies at the weekly Saturday night dances in the town hall. He and my Grandmother were excellent ballroom dancers and, I am told, won many prizes.

Living in a butcher's shop, the best quality meat was always available, and fresh cuts of pork, lamb or beef were at the heart of all main meals. Whilst still very young, post-war rationing was still in place but we were very fortunate to have our own supply. Then and in later years it was something of a luxury to be able to simply go out into the hanging room of the slaughterhouse and to cut myself a piece of very good steak for dinner. The centrepiece of the kitchen area was an AGA cooker. In this, not only was the daily fare cooked, but also hams and faggots prepared by my grandmother. These were all made on a Monday evening, ready for sale the next day, which was market day in Clun.

On one occasion, as teenage boys are wont to do, I fainted face down onto the uncovered Aga hotplate. Serious burns were only avoided by the quick action of gran who hauled me off the cooker and applied copious amounts of cold water-soaked towels onto my face.

Mum was very involved in the shop business with Dad. She served customers, and was responsible for the weekly takings, going out on meat rounds when needed; she also made several innovations for the business. Some of her ventures included the curing of sheepskins and selling them as small rugs. For a few years she began the intense farming of bantams, a breed of young chickens. The sight of so many baby chicks together was quite adorable. Their destiny I chose to blot out from my mind and simply enjoyed feeding them and cradling them in my hands.

In the early days after acquiring the business, my grandfather delivered meat to the farms round about by pony and trap. Although I never witnessed this, two horses were kept in a field just down the road from the house.

Across the road from our house was the Midland Bank, now a convenience store. Externally it is quite a formidable building with the appearance of a small fortress, fitting for a bank. Recent reading has revealed that in the late 1920s and early 1930s, the Midland Bank corporation was the largest bank in the world. In attempts to bolster the faded economy following the First World War the board, driven by Reginald McKenna, previously First Lord of the Admiralty, Home Secretary and Chancellor of the Exchequer, were persuaded to build impressive buildings to encourage depositors. With this in mind, they commissioned Sir Edward Lutyens to produce a template for their new building designs. Although the programme was not fully developed, because of the authority of the architect as well as the visual appeal, the neo-Georgian style he preferred was widely adopted. The Midland Bank had built and acquired 1,400 branches across the country, one of them being in

Clun. The head office on Poultry, in the City of London, was the flagship in style and commanding in appearance. The symmetry of the building, along with the large sash windows, grand entrance and large stone blocks are all features to be found in the Clun bank. The entrance and reception area of the head office in Poultry were beautifully tiled in large black and white symmetrical shapes. They can still be seen in what is now, the NED hotel, with a minor version on the floor of the old Clun branch. To think that our small-town bank had such lofty architectural associations makes me smile. It had always impressed me, and the musty smell of frequently cleaned and well-maintained buildings of good quality materials has stayed with me to this day. I remember clearly the day that my father took me, around my seventeenth birthday, to open my first bank account with Mr Marshall, the then manager. Dad, and therefore I, held him in high regard; after all, he controlled the money. Throughout my early career Mr Marshall was in post and was always supportive and helpful through mortgages and other advice. It was a warm and reassuring link with my home.

Regularly on a Saturday night just after closing time it was common for me to be woken by the droning of a speeding car heading up through the square followed by a loud bang and the splintering of glass as the hapless drunken young driver, slammed headlong into the bank. This would be followed by a real commotion as Mr Marshall ran out from his house, which was a part of the bank, to haul by his ear the stupefied driver to face the music. Some of the scars can still be seen on the wall of the building to this day.

We seemed to have 'proper' winters in the 1950s with frequent deep snow falls. Clun stands approximately 600 feet above sea level with the highest point of the hills around reaching 1,630 feet. Delivering meat to the farms high up in the hills was always an exciting experience in those winters. I remember being out with Mum in the dark one evening on the tops of the hills in deep snow when, even with chains on the wheels, we became stuck in a deep snow drift. Completely unphased by the predicament, out came the shovel as Mum dug us out; I was told to stay in the warm of the van whilst she did this. There was no means of communication at that time other than the rarely placed red phone box. The local farmers were always helpful, towing us out of the deep snowdrift with a tractor, and then taking us in for a warming drink by a blazing open fire.

On another occasion, Dad and I were taking a van load of sheep to the market in Craven Arms. It was early on an icy February morning. Just outside the village there is a sharp right, and then left-hand bend at a hamlet named after the big house set back from the road, The Hurst. We negotiated the first corner satisfactorily, but on taking the left hander we hit a patch of ice and skated off the road and through the hedge. When we came to rest there were sheep and sheep droppings all around us, with a big hole in the hedge behind us. Once we realised that we were all unhurt including, most importantly, the sheep, we couldn't stop laughing at our predicament. It only remained for my long-suffering Grandfather with Charlie to come and tow us out of the field before continuing our journey. The first stop was to go and apologise to the owners of the hedge that we had transgressed. There is still evidence of that hole in the hedge sixty years later.

Come rain, snow, hail, or sunshine the meat always had to be delivered on time. Parking in the farmyards we would walk with a wicker basket on our arm up to the house announcing our arrival with the loud call of 'butcher' and walk straight into the kitchen. If there was no one there, as was often the case, the door was always open and the meat was left on the kitchen table with the ticket headed Chas. E. Wells and Son High Class Family butchers, for later settlement.

At Christmas time every farmer would want to ply the driver, Grandad, or Charlie with some 'Christmas cheer'. Usually a 'small' glass of sherry. To this day I can see the very rosy cheeked and glassy eyed Charlie coming back to report in, before going home with an extremely big smile on his weather-beaten face and a somewhat rolling gait. The breathalyser had not yet been invented. However, greatly to Charlie's credit he never had an accident, although I suspect the meat round took longer and longer to complete as yet more sherry was consumed.

Danger and humour are never very far away in a butcher's shop and the slaughterhouse. We made our own beef and pork sausages which were covered with the cleaned intestines of the animal. After removal, the intestines were washed through thoroughly with a lot of water delivered with a hosepipe. When that was done, they were scraped with a wooden scraper on a wooden board to remove the internal mucosa. The result was a long tube of almost translucent edible natural tissue, not the plastic substitutes that are commonly used today. Once done, the intestinal tube was slid over a long tapering metal tube emanating from a cylinder with a large plunger driven by a metal hand-cranked wheel. The meat for the sausage was placed in the large barrel of the sausage machine and forced through the metal spout under pressure with one hand on the wheel and the other feeding the intestinal derived covering over the spout. It was cold and wet work.

To modernise, Dad decided to electrify the pump to drive the sausage meat into the freshly prepared intestinal tube. The first to use it was Grandad. On that occasion Dad and I walked into the sausage room to find, to our horror, Grandad with his right hand clamped onto the metal handle, shaking violently and jumping up and down as the electricity flowed through him. Our wiring had shorted out and with so much water around, the electrons took the easiest route, which was through dear Grandad, who was left demonstrating his dancing abilities, but unable to let go of the wet metallic handle. Thankfully on switching off the electricity he recovered quickly with no harm done. We laughed about it afterwards, but it could so easily have ended in tragedy.

We also used to boil our hams for sale in a very large circular gas fired boiler. The gas ring was at the centre of the base of the boiler. It needed to be lit using a long taper introduced through a small hole in a ring of metal at the base of the boiler. One day, Charlie was on ham boiling duty, as he was most days. Dad and I were in the shop fifty yards away, round the corner in the square. Suddenly there was a loud explosion. We dashed from the shop and as we rounded the corner, we could see the garage door blown open with smoke billowing out from it. We ran towards the garage where the boiler was housed to see a figure stagger out of the smoke with a blackened face and white rings where his glasses had protected his eyes, and the charred remains of missing eyebrows. His glasses were hanging from one of his ears. Shocked and confused, poor Charlie explained that he had attempted to light the gas. First, he turned on the gas. Then he found it difficult to light the rolled up soggy broad sheet newspaper that he was using as a taper. All the time that he was trying to light it, the gas was running, causing a considerable amount of gas to accumulate under the boiler. Finally, having managed to light the soggy newspaper taper, Charlie knelt to thread it through the small opening. With a huge boom, the now highly explosive gas mixture was ignited. Thankfully most of the blast went over Charlie's head blowing open the garage door. Health and safety were not much in evidence in those days.

Usually, the animals were bought in the market on each Monday and transported back to the slaughterhouse. When my grandfather opened the shop in the 1920s there were sheep markets in Clun. However, these closed soon after his arrival and he had to turn to buying the animals in Craven Arms, 9 miles away. At first, together with Charlie he would walk them, just as the medieval drovers would have done, the 9 miles to Clun. This would take half a day. By the time of my arrival, they were of course all delivered in lorries.

Occasionally, dependent upon the market price of the animals, sheep or cattle, Dad would buy some extra ones, usually of a younger age to put out to pasture for some months. We had a small field next to the old Norman castle in Clun. However, the sheep he bought were sometimes returned to the farm they came from to await their time. Their fleece had been marked with a red spot, to denote them from the others and allow easy identification later. I remember some astonishing feats of dog handling. Clun is surrounded by hills and is wonderful sheep farming country. At one particular farm that we used to go to, the sheep had wondered high up on to the hill, being like small white spots amongst the dark green of the hillside. After the farmer had pointed them out, I set off towards the hill to climb up and to round up the sheep. Before I had taken more than a few steps I could hear Dad and the farmer chuckling to themselves. They hadn't moved and the farmer then started to whistle to his Border Collie sheep dog, who sprinted away up the hill. It arrived close to the sheep, having slowed down and adopted a crouching position as it inched forwards so as not to frighten them. Their then followed a series of varied whistling tones from the farmer that directed the dog in different directions. Seemingly quite quickly, our sheep were cut out from the rest and driven steadily back down into the farmyard, where we loaded them into our trusty van to return home. Clun sheep are excellent hardy breeding sheep. They are found all over the world, particularly in Australia. Their black faces differentiate them from others.

By the time we had returned from the cattle market, late in the afternoon, the animals would arrive. The entrance was set just inside a yard, which meant they had to be steered through a right angle from the truck to the storage area. The sheep and pigs always tried to give us the run around but being smaller animals, we were able to guide them in the right direction. The much bigger bullocks were a very different proposition and occasionally, on a bad day, one or two would decide to go in the opposite direction and would charge past us onto the main road running down towards the square. This was when the fun would begin. Desperate shouts would be made to Charlie, who was around the corner in the shop, to head off the now errant cattle to prevent them running riot through the main square of the town. The cattle had a choice of turning left into the square, or right past the bank towards a lovely old house with a beautiful garden owned by retired Colonel Peppy. For some reason they always seemed to prefer the right turn and galloped headlong into the Colonel's Garden ending up trampling his cloches and ruining the vegetable patch. Colonel Peppy was very sanguine about it all but Mrs Peppy was not so amused, and a tirade of perfectly enunciated English would follow along with Dad and Grandad very sheepishly persuading the cattle, by now satiated on the potentially prize-winning vegetables, back in the right direction. I frequently thought that with what lay in store for them they had made an appropriate dash for freedom and secretly hoped they might make it to the open countryside.

The awful business of killing the animals then began. It is extremely hard work and went on until midnight or later. However, I suspect that if most people knew how the meat that they eat is procured, the world would have many more vegetarians. Although occasionally being roped in to help, I did my best to give the whole wretched business a wide berth. A positive spin off for me was that Dad's knowledge of anatomy was quite profound, and he taught me a lot. It was an excellent head start over others when we studied anatomy at medical school and helped in the dissecting room with some pre-existing knowledge of tissue handling.

Another influence on me was the fact that Dad studied for and completed his examinations to be officially registered as a master butcher from the Institute of Meat. To this day, it is a rare qualification with only fifty or so in the United Kingdom in 2023. Much later, this inspired me to work for my Master of Surgery as I thought that this had a nice ring to it and completed a family circle: Mr F. Wells Master Butcher and Mr F. Wells Master Surgeon. It was also shorter than the time taken for a PhD, and I was a man in a hurry once into the medical profession.

There was a great deal of family pride in the business and the way the shop appeared to the public was of the utmost importance. At the end of every day's business buckets of boiling water were brought down from the slaughterhouse to scrub the shop floor and the pavement outside. Fat from the meat would fall to the floor and become trodden in, making it unpleasant for the customers. Removing it took a great deal of effort, especially cleaning the surfaces on which the meat was prepared. The meat was cut up on a wooden block which needed scrubbing clean every evening ready for the next day. Both chores were hard work after a long day but kept us fit. There was no need for a gym in that business.

It was a tradition to dress the front of the shop on market days. As described earlier, the rosettes for champion animals were prominently displayed along with carefully dressed and prepared meat.

Dad was a Freemason and had an excellent memory; his ability to quickly memorise large chunks of text was demonstrated to me by memorising from the Craft Masonry books. I remember that, with his busy life, quite often he would be faced with a memory task with only a few hours to prepare but he never failed to complete it. Occasionally he would ask me to test him, and I couldn't fault him. Being a Freemason gave him great solace later in his life as practically his only escape from work and being primary carer for Mum so badly afflicted by multiple sclerosis.

The elder of my sisters, Rosamond, came along when I was three years old. Both of us attended the small primary school in Clun, as did our younger sister Charmian, who was born in 1963 when I was away at boarding school. Charmian was a complete surprise for me when I came home for an exeat weekend and was astonished to find Mum nursing her when I walked through the back door. No one had thought to inform me of this highly important new development in the family. Charmian was a wonderful addition. Sadly, being at boarding school throughout her early childhood, and then University, we didn't really grow up together.

This happy event had been preceded by a less fortunate one. As mentioned before, Mum presented the first signs of the debilitating disease multiple sclerosis when pregnant with Charmian. Sometime before, whilst helping to direct cattle into the slaughterhouse, some faeces from an animal splashed into her eye. A short while afterwards, she developed a white painless ulcer in that eye which lasted for several weeks. I have always thought that her eye contamination was the cause of the disease for her. During the pregnancy, she developed the first symptoms. It happened as follows. At that time, the closest ladies' hairdresser was 9 miles away in Craven Arms. Dad had driven her there during a lunchtime. As I remember from my father, being a Tuesday, it was market day in Clun so the butcher's shop had become very busy in the afternoon and there was no one to collect her. So, after completion of the usual 'perm and set', being of strong country stock, she set off to walk home. Having completed almost 7 miles, on reaching Clunton, the next village to Clun, her right leg gave way, and she could walk no further. A local farmer discovered her on the roadside and drove her home. This was the first presentation of the disease, which came to have a massive impact on all our lives. Multiple sclerosis, as with other degenerative diseases, rapidly becomes a family ailment as everyone must learn to cope with the consequences. In 1963, the clinical diagnosis was not easy, as computerised tomography (CAT scanning) and magnetic resonance imaging (M.R.I.) had yet to be developed. Therefore, it was a purely clinical diagnosis made from the history, that is the description of the symptoms by the patient, and thorough careful and detailed clinical examination. The understanding of the disease relied upon the symptoms and signs being correlated with post-mortem findings in the brains of victims. Thus, diagnosis in life was very much based on circumstantial evidence. The physical signs that Mum exhibited defeated our village GP Dr. Russell and were lost on the neurologists in Shrewsbury Infirmary. As a result, and as the disease progressed to affect all of Mum's right-sided muscular function, Dad made appointments for her to see neurologists as far afield as Birmingham and eventually Guys and St Thomas's hospitals in London. Finally, she was seen by the great pioneer in MS Dr Douglas McAlpine at the Middlesex Hospital who informed my parents of the diagnosis. His book Multiple Sclerosis became the seminal text on the subject.

MS seemed to be frequently localised in farming communities and recent work has identified a genetic relationship in the preponderance of the disease with cattle herders from the Mesolithic period to the Bronze Age. Recent work from geneticists and computer experts reviewing ancient genomic sets suggests that the genetic risk may have arisen among pastoralists from the Pontic steppe and been brought to Europe by migration approximately 5,000 years ago.[2] If there is any truth to this then the eye contamination from the bullock into a predisposed genome inherited by my mother may have been the cause. One day we may know more.

At that time there was no effective treatment. However, Mum was a fighter. She had been a teacher in Clun School and was made of stern stuff. She refused to give in to the disease and battled on as best she could; my Grandmother and Father provided the only help that she would accept. Depressing though the diagnosis must have been, she set about a detailed review of all that she could find on the subject. Her conclusion was that sunflower seed oil with Vitamin B complex were the best supportive treatments and so she embarked upon a daily intake of these to ameliorate the disease progression. Dad was tasked with finding every possible source of it. In the absence of the internet and health food shops, he had to track it down through newspaper advertisements and the few pharmacies that intermittently stocked it, buying in bulk where he could. Failing that, she would eat the seeds of a sunflower.

The disease often runs a remitting and relapsing course but is often a disease of thirds. One third have a mild attack from which the sufferer recovers and doesn't develop further symptoms, meaning that they can return to a normal life. In another third, the symptoms can be of varying severity with no recovery from the neurological insult that ensues. The final third run a relapsing and remitting course to severe physical limitations and sometimes an early death. That was the experience that my mother had. There was quite a fast initial deterioration, which then plateaued for a while before taking a new downward plunge. The loss of use of her right hand and arm followed quite quickly, only for the disease to seem to arrest again for a while. However, she would not give in to it and taught herself to write with her left hand in three months, so convincingly that it became almost impossible to discern the script before and afterwards.

Her gritty determination to continue as though nothing was happening to her meant that she refused the use of a wheelchair and would not countenance a blue invalid sticker on the car to access disability parking. She would proclaim that there were always more deserving people than her, but secretly I think that she did not want to admit to herself her serious disability.

This attitude, whilst praiseworthy for gutsy determination, made for great difficulty for my father, who was confronted with the law on occasions trying to park closer to venues when no general parking was available. It was also galling to see people with no apparent disability sporting the blue badge and taking priority parking spaces whilst my parents struggled to carry on as normal which was, of course, just not possible.

Perhaps the thing that I became most ashamed of was my immature embarrassment when we had to stand and watch and wait as our wonderful Dad would lift and manipulate Mum in and out of the car with insensible and uncaring passers-by staring at them, as is so inevitably the case. This was particularly acute in front of fellow pupils outside of school as everyone else was being whisked off speedily for half-term breaks. Mum was cared for completely by Dad and her mother. They had no outside help, and it was many years before she would allow a simple chairlift at home to get up the steep and narrow flight to the bedroom. She would shuffle from step to step on her bottom with Dad, a big man, 6 feet and 5 inches tall, squeezing into the small space to support and help.

His engineering brain came to the fore when it was decided many years later. After moving to a new and bigger house that Dad had built, he decided to put in a lift from the garage to the first-floor bedroom so that easy transfer could be made on returning home. After consulting several elevator specialists, he was told that it could not be done. This was because of the narrow access and the right angle that was needed to be negotiated at the upper floor level and with no elevation to accommodate the lift pulleys and mechanisms needed above. He could not accept this and so set about designing a system that could be laid out in the loft area. He designed a system of pulleys and wheels to transfer the direction of pull at a right angle. Having completed the design, and it being accepted by the health and safety agents, it was duly constructed and worked perfectly. An example of his natural engineering talent so sadly never developed as it should have been.

In the autumn of 1959, I had been given an exam paper to complete without realising what it was. Sometime later I was informed that I had passed a thing called the 'Eleven-Plus'. The outcome of this was that I was able to begin secondary school a year early, something that probably inhibited my development academically, but more of that later. Lessons always seemed to be enjoyable and clearly prepared us well for the future. I had wonderful support from our parents, especially Mother, who encouraged reading. Apparently when visiting other children's houses at weekends to play, I could often be found in a warm convenient corner browsing the books of the house.

Our Grandfather was an extremely generous and kind man. Birthdays and Christmas were always made special by him. On Christmas morning, he would arrive at the back door of the house with his arms full of exciting presents. On birthdays, he would arrange large parties of our friends in the grounds of the castle with a series of games followed by a birthday tea back at home provided usually by Granny.

Sometimes, we would visit Grandad's sister Great Aunty Dolly and her husband Uncle Fred in Norley Bank in Cheshire. Aunty Dolly was a tall and angular lady but so kind and amusing to us children. Fred was a genial man but very quiet. Grandad's brother, great uncle Frank was sometimes present with his wife Mary, although I never knew where they lived. These visits were always a daytrip back and forth with lunch together on arrival. Great Uncle Frank and Aunty Mary figured only a little in our lives. Uncle Frank was a tall, well-built and good-looking man. It is worthy of note how smartly dressed they all were, even into old age.

Frank had been a hero in the First World War. Very sadly other relatives on my father's side were more rarely seen. Betty and Barbara Babbage appeared to me to be very glamorous ladies, always laughing, and joking. They smoked and were quite the emancipated women, very unusual in quiet and staid Clun. They were warm, gracious and funny, but for reasons that I never understood, Mum didn't want to spend time with them.

Granddad's family came from Yorkshire. I know little more of them than that they lived in South Cave, near Hull. He had always been my rock and the one to whom I listened intently. His words were always sage and well considered. Some of my earliest memories are Wednesday afternoons, when Mum and Dad went to Wolverhampton as a break from thc hurly burly of the square and left us with our grandparents. On sunny days I would often sit on the front step with him and listen to his stories from the olden golden times.

Sadly, our mother's multiple sclerosis meant that there was limited socialising in our home. For Dad this was quite hard; he enjoyed being around people and loved to talk and to share. He was very proud of his Englishness and loyal to a fault. He would do anything for anyone in need or trouble. An example of this were his actions when Mr Blurton, the other butcher in Clun, died suddenly, leaving his wife alone to deal with the business. Without being asked, and although it was the competition, Dad immediately went to help. Neglecting his own business, he took over the running of theirs for over a month, and helped Mrs Blurton find her feet again. He went all day every day and ran the shop, ordered all the meat and other items that were needed for it to remain a viable business. Even after that he continued to support her.

Every family is unique, and most have tensions from time to time in some form or another. My mother's illness and the tensions of running a small business amplified an apparently already stressful marriage, although as children do, we never really knew what the dynamics of our family unit were. Dad was a lovely, kind and gentle man who did everything and anything that he could to ease our lives and to support us in our endeavours, providing the means for us to go away to a good school.

In 1967, Edmund Leach, a British social anthropologist, delivered the BBC Reith Lectures titled 'A Runaway World'. In them, he contended that 'the family, with its narrow privacy and tawdry secrets, is the source of all our discontents'. Perhaps too broad a generality, but there is no avoidance of the fact that the environment in which we grow and develop has a huge influence on who we become and our take on the world as we grow into it. The traumas at home were difficult for us all, but our parents' determination that we should succeed as adults superseded any of those difficult times. Their effects I have felt in more personal ways, perhaps reflected in my inability to choose rationally a sound life partner. However, quoting Salman Rushdie in his declarative account of his recent terrible trauma titled *Knife*, '...this is not the place to intrude too much on such narrow privacies or to spill tawdry secrets. I will say: we would not be who we are today without the calamities of our yesterdays.'[3] A sentiment I share.

Holidays

Holidays were taken only once a year and extended over four days and four nights. We would leave, usually late on a Saturday night after the shop had been shut and cleaned, returning on the following Wednesday evening. Wednesday was half-day closing in the village, thus the shop would only be neglected for that short period of time.

Our parents made sure that we saw a lot of the English country and seaside. We started in the far south-western part of England, Cornwall, Penzance to be precise. In those days there were no motorways and although traffic was far lighter than today, the drive from Clun was a long and tedious one. How Dad managed it after a long day in the shop and then a six- or seven-hour drive with two moaning children in the back seat I will never know. On some occasions we would arrive at the hotel at two or three o clock in the morning. Generally, the hotel receptionists had long ago retired to bed with only the night porter to allow us in.

Historical and natural highlights were always sought out for us to visit. They were not days spent languishing on a beach. Each year we visited a different location, gradually working our way around the English coastline to see as much of Britain as we could. In 1965, we flew from Speke Airport in Liverpool to Dublin in an old Aer Lingus turboprop aeroplane, our one and only flight together. It was very exciting. In Dublin, Dad had hired a Ford Anglia in which we proceeded to travel all around southern Ireland, stopping to kiss the Blarney Stone on the way. This was accomplished in six days.

On one trip to the Cornish coast we arrived late as usual and my sister Rosamond needed to use the toilet. I was asked to take her and to make sure she was alright. The toilet stalls in the ladies were surrounded by walls that were frosted glass in the upper half and open at the top. Rosamond managed to lock herself in and couldn't get out. She began to cry and was quite frightened. I managed to climb over the partition wall but once inside could not undo the lock either. In desperation after calling for help with no reply, Rosamond took control despite her very young age and smashed the glass with the lavatory brush. The noise attracted attention and someone let us out.

The most exciting holiday was a road trip to the south of France. After a rather stormy Channel crossing, we headed south via the Route Napoléon in our Ford Zodiac. I don't think that I had ever drunk 'proper' coffee before and the bowl of delicious coffee that we were served with fresh warm croissants for breakfast was delicious. The bowl with the coffee had no handles so one just cradled it in both hands to drink from. This seemed so exotic to this youngster from the Welsh borders. For our first night we had stopped somewhere in Burgundy. The following journey through the Alps, up above the snow line in places, was mysterious and wonderful. At one point we stopped very high up to admire the view, and whilst getting out of the car I inadvertently dropped my wallet which was left behind. The only thing of real value to me in it was a photograph of my earliest girlfriend Lynda in her polka dot bikini. On occasions, I still wonder who picked it up or whether it still lies abandoned in some ditch high up in the mountains. Lynda and I had met at a hotel in Eastbourne on another of our family holidays. A swimming competition had been arranged by the hotel staff for all the children staying there. Lynda and I were the same age and between us managed to win all the races in our age group. She lived with her mother in Cheshire and after the holiday, we began a long-distance friendship. Her father had died a few years before. We met infrequently but from time to time her mother drove her down to school in Newport so that we could spend some time together, something that my parents would never have contemplated. It didn't last very long as relationships at that age are wont. However, I had a huge surprise when ten years later I went into a hamburger restaurant at World's End on the lower reaches of the Fulham Road: there she was, serving behind the counter, hardly changed at all. Life hadn't worked out well for her at that stage. She was a single mum and had gone to London to find a new life. Sadly, I never saw her again and often wonder what happened to her.

Our French holiday was a wonderful adventure. Driving down the twisting narrow roads towards Monte Carlo felt truly romantic. The first sight of the azure sea as we emerged from the mountains is a wonderful memory. Once there I persuaded Dad to drive the Monaco Grand Prix circuit. I think that secretly he enjoyed it as much as I did. In Nice, we suffered a technical hitch whilst cruising the Promenade Anglaise. The exhaust fell off the car and began dragging along the road. The noise was horrendous. Faces turned and stared at 'Le Ros Bif family' disrupting their afternoon promenade. Being the engineer he really was, Dad had the car up on jacks and fixed the problem at the roadside whilst the rest of the family soaked up the sun and enjoyed ice-creams. An undiminished memory is of bowls of Cornflakes for most breakfasts and some other meals. Money was so short that the cereal became our staple diet.

The return journey was equally as exciting. We travelled along the toll roads past Paris and back to the channel port where we arrived with only thirty minutes to spare before the sailing. Once again Dad's extraordinary stamina was clear to see. He drove from the south of France to Calais in one day with only the briefest of stops for food, drinks and comfort. Once the channel crossing was complete, he drove back to Clun without any sleep. The next morning, he was back in the shop as usual by six a.m. Mum was equally as robust, as the cramps that she must have felt in her limbs being unable to move very much were borne without complaint.

Generally, life was very hard for our parents, with few light-hearted moments and little spare money and no socialising. Despite this, they seemed to be able to provide us with books, music and an ethos of hard work. Looking back now I realise just how fortunate we were to have lived and grown up in such a special and magical place. Any regrets that I may have are to do with leaving Clun and my family at such an early age. Whilst there were always the school holidays back at home, our mother's illness restricted so much of normal family life.

2

A Family at War

Dulce et Decorum est pro patria mori.[1]

Those of my generation who avoided the armed services as a career, have been among the most fortunate in history. We have not had to endure conscription nor go to fight in a war. For some of us, the only experience of the armed forces had been a taster experience in the Combined Cadet Force (CCF) at school, and even that was voluntary and mostly fun. Those who chose not to take part could spend the afternoon in the woodwork shed making wonky bookshelves. Our Geography teacher Mr Harding was our Commanding Officer.

Sheer accident of birth protecting us from the horrors of war was not so for my forebears. I have already referred to my paternal grandfather, Charles Wells, who served throughout the First World War in France and who survived, but contracted a malaria-like disease in the stinking dampness of the trenches, from which he suffered for the rest of his life. This would manifest as bouts of shivering and whole-body aches characteristic of the ague. My grandmother would wrap him in a blanket and sponge his forehead with a tepid cloth until the violent rigours had settled.

He had learnt to drive steam engines as a sixteen year old in Liverpool and then on to the Great Western Railway at Shrewsbury in 1911. In 1914, he volunteered for duty in the Royal Engineers. They were responsible for moving food, equipment, ammunition and the big guns. The big guns would be towed into position to fire four or five rounds on the forward German lines before being towed back into camouflaged sidings to avoid being spotted. Their route was from the docks in Calais and Le Havre up to the frontlines of the Somme, Ypres and Passchendaele, scenes of the most horrific loss of life in the history of human warfare. As with so many of these veterans, it was very hard to get him to talk about his experiences. One story he did recount was when his engine broke down crossing a bridge over the River Lys at the battle of Ypres. There were thousands of tons of ammunition trapped on the bridge that would not move. Whilst Grandad and his fireman were trying to fix the problem, a German biplane flew over them and, leaning out of the cockpit, the pilot began to drop bombs by hand onto them. With that, they opened fire with their Lea-Enfield rifles along with the engineer in the guards' van of the train. Luckily, the German pilot missed. In fact, everyone missed their target and after a few ineffective passes, the German flew away. At last, as they nearly had the train in working order again, back came the persistent German pilot, flying low over the cabin of the engine hurling bricks at them that he had obviously landed in a field to pick up. After that fiasco, they steamed on to the ammunition dump, but the German pilot had followed them and reported their position. Whilst they were unloading the ammunition, a squadron of German planes came over and bombed the dump, this time more effectively. As my grandfather reported it, they had to stay undercover for almost three days whilst the ammunition exploded. One of his lasting memories was the mud. Thick, cloying mud that sucked their boots off and sapped their energy and morale. Trench foot was universal. By the end of the war, compounded by the pandemic of Spanish flu that swept through Europe in 1918, illness of one kind or another killed more men than the enemy fire.

Most of the men helping with the running of the trains were Chinese. He spoke warmly of them and their good-natured hard work. They were referred to as the Chinese Labour Corps [CLC]. Around 140,000 labourers were recruited from Shandong province. They were vital in the area of Artois and the Somme, rebuilding broken track, maintaining the engines and resupplying the frontlines.

In lighter moments, he would talk about the impromptu music and songs generated by the soldiers despite the dire situation that they were in. A frontline publication, the Wipers Times and Salient News (Ypres being pronounced as Wipers by the squaddies and salient, salient being a play on the word meaning appropriate or to the point, and a military projection in a line of attack) gave a fillip to everyone that read it. This ingenious ad hoc publication came about with the discovery by members of the Sherwood Foresters, of an abandoned printing press. A sergeant in the battalion was a printer by trade and was able to get the press rolling again. Frederick John Roberts was editor. He went on to be awarded the Military Cross for bravery at the battle of the Somme. The sub-editor was John Hesketh. Satirical poetry and prose were the regular contributions, all taking aim at the stupidity of it all and the commanding officers. This ingenious invention, born of the innate humour of the men, inured by the unending slaughter and mental and physical exhaustion of the whole ridiculous exercise, kept the morale of many alive. It was celebrated recently by a play re-enacting the events, written by Ian Hislop and Nick Newman. There seemed to be an abundance of poets amongst the ranks, and at one point, Roberts had to limit their submissions in favour of 'more prose'. It was first issued on 12 February 1916. As the combatants moved base, the title moved with them, the Kemmel Times, the Somme News and at the end of hostilities The Better Times.

My maternal grandmother's brother, another Charlie, Charlie Griffiths, was as stated earlier, a runner during the Great War. These men delivered messages between the staff bases well behind the lines to those commanding at the front. Much of it demanded running across dangerous open ground under the constant threat of sniper and machine gun fire. Those, lucky enough to have motorcycles, ended up declaiming them as they constantly broke down, and were more of a hinderance than help. The central character of the contemporary movie, '1917' is based on the true story of Alfred Mendes, paternal grandfather of the film's director, Sam Mendes. Alfred was one such runner, taking messages from the generals to the frontlines to overcome communication difficulties in battle conditions. It was a heroic role, full of danger. Doran Carter, curator of the National World War I museum in Kansas City, USA, explained the importance of these men in communication in a usually confused battlefield.

> They were more reliable than other means of communication, and they could get to places inaccessible by other means. They were chosen for their fitness, reliability and ability to read maps. They had to be able to find their destination in all weather conditions and all circumstances. Of all the jobs in the infantry it was the hardest and most dangerous.

An article in the *Hartford Daily Courant*[1] stated:

> With the runner's job it was the hardest and the most dangerous, it was only a question of time before they were killed or wounded.

Alan Clark in his book, *The Donkeys*, describing the total chaos of the war as witnessed at the battle of Auber's Ridge, writes,

> By now the confusion within the British lines was so great that all movement was impossible. The communication trenches whose shallow depth had caused disquiet earlier were now proving to be death traps and the normal system was so overloaded with stretcher parties and walking wounded as to be unusable, despite this, however, some individual runners from Haig's HQ were able to get through to General Rawlinson with 'urgent instructions.[2]

Charlie's survival was little short of a miracle, but he would never talk about it.

The closest that I was able to get to Charlie's experiences were large brass ash trays in my grandmother's house that were made from shell casings from that time. They had the names of Arnhem, Somme, Arras and Ypres engraved around them. In the centre of each was a bullet casing and a round of ammunition mounted as a centre piece. Granny, just as with the others who lived through those times, never commented upon them. I expect that they were from her husband, long dead, or Charlie, her brother. He was a quiet and retiring, but exceptionally hard-working man and totally reliable, just as you would expect from a 'runner'.

There is a noble history to this role characterised by Pheidippides, the ancient Greek who is said to have been the runner that took news of the Greek victory over the Persians from Marathon to Athens in 490 BCE. The authenticity of the mortality of the wartime role is emphasised by the death of Pheidippides at the end of his epic run.

A terrifying aspect of life in the trenches was the introduction of chemical warfare in the form of gassing the opposition troops. Both Grandad and Charlie had direct experience of this abhorrent tactic but were lucky only to suffer minor damage compared to many. They described the clouds of yellow gas wafting over the trench and enveloping them in misery, with pain and death all around them. They were fortunate to have had their poor but partly protective gas masks with them at the time. This report from the war by Brigadier-General Charteris describes the chilling effects of this awful weapon.

> The horrible part of it is the slow lingering death of those who are gassed. I saw some hundred poor fellows laid out in the open, in the forecourt of a church to give them all the air they could get, slowly drowning with water in their lungs – a most horrible sight, and the doctors quite powerless.[4]

Words from the sixteenth Canto of *The Divine Comedy* 'Purgatorio' by Dante come to mind as an apposite description of the hell that those men endured on a daily basis for four years at the front,

> Darkness in Hell, or any night stripped bare of planets under impoverished skies [a pall of smoke as dense as these could be], has never formed, for me, as thick a veil as did the smoke that now surrounded us, or stretched a weave so rasping in its feel that eyes could not stay open in its feel.[5]

This passage evokes images of the nightmare of soldiers, literally drowning in their own secretions caused by the toxic gas, in the dank and darkness of those trenches amid the barbed wire and exploding shells. The hell of the trenches in that war cannot be imagined by most of us in these times other than by the front-line troops in Ukraine, which has produced similar conditions.

Another close family relative who was involved in the First World War was Great Uncle Frank Wells, my grandfather's brother. He was an infantryman with the Cheshire regiment fighting alongside the Australians and the New Zealanders (ANZAC troops). They were involved in the Gallipoli campaign, which was ordered by Winston Churchill, then first Lord of the Admiralty. The idea was that through a second front in the underbelly of Europe it would be possible to ease the challenge that Russian troops were facing to the north and to use the navy to aid in the various land battles. To that end Churchill first planned a purely naval assault on the Dardanelles. He was aware of the dangers in approaching the Dardanelles through the straights of Marmora, less than one mile wide at their narrowest, made extremely hazardous by large numbers of mines and with Turkish forts heavily armed on each side. However, he was of the opinion that the Turks could be overwhelmed by sea power alone, something that some other cabinet colleagues of the time disagreed with. Indeed, to secure success, it was felt that an assault army 200,000 strong would be needed at the same time as the naval bombardment. The Greek army could not provide sufficient troops and Lord Kitchener stated that he didn't have enough troops under his command to allow that. Also, Churchill in his role at the Admiralty and with his passionate love of the navy, wanted a significant naval success as most of the British fleet at that time were tied up in the North Atlantic carrying out protection and prevention manoeuvres. Earlier in the war, two large British naval battle squadrons had failed to prevent a major German battleship, the *Goeben*, and a lighter vessel from slipping through the straights of Marmora from the eastern Mediterranean. Churchill had taken the flack for that. Despite fierce cabinet level battles and the obvious danger of failure, Churchill pushed through the plan. Amongst the opposition to the plan was the First Sea Lord Admiral John Fisher. He threatened resignation over the affair stating that, 'the damned Dardanelles, they will be our grave'.

Finally having decided to go ahead without the necessary simultaneous land assault the adventure began with a heavy naval bombardment on 18 March 1915. It was a disaster with several ships sunk and little impression on the Turk emplacements. It was followed a month later by the land assault on 25 April. That too was a disaster of immense proportions. At the failure of the naval assault, Admiral Fisher resigned his post, which began the slippery slope to the removal of Churchill. This was perhaps Churchill's most disastrous and dark moment and damaged his reputation for a long time afterwards.

Little is known of Uncle Frank's own escapades, other than he survived some horrendous battles in the Suvla Bay landings. A major assault was supposed to be on the ridge of high hills surrounding the horse-shoe shaped bay of the peninsula. The fourth and the seventh Cheshire regiments were there with the Manchesters and the Anzac troops.

The 4th and 7th battalions left England in the middle of July 1915. In the months before they had been very badly managed with muddled and disorderly training. To add insult to injury they were not told where they were going other than it would be a hot climate. They also sailed without battleship escort and not in convoy. All lights were out by 7.30 p.m. leaving nothing to do but to go to bed. Preparation for what was to come was not possible as they didn't know their destination. Their arrival in the port of Alexandria yielded some amusement as they were met by an embarkation officer dressed in shorts and wearing enormous spurs.[6] They were not allowed to disembark and sailed on to Port Said. Finally, sailing after dark, they dropped anchor off Mudros Harbour. It was as daylight arrived that they could see that they were in a curved bay enclosed by high rocky boulder-strewn hills. They had to capture the hilltop fort named Tekke-Tepe, a formidable task. Already the ANZAC forces were taking heavy casualties with fire reigning down on them from all sides. In front of the hills was a salt-lake plain with no cover. Astonishingly, they still had not been told where they were, and it was only when someone found a box containing maps that their position was revealed to them. Worse still, the surviving troops already there were exhausted and completely demoralised. Added to that, the only ammunition that the newly arrived troops had was that which they had managed to bring ashore with them. With little food and no proper rest it is easy to see just how demoralised they would have become.

No organisation was seen and they were sent directly into battle with wounded troops streaming between them in the opposite direction and having to weave amongst the dead left lying on the salt pans. It must have been a scene of horror for those men having just arrived after being couped up on a ship for three weeks. There was dissonance between the officers, with some ordering the men to certain death and others refusing to obey the order.

As the assault progressed, little was seen of the Seventh Cheshires as reported by a Captain Crookenden of the 159th Brigade headquarters, suggesting that they had been all but wiped out. We do know from personal reports by Frank to my father that on one assault, his battalion were charged with scaling a cliff under heavy enemy fire from Turkish soldiers entrenched on the summit. In the initial landing, they had been ordered to fight with their bayonets and not to fire a shot so as not to call enemy fire onto them. There was intense hand-to-hand fighting and of more than 500 men in Frank's battalion only 70 survived. In the general assault there were 18 officers killed, 16 badly wounded and over 800 men wounded, lost or killed. Overall, over 30,000 British Empire men were killed on this atrociously planned and poorly executed exercise. This whole debacle was a major catastrophe, which exemplified the very poor command and control of the unfortunate troops on the ground and left Winston Churchill's reputation in tatters.

Again, like the others, Uncle Frank never spoke about the war, but as with my other family members, he served for the full four years. He and his surviving colleagues went straight from those death ridden battlefields to Mesopotamia where further massive casualties awaited them. The survival of any of them seems miraculous.

My father's maternal aunt Hannah Babbage (nee Brookes) had three children: Betty, Barbara and Cyril. The families spent quite a lot of time together as both had butcher's shops and lived quite close together. Indeed, on discharge from the army, my grandfather had worked with Mr Babbage senior in his shop in Ludlow. Cyril, born in 1917 was ten years older than my father, but Cyril, Barbara and Betty were very close. Dad frequently told stories of the wonderful times they had shared in Ludlow and latterly in Ross-on-Wye.

Cyril, later known as Frank, like my father, joined the Royal Airforce Volunteer Reserve, [R.A.F.V.R.] in October 1938, as a pilot officer. He learnt to fly Hurricanes and Spitfires and was a moderately experienced pilot at the outbreak of war in 1939. He was called up in September of that year and joined 602 Squadron [City of Glasgow squadron] first based at Drem in Scotland before moving to Westhampnett, now Goodwood, in August of 1940. Westhampnett is very close to RAF Tangmere and the squadrons seemed to have used both airfields on a convenience basis.

Immediately embroiled in the Battle of Britain, he was 'one of the few' immortalised by Winston Churchill in his now famous speech, delivered in the House of Commons on 20 August 1940, during which he said,

> Never in the field of human conflict was so much owed by so many to so few.

Cyril, whose nickname became Cabbage (for obvious reasons), rapidly made his mark in the squadron, claiming a Junkers Ju 87 on 18 August and a Ju 88 the following day. He then won a battle between himself and an Me 110 and destroyed a Dornier Do 17 on 25 August. The following day, he shot down a Bf 109 over Selsey Bill. At that point, his luck ran out and he was shot down by Hauptmann Mayer of 1/JG53 squadron. He was able to bail out and was picked up after several hours in the sea by a rowing boat and landed at Bognor Regis Pier. Perhaps the putative last words of King George V who, on being offered the opportunity to recover in Bognor Regis were, 'Bugger Bognor' might also have run through Cyril's mind. More likely though, he was probably pleased to see the coastline there on being recovered. His Spitfire X4188 crashed into the sea.

The coolness of these young men under fire can be seen in this extract taken from the combat report of the incident written by Cyril in his own hand on 26 August 1940:

> I was Green 2 and took off from Westhampnett at 16.13. I followed Green 1, climbing to attack fighters and got separated. I saw ME109 on tail of Spitfire and attacked from dead astern and as he turned away used a deflection shot. [Firing ahead in anticipation of where the aircraft would be]. He fell into a spin from the turn and went down with large quantities of black smoke coming from engine. I am confident that this enemy aircraft was probably destroyed. I then attacked centre aircraft of 3 Dornier 215's in 'V' formation which was one of several such formations making out to sea, adopting a dead ahead attack, opening 300 yards and firing until my ammunition was exhausted. I saw my bullets striking this enemy aircraft but observed no damage. Heavy crossfire was experienced from all the bombers and as I broke away downwards to the left, I was struck by a cannon shell probably from an ME109 and had to bail out because my aircraft was on fire. Signed C.F. Babbage 602 squadron.

He had shell splinters in his legs, which needed hospitalisation, but after two days he was back in the air. His commanding officer was Squadron leader Sandy Johnstone. He collected him from the hospital with the base medical officer the same day as the accident. His clothes were still damp from his immersion in the Channel, so he was driven back to Westhampnett in a coat borrowed from a hospital porter. Such was the spirit of the times.

The irony of this story is that one of those who rescued him was a commando with whom he became great friends. They used to meet in London whenever they were on leave. On the last occasion that they met, the friend was driving back to Aldershot when his car was struck by a stray German bomb and he was killed. The terrible vicissitudes of war.

An important victory was over a serious German ace, Hauptmann Walter Adolph. He was flying an aircraft superior to the Mk V Spitfire, the Focke-Wulf 190. It was a faster aircraft, and it could fly higher than the Spitfire, which was only superior in tight turns. To win this battle against one of the top fighter pilots in the German air force was a major victory showing great skill and courage. These air battles were latter day duels in the sky, and excellent airmanship and a considerable degree of luck was usually the deciding factor.

Cyril shot down several other aircraft and shared in the destruction of many more. He was shot down a total of five times himself during the whole of the war but survived them all.

He was awarded the Distinguished Flying Medal (DFM) for bravery on 25 October 1940. This was the citation in the *London Gazette*,

> Sergeant Babbage has shown consistent keenness and ability in operations against the enemy. He has personally destroyed six enemy aircraft and probably one other.

He spent time as a flying instructor at the operational training unit at Grangemouth and was commissioned flying officer in December 1941. In June of that year, he had been posted to 41 squadron at Merston, just north of Bognor Regis. With that squadron he flew operational tours on what were originally referred to as mosquito and circus operations. Mosquito ops. were daylight raids on selected targets in northern France. The Circus ops. were joint attacks with bomber command acting as fighter cover for mid-range bombing raids. The name of Mosquito raids was changed to Rhubarb operations because of confusion with the aircraft of that name. During these very dangerous operations his aircraft were hit but he survived these intact. These were often low-level attacks with just one or two fighters flying into enemy territory under significant cloud cover. The low cloud cover and often squally conditions made the flying dangerous in addition to the danger from flack and enemy aircraft. During these missions many skilled pilots, who had survived the Battle of Britain, were lost. They were seen by those in charge of running the RAF fighter division as important elements of the forward attacking force as the war was taken from the defensive, as in the Battle of Britain, to the offensive in Europe. However, it is questionable just how effective they were when measured against the serious losses that they sustained.

Following this episode Cyril was transferred to 9 Service Flying Training School at Hullavington.

Cyril continued in the RAF after the war and became a senior instructor doing tours in Greece and the USA. He retired in 1964 having achieved the rank of Wing Commander. He died in 1976 with a form of dementia and part of the cause was said to be the effect of high altitude flying without supplementary oxygen at the beginning of the war. As mentioned earlier, it was the way that the skilled pilots avoided the Bf 109s and FW 190s. It was said that they would climb as high as they could until they blacked out, hoping to gather the aircraft as they fell to lower altitudes regaining their consciousness.

Needless to say, Cyril was quite the hero in our family. Father recounted how on one occasion, he appeared over Clun doing low passes and victory barrel rolls to the great delight of the town folk, Dad in particular. He was the archetypal Battle of Britain pilot with the black Labrador dog and a British racing green open-top MG sports car. I never met him but as a youngster glowed with pride in his reflected heroism.

With the advent of the Second World War, Grandad had already made himself a significant person in the town and was very well-known. He seemed a natural choice to head up the A.R.P. [Air Raid Protection] wardens, colloquially known as Dad's Army. It may seem ludicrous to think that Clun, such a sleepy backwater could be of any interest to the German war machine, but it turned out that there were things going on that did attract attention. On the hills above Clun, large amounts of ammunition were being stored in covered shelters under the hedgerows, and Grandad and his fellow wardens were charged with their safe keeping. A stranger appeared in the town quite early in the war and kept himself very much to himself. Grandad and others noticed some suspicious behaviour in the walks that this man was taking, especially after dark. One evening they followed him at a discreet distance and found him making notes on the dumps of ammunition and taking photographs. They seized him and handed him over to the police who passed him on to the secret service. He was spying for Germany, preparing to report the whereabouts of those dumps so that they could be attacked.

The other stark reminder of war was that from the tops of the highest hills, Grandad reported that they could see the ominous glow in the sky to the north where Liverpool docks were being bombed. At the same time, my mother to be was living in Llanelli with her family. They were very close to the bombing of Swansea and Cardiff. It was a terrifying sight to see Swansea Docks ablaze after enemy bombing. There was a Royal Ordinance factory in Llanelli, which was also the target of heavy enemy bombing.

My father, being only eleven years old at the outbreak of war, was spared that terrible ordeal. However, in 1947, he was called up for the Palestine campaign. He joined the R.E.M.E. (Royal Electrical and Mechanical Engineers). After a period of training, he was shipped off to North Africa. First to Tripoli and then to Palestine. It was another squalid affair and rarely spoken about in the campaigns that Britain was involved in. Many British troops were killed and often in awful circumstances. Kidnap and murder were common.

After the First World War ended, the League of Nations passed the mandate for Palestine to the British. The Balfour declaration from the British government promised to establish a Jewish national home and the Arab nationalists a united Arab country covering most of the middle east if both groups would fight with the British to defeat the Ottoman Turks. Britain failed to deliver on either promise. This led to the Arab revolt from 1936 to 1939. As a realisation of the absolute horrors of the holocaust struck home, Britain limited Jewish immigration to Palestine to European Jews to help them escape the terror of Nazi persecution. The numbers were limited in

1939 in an attempt to appease the Egyptians and the oil rich Arab countries. There was a serious Jewish reaction to this and the Haganah began to use terrorism against the British. Dad and his fellow troops were tasked with capturing their leader. The main terrorist group was the Irgun Zvai Leumi led by the future Israeli prime minister, Menachem Begin and the Lohami Heruth Israel, fighters for the freedom of Israel (LHI). The British called the LHI the Stern Gang. In November 1941, the LHI assassinated the British Minister for the Middle East Lord Moyne. At the end of the Second World War, President Harry Truman made repeated requests for the ban on immigration of Jews to Palestine and to limit the numbers to 100,000 Jewish people. The British refused and the terror campaign intensified. The Hagenah that had restrained from attacking the British whilst they were fighting the Nazis then joined forces with other underground groups and began to attack the British troops. In 1947 the number of British troops there had reached 100,000 and the majority were National Servicemen like my father. They were of the 3rd. Infantry division and they needed a great deal of mechanised support. Tank transporters, tanks, scout cars and troop carriers all needed continuous maintenance. The army could not operate without the support of the Royal Engineers.

I remember Dad talking about the Hagenah and the Stern Gang. Elements of them would lure the troops with apparent friendly banter into local hostelries and then murder them after a few drinks. Whatever the rights and wrongs and the politics of these wars, major or minor, it is the men on the ground who must follow the orders of their commanders who in turn are directed by the politicians. It was in this hot bed of revolt that Dad found himself immersed. Several of his friends were killed, some of them by his side.

A highlight spoken about by many of the soldiers was (and still is) the Lady of Gharyan. In a former Italian barracks there is a mural of a naked woman painted on one of the walls. The upper outline of her torso is supposed to represent the form of the North African coastline. Certain points of her anatomy are marked with the towns of North Africa. It was drawn by Clifford Saber in March 1943. Saber was a volunteer American ambulance driver with the British 8th army. The Lady adorned the wall of Dad's workshop in Gharyan. It continues as a tourist attraction.

That ugly war seems to have largely been forgotten in modern times, but many good men were lost. Once again, the artificial division of native lands by foreign powers set the scene for the following decades of despair, war, death and destruction, which continues to this day. I am truly grateful that neither I nor my son Nicholas have had to endure what earlier members of our family had to live through.

3

School Days

Wisdom is the daughter of experience[1]

St George's Primary School, Clun

My memories of Clun school are mainly pleasant, if dimmed with the passage of time. When I cast my mind back to those distant and dreamy days, images of the tall and angular Mr Guppy the headmaster predominate. Always with a ready smile and the aroma of pipe tobacco, his genial manner was very reassuring. Mrs Guppy, his somewhat rounded and jolly wife and deputy head, seemed more in the background. I have little memory of the other teachers.

The school day began with a walk from our house in the market square down to the old bridge over the River Clun, past the blacksmith's forge, and then up the short steep hill towards the church and then right along School Road. This took around ten minutes without stopping along the way; however, the desire to throw stones into the river and to play Pooh sticks was often irresistible. At the ages of five or six my grandfather would walk us to school, but thereafter we walked with friends or my sister Rosamond who was enrolled three years after me.

The return journey was often highlighted by persuading my grandfather to buy some sweets from the strategically if somewhat cynically placed kiosk at the corner of School Road. If the blacksmith was at work, we would stop to stroke the horses and to watch the dramatic performance of heating the metal shoes and then the shoeing of the horse. The smell of the burning hooves and the rising smoke and steam added to the drama. At the sight of the horses, Grandad would recall stories of delivering the meat to farmers up in the hills by pony and trap.

The first classroom that I can remember was dominated by a tall, circular, iron coke burning stove with an angulated metal narrow chimney venting somewhere through the roof of the classroom. I can still sense the smell of the acrid fumes that arose from it in the winter. They made me cough and could be quite overwhelming. Today these fumes are classified as a class A risk for lung cancer and other respiratory illnesses. They contain methane, carbon monoxide and ethylene and I think that it was the ethylene that caused the bronchospasm and coughing. There was no talk of health and safety in those days. We were just thankful to be warm.

At 11 a.m. each day a glass bottle of milk would be given to each of us: the original free school milk. In the winter the bottles were placed around the top of the stove to warm the milk, the heat from the bottle warming our hands in turn. We were always provided with a hot lunch which was usually quite edible apart from the ubiquitous school overboiled cabbage stinking of sulphur.

The subjects taught were quite widely spread but with a firm focus on the three 'r's: reading writing and arithmetic. A heavy emphasis was placed on being able to write legibly and neatly. This instilled in me a love of handwriting that I still have. In this time of e-mail, text messages and social media, it gives me great delight to receive a letter and I continue to hand write thank you letters and some of general information. I think that it is possible to tell a lot about someone's character through their handwriting and the fact that they take the time and trouble to communicate in that way. I still have many letters from people that I have cared about, from parents, grandparents and other close relatives and friends. Re-reading the letters and cards, and the tactile experience of holding the paper that they wrote upon, makes me feel close to them again. Especially now that many are no longer here and there is little other tangible connection with them.

Rudimentary biology, geography, history and religious studies were favourites of mine. The stories of the Plantagenets and the Tudors sparked a lifelong interest in medieval history. As a result, years later I visited the Abbey at Fontevrault, near Tours to pay homage to Queen Eleanor, someone that I had first learnt about at Clun school. Seeing the tomb of Eleanor of Aquitaine lying next to her husband Henry II, with her son Richard I close by was a most moving experience. As I approached the tomb, sunlight was beaming powerfully from a window high above, spotlighting Eleanor's face. Of all the women that I admire, Eleanor has pride of place having led a most extraordinary life. She married two kings, first Louis VII of France and then Henry II of England, and gave birth to two future kings, one the romantic idol Richard the Lionheart and the other King John, a wretch, but the author of the Magna Carta. It is extraordinary to think that Henry and Eleanor ruled from the Scottish border to the Pyrenees. The enthusiasm with which we were taught back then was infectious.

Maths was always a trial for me. Any ability that I might have had was probably compromised by mild dyslexia. Something I came to study later during my early years as a medical student at the Helen Arkell dyslexic centre at Parsons Green. Susan Hampshire was an early patron and made several visits to the centre and volunteered to be part of the study that I arranged with Dr Hugh Jolly, paediatrician at Charing Cross.

Being something of a talkative youngster, my earliest school reports are replete with comments such as 'Francis is interested in everything, but he talks too much in class', and in another entry, 'Francis is a chatterbox'. I loved to ask questions, a feature of my character which persists. I must have been an annoyance to the rest of the class. However, I remember the patience of the teachers in answering me. Perhaps I was more destined for a life in politics than medicine.

We were brought up to be polite and respectful, particularly by my grandfather. Probably because of this, in one end of term report Headmaster Guppy commented that I was a good little boy (who is very young). On re-reading my old school reports, assiduously kept for me by my mother, I find that in the springtime of 1960 I was top of the class. There is an amusing comment on my spelling which reads, 'spelling a little original'. It hasn't improved with the passage of time. However, this relative academic success was short lived.

These results led to an early sitting of the Eleven-Plus examination. All that I can remember of that is one day being told to sit quietly in a room on my own and answer the questions on the paper placed in front of me. This turned out to be the aforementioned exam, which somehow, I managed to pass. When I received the results, I was allowed out of school to tell my parents. I think that it was in the middle of a busy Tuesday morning, market day in Clun. On my return I fell over on the gravel path badly grazing my knees. I went back home to be cleaned up and receive some T.L.C. The event stands out so clearly in my mind as in the excitement of the moment, Mum managed to confuse a tube of toothpaste with Savlon antiseptic wound cream. The sharp sting of the toothpaste smeared on both knees ensured the memory was long-lived.

My success in the Eleven-Plus led to premature entrance to secondary education. The only school close to us was the secondary modern school in Bishop's Castle that Dad had attended. Although the school's certificate had been replaced largely by GCE O levels in 1951, there was little or no progression to higher education. All the children progressed to practical forms of work, mainly on the surrounding farms or into associated jobs, which were plentiful. At that time manpower was still essential to bring in the harvest and to look after the animals. No one in Clun was out of work as far as I can remember. At that time, farm machinery was simple, and each farm needed many employees. Few moved away. Perhaps more striking was the statistic that no one had reached university in our town. My mother knew that she wanted better for us and so the search began for an appropriate school for each of us. This inevitably meant some form of boarding school. The exact process that they went through in trying to find an adequate place we were never told. It was going to be an enormous financial commitment for a small country butcher business. This must have been a factor in the very limited holidays that we had.

I remember being entered for a choral scholarship at the Hereford Cathedral School where, similarly to King's College School in Cambridge, scholarship places were awarded to pupils with a good singing voice. The passage from Handel's *Messiah*, 'How beautiful Are The Feet' was chosen as suitable in length and pitch. I was tutored in this by my piano teacher. The day of the audition arrived, and we drove to Hereford for my performance. I remember very little other than standing alone in the nave of the cathedral and singing my heart out. How it really sounded I will never know but, surprisingly, I was offered a place. However, when I was informed that it would mean being away from home for much of the Christmas and Easter holidays, I made it known that was not what I wanted to do. I suspect that my kind-hearted father felt the same and so this option was closed.

I think that I must have expressed concern about being sent away from home as I remember that attempts were made to persuade me how wonderful this would be. I had been given books such as *Tom Brown's School Days* and the escapades of Billy Bunter to encourage me. Gradually the mythical possibilities of boarding school began to infiltrate my mind. The schoolboy pranks described therein began to appeal to me. I remember phrases such as 'I say you fellows' and 'Crikey, you beast'. All sound so archaic now. Slowly I warmed to the idea. Little did I know how close to the truth the darker elements of these books would become. Thrashings by both prefects and masters, as well as long periods of detention would become common place.

Then one day, I was whisked off to Adams' Grammar School, a Haberdashers' school in Newport, north Shropshire, approximately 70 miles from Clun. The eldest son of a very well to do family of farmers further down the Clun valley had already attended the school and his parents were delighted with his progress. He had become a very successful auctioneer, a profession that my father knew well through the cattle markets, and for which he had respect. Dad drove me there in our cream-coloured Ford Consul. We were met by the school secretary and ushered into the headmaster's study. Jeff Roberts was headmaster throughout my time at the school. He was a lovely man whose attitude towards his pupils and pastoral care afforded was excellent for the time. He had a wonderfully gentle and reassuring voice. Another pipe smoker like Mr Guppy, that genial man left a wonderful impression on me. We remained in touch until recent times. Later when I was in the lower sixth form, he took up the cloth and every Sunday he was seen leaving for a seminary in Lichfield in preparation for the priesthood.

The interview with Mr Roberts was in the presence of my father. I can remember little of it except that there was a step down from the hallway to enter his dimly lit study in which one was enveloped by the fug and aroma of pipe tobacco which hung in the air. It was a quiet, book-lined room with a large desk in front of an even larger window, behind which Mr Roberts sat with a most congenial smile, rising to shake hands with us and to welcome us to the school. He had an extremely quiet but authoritative voice. Clearly all went well, as I was offered a place to start in the autumn of 1960, and a scholarship to cover all my books and a proportion of the boarding fees. Despite that, if my memory serves me well, it was going to cost my father £75 per term which, considering subsequent devaluation of the currency and inflation since 1960, was roughly equivalent to £1,500 today. This was a huge amount for them to find and then to do the same for my two sisters, for they were intent on treating us all the same. It meant significant restrictions for the family.

One of the saddest things about going away to school was that once my elder sister Rosamond followed suit it felt to me that family life really evaporated. We saw little of each other and Charmian as our younger sister was a generation apart from us. There were exeat weekends when we could go home from the Friday evening until Sunday afternoon. But for me, they were more unsettling than reassuring as the return to school was quite traumatic. I suffered badly from homesickness in the early years, exacerbated by my concern for my mother because of her illness.

Adams' Grammar School

As the time to start at school approached, we had to buy the school uniform in Newport. I can still remember the excitement of these preparations for my departure. One Wednesday during half-day closing in Clun, we drove to Newport to the school outfitter T. Whitmore in the high street. It had a deeply ingrained characteristic smell of new clothes and leather in a long-existing setting. Dust hung in the air, highlighted by the rays of sunshine. Blazer, cap, tie, and short trousers were duly bought in the regulation amounts, all a size too big so that I could 'grow into them'. We returned home, where Granny sewed into them the necessary name tags. The excitement was building.

It was in September of 1960 that my time at Adams' began. My grandfather talked to me about the way to behave towards others and always to respect Mum and Dad, remembering that they wanted us to succeed for ourselves and not for them. He was such a good and honest man who always thought of others first. I miss him and his songs and humour.

Being ten years old, I was significantly younger than the other boys in my year. This immaturity probably contributed to my poor start. I had been placed in the 'A' Stream on the basis of my results at Clun primary school. This was not to last.

The first two years were spent in the junior boarding house Aston Hall, on the outskirts of the town, approximately half an hour's walk away. This had to be undertaken whatever the weather, not terribly comfortable in the winter as we had to always wear short trousers, without exception. Boys from the year above could cycle, but few boys had bikes at school. During that year, one boy was hit by a car and killed.

Perhaps going away to school so young was a mistake for me. As the first months passed by very slowly, the romantic visions derived from the children's books receded into an idealised myth and the homesickness began to set in. The freedom of the Clun countryside was replaced by the restrictions of the boarding school. Rules were tight, and the rigour of fixed mealtimes, set prep times and lights out felt claustrophobic. I found myself existing from exeat weekends to the end of term, to be able to return home.

Fellow boarder, Desmond (Dessie) Shaw became a very good friend with whom I shared a lot of free time. Dessie was a very bright boy and was top of the class in Maths and other subjects. It all seemed to come very naturally to him. On the other hand, I struggled badly and seemed to drift down the class order with each successive term. I can still remember being on a walk one sunny Sunday afternoon with Dessie expressing my depression at being such a failure. His mature kindness towards me was quite inspirational and he managed to spur me on to continue to try. I seem to remember him trying to reassure me that I was not really as stupid as I had expressed myself to be. Perhaps he was partly correct as once out of the boarding school environment and away at university I seemed to achieve good results without too much difficulty, but I had great difficulty concentrating and really didn't know how to work efficiently.

Leaving home each time was a traumatic event for me. I can vividly remember the cauldron of emotions churning inside me as we set off back on a Sunday evening. Before leaving I would visit my grandfather and grandmother in their next-door terraced houses in Castle Street for some quiet time. It was always to Granny Mold first, and then to Grandad next door, where he would spur me on for the next bout of school. The drive back would take about one and a half hours. As we approached Newport we passed through the moderately sized industrial town of Wellington, where there was a steel works. In the winter darkness or the half-light of a late summer's evening, you could see the molten steel flowing from the blast furnaces in bright yellow rivulets. I always felt foreboding at that point in the journey, as drop off time was only fifteen minutes away. I unashamedly admit that my parents' departure, especially that of Dad, caused serious tears to flow, which often needed the help of the Matron to calm me. On one occasion seeing me in such distress, meaning well, but doing the worst thing possible, Dad drove around the block and returned to Aston Hall. I was standing in a tall window hoping, but not expecting that they would return, when suddenly the car reappeared. I rushed down to the entrance and after a period I had to be pulled away so that they could leave again. My mother was steely hard in her determination that I should stay, but I think that if Dad had had his way, I would have been removed from the school. Who knows where I would have ended up then. I suspect, as I have matured, that she suppressed her true feelings knowing that that was the only route out of a mundane future life in Clun. She persisted, and I stayed and as they say the rest is history.

The boarding house, Aston Hall might have been a lovely old house in its day, but this was largely lost on us pupils. Built in the late, somewhat austere Georgian style, the grounds were quite extensive with a somewhat foreboding wooded perimeter.

On arrival we were met by the Housemaster, who greeted us and our parents. Mr Anderson, a very caring man bore, for obvious reasons, the rather unkind nickname of 'Flapper'. After the parents had departed, leaving us with our cases and tuck boxes, we were given a tour of the building, something that I have little memory of.

As in many groups of boys and young men, there were rituals that had to be passed through for full acceptance in the group. In the garden was a large Holly Bush with a narrow opening at its base, the cause of which we soon discovered. The ritual that we all had to pass through as a rite of passage was to be thrown backwards into the bush. Few complained as the more senior boys took revenge for their own traumas and threw us in with a vengeance. A few cried but not for long. With courage and a maturity beyond his years Dessie refused to take part and after several attempts by the seniors to hurl him into the bush they desisted. This was not the 'done thing', but I soon began to learn the importance of collegiate support for your peers.

We were housed in dormitories of varying size, and I remember that my first one slept eight of us, along with a dormitory prefect. He was a senior boy from the upper sixth form of whom I have but few memories. Lights out was at 9.00 p.m. and there was a strictly enforced no talking rule. If caught reading under the bedclothes with a night light, chatting or wandering around, we were issued with capital punishment dealt out by the prefects with the use of a sports shoe, often with a hole cut in the sole to trap the air and increase the pain factor. The prefect's room was at the top of an old sweeping staircase. Whilst awaiting capital punishment, we had to stand patiently in the hall outside, waiting to be called in. Thrashings were quite a regular event but were too much for some of the quieter boys. It was not unusual to have the more robust of us offer to take the punishment for them. Despite those threatened traumas it was common, on return from home after exeat weekends or at the beginning of term with full tuck boxes, to hold midnight feasts by torchlight, and occasionally candlelight. How there were no fires I will never know. During one such feast, we were discovered and two of the boys leapt into a large wardrobe swinging the door closed after them. Their weight distribution was uneven and slowly but gaining momentum we could see this large piece of furniture with the two boys inside collapse door downwards with them trapped inside. The loud bang followed by the muffled cries of those trapped inside rather gave the game away. Yet another thrashing ensued.

The staff to pupil ratio at the Hall was very low, with just the housemaster Mr Anderson, the two sixth form prefects and a long-suffering matron. There was a small sick bay reserved for boys who succumbed to 'flu or some other lurgy but mainly occupied by boys impersonating illness to avoid an exam, a cross country run or some other event. My one short stay there with a heavy cold or 'flu was treated with regular aspirin, unpalatable soup and the rather lovely motherly matron regularly taking my temperature.

Adams' school was founded in 1656 and named after William Adams who was himself born in Newport. He became a wealthy London merchant and made his fortune in Haberdashery. In addition to the school, he built the alms houses situated on either side of the school frontage.

It was a direct grant grammar school. Direct grant schools, abolished in 1976, were schools largely paid for by the parents, but which were allowed a government grant in exchange for taking non-fee-paying pupils. We had a significant number of 'dayboys', as we called them, who filled those places. Since the death of William Adams in 1661, the school has been sponsored and soundly supported by the Haberdashers' company, a prominent member of The Great Twelve livery companies of the City of London, where wealth dictated power and influence. In the medieval period, the Haberdashers were in competition with other prominent livery companies, particularly the Merchant Tailors, being initially known as the Merchant Haberdashers. A charter by Henry VIII forced them to drop the merchant part of the idiom but in return the Merchant Tailors had to pay a sum of money to the Haberdashers. At that time, there were quite violent disputes between the two livery companies which resulted in rioting in the streets, so much so that the king declared that the two companies would alternate in their hierarchical positions in The Great Twelve. One year, the Haberdashers would be number six and the Merchant Taylors number seven. This ranking was very important to their status in the city. The higher ranked company would then have to entertain the other to a feast once a year. This would then rotate the following year. This gave rise to the common saying of being at sixes and sevens still used today. Other common terms originated from those times. The phrase 'pin money' alluding to some cash given to the spouse for household purchases came from the money given to wives to purchase exuberant hatpins, usually imported from France. The term pin money is still in common use today.

Some of the classrooms that I remember were quite austere. The old wooden desks with the fold up lids were rickety and often smelt of strange things stored within from the past. In the summer we would place our little self-made radios into the closed desk, and run a wire attached to an earpiece up our sleeve to emerge at the wrist. One's head would then be rested against the hand and the earpiece placed discreetly into the ear. We could then listen to the test match in the summer, preferring the dulcet tones of Brian Johnston, Richie Benaud or John Arlott, over the boring Geography, Latin or Maths master.

I remember little of what of was taught in those early years and my school reports reflect this lack of engagement. My school report from the end of my first term in December 1960 placed me 28th in class and 31st in the overall examination results with only thirty-one in the class. The headmaster's report says it all, 'His positions are rather disappointing. He must work hard to improve.' This, from the man who had offered me a scholarship on perceived potential and a place one year earlier than was probably wise. His disappointment is palpable in those words. These poor results led to me being demoted from the A stream 1A to Class 2B for the following year. I managed to find some comfort from this, as it was the class of the Bash Street Kids in the *Beano*, my journal of the time.

My school reports for the rest of the year changed little, with comments such as:

> ...very fair, but needs to be driven, in Latin and French. Seems to do his best but is inclined at times to find unexpected difficulties in Maths.

Life settled into a rhythmic routine. The wake-up bell was rung around the houses by the duty prefect at 7.00 a.m. The usual ablutions were followed by bed-making and then inspection of the neatness of the bed, then hands, hair, shoes and blazers, front and back by the house prefect. Breakfast was at 8.00 a.m. in the dining hall followed by the twenty-minute walk from Aston Hall to the main school or a short fallow period prior to the beginning of lessons.

The day's lessons were timetabled into single and double periods. Games were scheduled for every Wednesday afternoon. Rugby or hockey in the winter and cricket in the summer. In addition there were physical exercise lessons twice a week and from the late springtime through to the beginning of the autumn term in late September there was compulsory swimming in the outdoor pool. In the gym we were subjected to rope climbing with the teacher standing beneath us with a sport's shoe in hand to hit us on the backside if we didn't make to the top of the rope. Circuit training and a lot of running around with medicine balls was commonplace. In the latter years, the school obtained a full-size trampoline, a sport that I began to enjoy enormously. At the end of the session there was five minutes to shower and dress. As we left the changing rooms for the next lesson, anyone over the five minutes would receive a further wack on the backside with a tennis pump, delivered by the teacher with a sardonic grin on his face and calling after you, 'next time you will be quicker'. Frequently and probably sadistically, the pump would hit the back of the thigh, which stung much more. To achieve the shower and get dressed in the time with thirty boys all crammed into a small shower and changing room area, meant getting dressed whilst still wet with our clothes sticking to us most uncomfortably. Usually you got your leg jammed half way into the trouser leg and found yourself hobbling out half-dressed to avoid the attack. If that was the case we were dragged back and given two more hits for our pains. This was all done in the name of discipline.

Something that bothered me on the games field, beginning at that time, was my name: Francis. At that stage in my life it seemed very cissyish and not at all what was expected of a rugby forward. It was then that I took on the name of my father and great uncle Frank. It stuck through much of the rest of my life, although as I grow older my actual name seems to be becoming more natural. It is surprising how difficult it is to reverse the habit for friends around me. However, it has to be said that most seem to prefer my given name these days.

At the end of the school day the day boys would line up by the school gate with a bus prefect making sure that there were no high jinks. We boarders would then go on to after school clubs such as chess, woodwork or art with the regular cross-country run thrown in for good measure. Dinner was at six followed by invigilated prep. Its duration depended upon the year that we were in. On Friday evenings, there was a film club that would show films selected by the masters. I remember *Battleship Potemkin* particularly well for its harrowing scenes such as the baby in the pram running away from the mother down steep steps and the mutiny of the crew, through which we lived vicariously, rebelling against the masters in our own minds. Rarely would the film be entertaining but more with the attitude of cultural expansion.

It was in the middle of one of these showings, the evening of 22 November, that Mr Humphries our house master entered the hall to tell us to stop the film and to switch on the television to watch the breaking news of the shocking death of President Kennedy. We were all stunned into silence. We were allowed to follow the news avidly over the weekend for the momentous event that it was.

Saturday morning was a further prep period and more time for club activities. In the afternoon, those of us in school teams would play at home or away matches against other schools and clubs. Saturday evenings were free. Sundays began similarly but included compulsory church service at St Nicholas Church, a grand sandstone building just across the road from the front of the school. Those of us in the choir were required to attend choir practice regularly. Sunday afternoons were free, and exeats could be obtained from the house master to escape the cloistered life and roam the countryside for covert meetings with girlfriends or long cycle rides. Following dinner in the evening we were expected to write letters to our parents in a formal quiet period followed by more prep and bed.

Despite my poor performance in the mainstream subjects, in the arts I was flying along and doing well. Our art teacher Mr Jerry Chambers seemed very pleased. He wrote in my report, 'He is very interested with good results'. Chambers was a member of the jazz group The Temperance Seven, playing the trombone. His attitude was liberating. As many know, the sight of a blank sheet of paper can be intimidating. To get us over this, he would wander around the classroom declaring that we should, 'Waste paper, boys. Waste paper'. Occasionally, he would bring out his trombone or trumpet and stroll among us playing jazz. A wonderful man whose memory still produces a smile.

There was an annual arts and music competition between schoolhouses, of which there were five, Adams, Clive, Darwin, Talbot and my house, Ward. This was called the Dixon Cup Art and Crafts Competition. It was founded on high ideals. As Mr Chambers summarised in his commentary on its aims,

> It should be seen as an instrument of expression for human aspirations and emotions through the Arts, and that the Dixon Cup competition is also all about communication. The House which satisfactorily communicates within itself is the House which is poised and confident.

High ideals indeed.

In the fifth form, I was put in charge of organising Ward house's entries. I was determined that we should win it. There were two parts. The first was a concert in which we could stage whatever we wanted to. I had been practicing Rachmaninov's prelude in C sharp minor and we had a madrigal choir that I had pulled together and conducted. Other boys played violin pieces, and we had a string quartet. We had made a film of a group of boys on a fishing trip and recorded Schubert's Trout Quintet as the soundtrack. Filmed in the sunshine of the previous summer term, it was great fun recording clips of friends cycling on the tow path of the Shropshire Union Canal, falling in and other riotous events. The rendering of the music was a bit ropy but the movie, filmed on 35-mm film, was a great success.

For the theatrical part, we constructed an artificial trench to simulate those of the frontline in the First World War and had recorded the sounds of exploding shells from our cadet force exploits at Sennybridge. In that setting, and over the background hullabaloo of live fire, we recited extracts from the great poets of that war, Houseman, Rupert Brooke, Robert Graves and particularly Wilfred Owen. Dressed in our army uniforms with blackened faces it was a great success.

Part two of the competition the following week was an art exhibition. I wanted it to be as spectacular as possible. I had designed a form of an Arabic tent with a large centre piece. This was comprised of a wonderful 5 feet tall old Yew tree trunk which we had found along the side of the Shropshire Union canal. This we dragged back to school and set about stripping parts of the bark and leaving the rugged surface in others. We then polished the smooth bits and varnished them to bring out the glorious colours of the wood. The father of one of my friends Tim Summerfield was a coal and building contractor's merchant from whom we scrounged large quantities of sand and a large sheet of stainless steel. The polished trunk was to be stood in a pile of sand. The broad strip of stainless steel was to be wrapped in a spiral around the trunk, producing beautiful and distorted reflections of the wood, brought out with several spotlights directed at the installation, one from above. Mr Summerfield was very supportive and kind and duly had the materials delivered to the school under cover of darkness. For the roof of the tent, I had envisaged a series of triangular white sheets, with the bases of the triangles forming the periphery of the roof and the apex fixed to a central pole, all at staggered, alternating heights. The only readily available sheets in the quantity that was needed were those on the beds in the dormitories. For that reason, construction had to be overnight in time for the opening of the exhibition the following morning. You can imagine the looks of surprise and horror on the faces of the more junior pupils in our house as their beds were stripped of their sheets following lights-out and they were all co-opted into helping with the construction. At sunrise the installation was complete. An introductory review in the school magazine the *Novaportan*, written by Mr Harding, the history teacher and our housemaster, states, 'Clearly Ward House were determined to win and had prepared accordingly.' Mr Jerry Chambers, the art master, in his review of the exhibition wrote:

> The winning Ward House exhibition .... Will long be remembered as a model of efficient organisation and dynamic leadership. Monumentally, in the centre, stood the main sculpture piece: 'Experiment in Contrasts'. The wrapped-round polished metal sheet reflected the exhibits in a kaleidoscope of extravagant shapes and colours. On the inside the mirrored texture of the timber moved intriguingly as the spectator moved and produced a non-mechanical kinetic effect. Wells and Randall are to be congratulated on scheming up this imaginative and 'moving' sculpture. Movement was also expressed in the sensitive line drawings of Wells and the sinuous contours of Randall's 'A Futuristic Look at Womanhood'.

In addition to the fine arts and music, the school had a very healthy dramatic programme with an annual school play performed before the end of the winter term. I really enjoyed taking part in these and had roles in several of them. In December 1961, before my voice broke, I played Calpurnia, Caesar's wife in Shakespeare's *Julius Caesar*. A couple of weeks before I had stubbed my right big toe heavily on the rugby pitch and, as my boots were too small, fractured my first metatarsal. This rendered Caesar's long-suffering wife with a serious limp. Having declared the words, 'Your wisdom is consumed in confidence', the performance took something of a downturn, when about to deliver the line trying to dissuade Julius from going to the forum, I caught my foot in a fold of stage canvas and let out a loud yell, followed by 'Do not go forth today: call it my fear that keeps you.' Howls of laughter burst from the assembled parents and teachers. Now prostrate on the stage I manfully continued, 'We will send Mark Anthony to the Senate house, and he shall say you are not well today.' Managing to salvage something of the momentous dramatics, I hoisted myself onto one knee to declare, 'Let me upon my knee prevail in this.' By now, all were in hysterics with tears pouring down their cheeks. Quick as a flash, Lowe, a boy in the fourth form playing Caesar said, 'Mark Antony shall say 'YOU' [instead of 'I' am not well] are not well and for thy humour I will stay at home.' I had one further line, which should have been, 'Say he is sick,' and following the cue from Caesar said, 'Say I am sick' as I crept from the stage prematurely in great embarrassment. Apparently, it rescued an otherwise pedestrian performance.

Another catastrophic entrance on my part was playing the Reverend Anderson in the play *The Devil's Disciple* by George Bernard Shaw. The play is set in the British colonial period of 1777 during the Saratoga campaign. The Reverend Anderson saves the central character Dick Dudgeon from the gallows at the last minute. Towards the end of the play with a rope around Dudgeon's neck I had to burst onto the stage and stop the execution. This was staged with me running the length of the central aisle of the gymnasium, through the audience, and to leap onto the stage with drawn sword shouting, 'Amen, and stop the execution. I am Antony Anderson, the man you want.' However, two rows back from the stage sat Dad with his long legs splayed out into the aisle, which I couldn't see in the darkness of the unlit hall. With thigh high jackboots, long flowing overcoat and sword raised high, I tripped over his legs and sprawled onto the apron of the stage. Not to be deterred by the calamity, somewhat bedraggled and dazed I rose to my feet, I thrust my sword, loftily into the air only to find it now bent at a right angle. I tried to carry on as though nothing had happened. Inevitably, another moment of high drama was lost in howls of laughter from all present, including those on stage.

Dramatic events such as these were quite commonplace. In an earlier year in a production of *Midsummer's Night's Dream*, during the dance of the fairies with Titania the fairies were played by us in the first form. We were all sporting lighted tapers for dramatic effect. Things got out of hand when one of the fairies lost concentration and managed to let his taper droop onto the hair of the fairy in front, causing it to catch fire. Pandemonium erupted with screaming parents and shouts of 'Fire, Fire'. The hapless child just in front of me, at first unaware that his fairy headdress was on fire, suddenly felt the heat and began running around the stage like a headless chicken. I remember reflecting on how quickly a fairy's headdress and hair could ignite. The moment was rescued when a parent, again Mr Summerfield, grabbed a nearby fire extinguisher, leapt onto the stage and doused the poor fairy's head with a blast that nearly blew him off the stage.

Somewhat more civilised productions of Gilbert and Sullivan were achieved, in which I played the Pirate King in *The Pirates of Penzance* and Sir Joseph Porter KCB in *H.M.S. Pinafore*. I thoroughly enjoyed polishing up the handle of the big front door on three consecutive nights!

The William Adams society was the school debating society. It was quite active, with at least three debates per term. Topics for debate were wide ranging and included such topics as 'This house opposes any merger between the Newport Girls High and Adams' Grammar School', motion carried. 'This house deplores the taking of drugs by pop personalities', motion carried, notably by the chairman's casting vote [the geography teacher], 'This house considers censorship necessary', surprisingly the motion was carried. At the time of the 1965 election, 'This house approves of state control of major industries'. Not surprisingly, Old Novaportan and highly contentious future leader of the Labour party Jeremy Corbyn spoke for the motion, blaming the Tory party for all the ills of the country. This was accompanied by a school mock election with Jeremy standing as the leader of the Communist party and its sole member. He managed to attract only 16 votes as opposed to 185 for the Conservative Party, 82 for Labour, 43 for the Liberals and 15 for the National Teenage Party. Something of a loner at school, it is clear that he has never deviated from his deep socialist principles.

As described earlier, in the sixth form we were expected to join the Combined Cadet Force. Those who didn't were condemned to spend the equivalent hours in the woodwork room or doing extra Latin or Calculus. There were two branches of CCF: the Army and the RAF. The majority of my year opted for the Army section, and I followed suit. There was a lot of square bashing accompanied by a lot of shouting. The master charged with organising us seemed to get a great deal of pleasure from striding up to one of us and then screaming in the unfortunate victim's ear as loudly as he possibly could with a great deal of unconcealed aggression. In retrospect and with a better understanding of human nature, there is little doubt in my mind that several of those with authority over us were using their position to work out their own personality disorders. Similarly, some of the senior boys could be seen to express the aggressive side of their nature. The passage of time has revealed many stories of bullying and aggressive behaviour flourishing in boarding school settings in particular. A recent book by Justin Webb, *The Gift of Radio, My Childhood and Other Train Wrecks*, vividly describes the traumas experienced in his Quaker school, experiences shared by my direct contemporary surgical colleague Stephen Large, who attended the same institution.

There were some high points. We learnt to use an army issue .303 rifle, fire flares, and have fun on field exercises, usually in some deserted region of Wales. A highlight of the year was a week-long army camp at Sennybridge, 31,000 acres of Ministry of Defence land in the Brecon Beacons, South Wales. The week consisted of early rising, cold showers, lots of square bashing under the command of a regular sergeant major with the voice of a foghorn. He seemed to get his thrills from terrifying us. Practical jokes were rewarded with a 5-mile hike at the double, with a fifty-pound backpack and a local SAS trainee to urge us along. Needless to say, the form jokers were rapidly silenced. Target practice on an open-air range with rifles and Bren guns was entertaining. I remember the army food was solid but good. The high spot of the week was a night exercise. We were split up into squads of five boys, with one chosen as leader from his performance during the week. We were dropped off somewhere in the hills armed only with an ordinance survey grid position, a compass, map, torch, .303 rifle with blanks and a thunder flash or two. These were devices which, when thrown, would explode with a loud bang, lots of smoke but no explosive damage unless detonated very close to the target. We were also given some bare rations of water and a little food. We had to trek about 5 miles across open country with heavily camouflaged regular soldiers entrenched along the way. Should we manage to negotiate the route without being caught, our target was an encampment where the regular N.C.O.s and our teachers were based. The idea was to capture them to win. We heard other squads being challenged and roughed up a bit when captured, but somehow we slipped through the defences and found ourselves behind a hedge next to the masters' camp. Our attention centred on our Welsh P.E. teacher who loved to bully us. After deciding our plan of diversionary tactics, we set about the assault. Thunder flashes were set off by two of our number on the opposite side whilst the other three raced to the back of the army wagon where the masters were sitting drinking tea and joking with each other. The look of surprise on their faces, when three of their boys suddenly appeared and held them at rifle point was worth staying up all night for. With great delight we tied their hands and feet with some rope we found in the truck; probably a little tighter than was necessary in a form of mild retribution for the low grade trauma inflicted on us on a regular basis. Game over and triumph for the boys' army squad.

Despite those high jinks, after a few months I decided that the seemingly more cerebrate R.A.F. was for me. After the first year in the fifth form I moved to that section in anticipation of learning to fly a glider and possibly a light aeroplane. For a while, I had ambition to become a pilot flying fast jets and went to Biggin Hill for an aptitude test for a flying scholarship. I managed somehow to pass the tests, but my significant astigmatism disqualified me from the flying scholarship programme. However, I was invited back to Biggin Hill in an attempt to encourage me to join the non-flying ranks, in particular the medical research limb of the service. This entailed going to medical school to train as a doctor in the usual way, but with the added attraction of being paid whilst I did so. It seemed very appealing. As an inducement, I was given a tour of the facilities among which were several testing chambers. I remember the shocking sight of a non-commissioned officer being exposed to sudden decompression with the spattering of blood from his nose on the window of the chamber, from which I was hurriedly moved on.

Whilst there, I was shown the capsule from Apollo 1 which had been sent over for analysis following the disastrous and tragic loss of the lives of three of the early astronauts – Gus Grissom, Ed White and Roger Chaffee. An electrical short in the cabin ignited the 100 percent oxygen atmosphere that the Americans had been using. This had been against the advice of their British counterparts at Biggin Hill. I don't think this exchange was ever revealed. The first brave men to launch after this tragedy were Walter Cunningham, Wally Schirra and Don Eisele. The courage to step up for this potentially fatal mission was typical of the men selected for these hazardous flights. Years later, I would meet and spend time with Walter Cunningham.

A trip on the centrifuge to generate supra-normal gravity was very uncomfortable and I realised then that the space programme was not for me. At that time, Britain had a significant research role in advanced supersonic and space flight. For a while, just after the war, Britain held the world air speed record when a Gloucester meteor raised the record from 469 to 606 mph. Breaking the sound barrier became a golden egg for which both the British and the Americans vied. It was thought to be impossible, as Geoffrey de Havilland, son of the aircraft designer, had tried to do it in a de Havilland 108, but the aircraft broke up in the attempt. It wasn't long after this that Chuck Yeager, the all-American hero fighter pilot achieved this in the Bell X-1, really a rocket engine with tiny wings. Being a man of few words but a giant ego and huge courage, he succeeded in a very understated way. In 1952, a British movie called *Breaking the Sound Barrier* starring Ralph Richardson, gained huge international success. However, the claim in the movie, that the British had achieved the goal before the Americans and defined the way to fly safely through the barrier by reversing the direction of the controls caused an angry kick-back from the flight jocks at Edwards Air Force Base in California. They knew that this was not true. The salt was rubbed firmly in the Americans' wound when Chuck Yeager was invited to the first screening of the movie. He managed to sit through it with clenched teeth. The British space programme was modest in comparison to that of the Americans, fuelled by a race against their nemesis the Soviet Union. The British never stated the aim of their programme in manned space flight but their Arrow programme, launched in Australia, succeeded in placing a single satellite in orbit in 1972. It appeared to me, however, that there was serious work going on at Biggin Hill as well as other places.

As a result of my expressed interest in a career in the Royal Air Force, I was invited to go to RAF Waddington to see the Vulcan bombers, part of the celebrated V bomber force. These are immense machines, quite beautiful with their swept back 'V' shaped wings and tapering nose. My exuberant enthusiasm exhibited on a guided tour of the cabin of one of these majestic aeroplanes resulted in a short flight out over the North Sea. I found myself being seated in a cramped space on a small step, which doubled up as an extra seat, behind the pilot who sat raised up next to his co-pilot with the engineer across the cabin from me and the navigator next to me with his radar table. It was one of the most exciting episodes of my life. As we cleared the coast, the pilot had great fun in informing me that if 'the balloon went up' our next stop was Moscow. More adventures with the RAF would follow later in my career.

We had the chance to learn to fly gliders at a nearby airfield, RAF Cosford. The aircraft were very clumsy machines, not the sleek craft that are seen at gliding clubs these days. It was either a Mk IV or a Sedburgh glider. Both heavy by modern standards. They were launched by a cable attached to a winch. We had to learn how to react if the cable broke when the nose of the glider would rocket towards the vertical, precipitating what was comfortingly referred to as a death slide where, after losing all lift, it fell back along its own axis and crashed. The correct response was quickly to push the joystick forward and aim at the ground! A rather nerve-wracking manoeuvre at first. These we had to practice and after a number of launches the instructor would simulate a cable break by pulling the release handle prematurely when the glider was at a very steep angle with huge force on the cable. All a lot of fun.

When we had reached a sufficient standard, we had to complete a solo circuit to gain our A & B certificate. After several weeks of training on a Sunday afternoon the fateful day arrived. We were duly bussed out to Cosford and after a briefing the flights began. We all succeeded in taking off satisfactorily, staying inside the projected height and distance parameter so as not to wander outside the window for landing at the airfield, and landed safely. Finally, it was the turn of our Latin teacher, Mr Whiteley. All of us gathered expectantly outside the dispersal hut hoping for some excitement. Sure enough we didn't have to wait long. There were huge cheers as Seymour cleared the perimeter fence and sailed up into the clear blue sky. The circuit was completed satisfactorily, and we all began to feel a little disappointed, expecting a boring landing and end of the solo flight with Mr Whiteley waltzing up to us with words such as, 'there you are boys that is how you do it'. However, as we watched keenly it became obvious that he had left his landing too late. At 100 feet or so he was over the middle of the grass runway and rapidly running out of space to get the glider down safely. Excitement in the group grew rapidly as his glider hit the ground hard and shot straight through the perimeter fence, disappearing into a hedge with just the tailplane sticking out. Initial quiet concern gave way to loud cheers, and whoops erupted as we saw Mr Whiteley emerge from the foliage looking very straggled and with bits of tree in his hair.

Other exciting events were flights in Chipmunks, one of the air force's training aircraft. The radio and oxygen mask stank heavily of old rubber and vomit, inducing quite a lot of air sickness in us. The paper bags were always displayed prominently and used frequently. The metal seats in the aircraft were softened by the parachute that was positioned behind your backside. It made walking out to the Chipmunk highly entertaining for those watching as we looked like ducks waddling to the edge of the water. One can see why the Second World War fighter pilots dashed to their aircraft often carrying their 'chutes.

My association with the RAF did engender a respect for the professionals and it gave me a great deal of pleasure to be able to keep career pilots in the air by reconstructing their heart valves years later.

As the years rolled by, Mum suffered more from multiple sclerosis. This was quite understandable as she had an active and agile mind. By 1966, the whole of her right side was paralysed, but she battled on and would not allow any assistance other than that which was essential. This made life for Dad so much more difficult as, other than my grandmother, she would have no help in the house. There were moments of levity and I think we all felt huge joy at those moments when Mum would smile and laugh. There was a good sense of humour hidden beneath the pain of the disease, and pain there was, although she never complained of it until it became unbearable. The severe muscle spasms could be seen in her face. There was no meaningful medical help at that time, but she would not give in to the disease, forcing her to do everything that she could to keep going. In this endeavour her mother, our grandmother, was a rock for the whole family and my father frequently referred to her as just that, his rock on whom he could always depend. Even with a broken wrist after falling on some ice outside the backdoor aged ninety-two, she kept going without telling anyone and concealing the injury with the long sleeve of her cardigan which she always wore. When we finally saw it, it had set at an angle, but never once did she complain. Charmian, our younger sister, later with her partner David, was constant in her support when at home. Although that terrible disease distorted the family relationships, we were extremely fortunate to have parents and grandparents who were so very supportive and caring of us. The example of the discipline of hard work, caring with courtesy for others, and taking care of one's appearances were the standards that they set for us. I owe all of them a huge debt of gratitude. I came to know later, as it was never expressed to me that most of my mother's pleasure in life came from seeing us succeed.

Mum's determination to ensure that we all succeeded in our careers was unstinting even though it was painful and difficult a lot of the time. I think that her considerable intelligence found the environment of a small country butcher's business very constraining, and this simply compounded the emotional problem for her.

For reasons that I still do not understand I found going into the shop when customers were there quite intimidating. Similarly, being asked to go much further than the boundary of the square into the rest of the village produced a slight sense of foreboding. I suspect it derived from the lack of real social interactions that we as a family experienced, other than in the shop with customers.

Naturally my parents' attendance at our school functions was very limited. By then, Rosamond was at Dr. Williams' school in North Wales and Charmian was growing fast. Picking us up from school or returning us became a marathon trip to Dolgellau, then over to Newport before returning home, a round trip of 200 miles, all in an afternoon and evening. The pressures in the family were building. This became obvious in my school results. Whereas improvement could be seen in the middle years, my GCE O level results were just about acceptable but not at all outstanding, other than in Biology and English. French was a disaster. Enough was achieved, however, to see me into the sixth form and the subjects of my choice.

Sixth form, Year Twelve in modern parlance, began for me in 1966. What made me choose Science subjects, I am not entirely sure. My strongest subjects were English Literature, History, Art, Biology and, surprisingly, Religious Studies. I had no allegiance to any particular religion but found the history of the early Christian era interesting. I suspect that my mother had a strong hand in my choice of the Sciences and perhaps an occult plan to steer me towards the medical profession.

And so a rather painful two years began, studying or, more accurately, sitting through Physics, Maths with Physics, Chemistry, Biology and something called General Studies. In the latter we were supposed to read and learn about world affairs and I seemed to excel at that. The only thing that I can remember about Physics was the teacher, a wonderful bear-like man with a huge black beard, rather like Desperate Dan in the *Beano* or Captain Haddock in *The Adventures of Tintin*. Despite his size he was gentle and softly spoken. I did rather test his patience one day when he caught me rolling a five kilo cylindrical weight from the back of the classroom to demonstrate the effect of energy dissipation determined by velocity and mass, something to do with a chap called Newton. The case was made for both Newton's Second Law, that force is equal to mass times acceleration, and the Third Law that for every action there is an equal and opposite reaction, when the cylindrical mass of iron smashed through the front of the teacher's desk, only being arrested by the opposite reaction of his shins, behind the desk. This resulted in detention and the writing out of Bill's Will many times; this was the last will and testament of William Adams, the founder of the school. Written in old English script it was a painful exercise to reproduce. There was a side business that one or two of the entrepreneurial boys had set up whereby they had made multiple copies which they bartered for the best bits in your tuck box. All was well until the sharper masters recognised the dissimilarity in the handwriting to yours. This just doubled the number of times that it had to be written out and was often accompanied by a thrashing with the dreaded 'holey' pump.

Instruction in the ways of the birds and the bees was carried out in the fourth form to embarrassed giggles and clowning around by the jokers in the class. How much was absorbed I am not sure, but girls really had yet to be invented and remained an enigma to most of us. The only contact we had was when we were allowed a written pass to walk up the High Street on a Saturday morning for any shopping essentials, or in the sixth form to visit the local 'caff'.

The sexual highlight of our year was the annual sixth form ball. This took place at the end of the spring term. The sixth form of the Girls' High School was invited to make up the female contingent, or, as cannon fodder for the testosterone fuelled boys. In preparation, we had dance practice on a Thursday evening after prep with the rugby second XV playing the girls and the firsts the boys. These were hilarious events with several injuries. It didn't bode well for the girls. My first experience of the ball resulted in a long snogging session behind the gymnasium against the bike sheds (didn't everyone's?) with my partner for the evening. I cannot remember her name now but at the time she was Aphrodite and Marilyn Monroe all combined in one heavenly body. However, because of the passions aroused, tragedy struck. A serious overproduction of testosterone was fired up and over the following Easter holiday my face broke out in the most horrendous attack of acne. This persisted well into my early twenties. It was so bad, that I was sent to the local hospital in Wellington every Monday for three months for ultra-violet light treatment which was supposed to cure the problem. I can still remember the smell of my burning flesh as I sat under the lamp with large sunglasses protecting my eyes. This drastically cooled my ardour, and Aphrodite went off with a far more adventurous boy. His excessive passion resulted in expulsion from school. The girl's parents returned prematurely from a foreign holiday to find them cavorting around the house naked and well-fuelled by her father's wine cellar. The inevitable pregnancy followed but I believe that they went on to a happy and settled life together.

Meanwhile, the acne took its toll and became a source of severe embarrassment for me. When at home my mother used to try to squeeze pus out of the inflamed masses on my face and back. She would drape flannels soaked in boiling water on my skin first to attempt to draw out the poison. The pain was excruciating, and the result only made things worse. The experience has made me very empathic towards teenagers who have to suffer that same curse.

In the sixth form I switched from rugby to hockey which I enjoyed much more. This matured to a trial for the county team. We were encouraged to play in mixed sex matches with the Girls' High School, a lethal sport as I was to discover. I was knocked unconscious in a mixed hockey match with the girls. All was going well until I was scythed down by one of the girls who ignored the rule limiting the height to which the stick could be raised.

From well above shoulder height the stick hit me on the point of the chin and the lights went out. I woke on the way to the accident and emergency department in Wellington, already well known there by my acne visits.

That was not the first occasion when I was rendered unconscious. This occurred when I was twelve. As part of the annual summer swimming gala, there was a diving competition. A representative from each year was chosen for a diving display in front of the parents. We were lined up along the edge of the pool. Despite my young age, I was already very tall. Being in the lower form I was placed at the shallow end. On diving in, my arms and then head hit the floor of the pool before my waist had entered the water. My parents watched as I crumpled under the water, clouds of blood swirling upwards. It was a bit of a dampener on the proceedings, and I was dragged out and taken off to matron's quarters.

Finally, in June 1967, the 'A' level exams arrived. Perhaps the most memorable event of those anguished weeks of toil was a musical one. As we turned over paper one in Biology, the mellifluous strains of Procol Harem's *A Whiter Shade of Pale* floated into the gymnasium. We all put down our pens and listened until it ended. We then settled down to complete the exam. The main exams extended over three and a half weeks. These were followed by the General Studies paper and scholarship level Biology.

Speech day marked the end of term. The usual platitudes were expounded by an elderly distinguished person, always seemingly a man in high moral dudgeon, droning on about success and failure and the vicissitudes of life. This was followed by the prize-giving. The whole programme lasted for about two hours. Those years always seemed to have hot summers, making the event quite uncomfortable. As soon as it was over it was time to leave for home to begin the summer holiday.

For me there was no prospect of a glamorous holiday abroad or lazy days stretched out in the sun somewhere. The time was spent working in a garage in Knighton, cleaning cars ready for sale, and sweeping the forecourt endlessly. The highlight was a ridiculously fast trip to and from work on the back of a friend's motorbike. How my usually careful parents allowed this I do not know. To their faces, he was a mild-mannered young man, but once on his motorbike he was a maniac. The 7 miles from Knighton to Clun were simultaneously exhilarating and terrifying.

In early December 1967, the weekend of the 7th to be precise, I was home on an exeat weekend and my mother asked me what I really wanted to do with my life. I answered honestly that I would really like to do something in the arts as the science subjects didn't seem to be suiting me. 'Such as?' she queried. 'Well, actually, be an artist,' I replied. I had enjoyed drawing and painting since very young. 'You will never make any money from it, and you can always do that in your spare time,' came the reply. 'Alright,' I said, 'then what about architecture?' Again, came the rejoinder that I would probably end up doing loft conversions and patio extensions. That vote of no confidence stung somewhat as I had imagined being someone like Richard Rogers or I. M. Pei designing wonderful structures that would last for centuries. At that moment it was announced on the television news that Christian Barnard had just completed the first orthotopic heart transplant in Cape Town South Africa. Without drawing breath, and with little conviction I stated, 'Ok, I will do that then', to which Mum replied, 'That's fine.' And so, it turned out that I did. Now I had a goal and that was to get into medical school to become a doctor. Little did I know then that that would come to pass and that in later years I would meet Professor Barnard. However, before that could happen, there were a few hurdles to clear, such as improving my 'A' level grades.

All the time, in the back of my mind, was the dreaded arrival of the school report and the examination results. Eventually, the feared envelope arrived. The results were not what was needed to get me into medical school. My mother was understandably beside herself with anger. I was offered a second chance with an extra year at school, not something that I relished but a necessary evil to ward off working in the shop amongst the flayed and quartered animals. On reflection, I can see that the extra expense that incurred was significant, but another demonstration of their determination that I should succeed in life.

I had begun to learn to drive in the fields of friends' farms when I was fifteen, and when sixteen on the back roads in the hills around Clun. The only other road users we met were the occasional horse-drawn cart, or tractors. As soon as it could be arranged after my seventeenth birthday, I sat my driving test and passed. Not long afterwards, Brian, a young man working in our shop had bought a Mini Cooper-S of which he was very proud. We had driven together to Craven Arms to pick up some extra meat from the local abattoir. It was the time of a severe epidemic of foot and mouth disease in cattle. Where the animals had to cross main roads, the farmers had laid down straw sprayed with antiseptic to try to limit the spread. Brian had invited me to take the wheel and to drive home. Slipping into amateur racing driver role we were motoring quickly back, when I entered a corner sharper than expected with antiseptic dowsed straw across the road. We hit it and we left the road shooting through a low thin hedge into a field where we skidded to a halt. We were very lucky that there were no significant obstructions in the way. Damage was slight and we were unharmed, but my ego was badly bruised, as was my backside when I reported the accident to Dad. He of course paid for the repairs, and I was not allowed to drive Brian's car again. However, with the freedom of a driving licence, I was able to spread my wings. For this I had to be satisfied with one of the old delivery vans smelling strongly of old meat and fat. Girlfriends were not only frowned upon but positively embargoed. Hence surreptitious trips into the countryside were only possible in this most unromantic of vehicles. On one occasion, I remember having to steer with one hand whilst using the other to hold the driver's door in place as it had fallen from the upper hinge.

My parents' commitment to the family business and their work ethic was so strong that there was little time left over for family things. I remember one precious summer's evening being taken fishing by my father on the River Clun. Precious because it was unique. There were few other shared events; a trip to the races at Brands Hatch, and once to Silverstone allowed us to share one interest. Other than that, all other memories revolve around 'the shop'.

My quest to gain entry to medical school was set back once again by what followed next. In 1968 I was made head boy and school captain. During that year the school was visited by Princess Margaret, the Queen's sister. Her Royal Highness had just been made an honorary Haberdasher and was the first woman adopted by the livery. Unfortunately, I allowed the demands of being school captain, captain of house and the arrangements for the Royal visit to dominate my school year, with deleterious effects on my studies. I think, in retrospect, that I was happy to have interesting distractions from what should have been my main task of passing A levels with good grades. The sad consequence of these distractions unfolded as the year passed.

Now in a position of some authority as head boy, my priority was to stop the physical punishment of fellow pupils. I had suffered under it a lot through the years. Thrashing by prefects and masters was used liberally, causing significant scars both physical and mental to many of the pupils, including me. I made the case as strongly as I could to Mr Roberts, the headmaster. After a short discussion, to my amazement he agreed. This made a huge difference to relations between pupils, prefects and masters. It was notable that the wife of our housemaster Mrs Humphries, my lovely English teacher, never dispensed physical punishment and vociferously supported me in my efforts to ban it.

One day, the headmaster summoned me to his office to inform me that in Her new role as honorary Haberdasher, Princess Margaret had asked to visit their schools and that ours, being the oldest secondary school was to be the first. Moreover, rather than spend much time with the teachers she wanted to meet the boys and, as the head boy, I was to be her principal host for the visit.

The great day dawned, and the Princess arrived by helicopter with her lady in waiting in a bright green satin suite and Sir Ian Bowater, the then Lord Mayor of London, and Master of the Haberdashers. The Lord Lieutenant of the County along with the governors of the school and the headmaster were there to meet her. The company had recently bought a medium sized stately home, Longford Hall to replace the lesser Aston Hall as a boarding house. The tour began there. After inspecting the Hall and the boys at Longford, we all moved over to the school for the visit proper to begin.

I had been formally introduced to her when she arrived at Longford Hall and was reintroduced at the main school gates and then accompanied her on her trip around the school. She was utterly charming and fun to be with, making my task very easy. We went from room to room where classes were going on. After the tour the plan was for me to guide Her Royal Highness to the dining hall where she would be given tea and whilst seated I would introduce her to a chosen representative from each year. All had gone well to that point. As I began to excuse myself to bring the first boy, Margaret turned to me and insisted that I sit next to her at the tea table. That meant that all the dignitaries had to move up one place for me to be able to sit down. I flashed a desperate look at the headmaster conveying the question 'What do I do now?'. He gesticulated to me to obey and to sit. Sir Ian Bowater moved down a place and was seated to my left with the Princess to my right. Conversation flowed easily, although now I cannot remember the content. There was much laughter, and her lighter side showed through, amplified by a bright blue satin suit and a large Mickey Mouse watch that she sported on her left wrist. Then, Sir Ian managed to drop a pair of sugar tongs onto the floor, landing exactly in front of the feet of the Princess. What to do? I was sure that I did not want to squat down to pick them up as H.R.H. was wearing a very short skirt. Completely unphased, Sir Ian crouched down onto all fours and reached for the tongs. What I saw next was hilarious. Just as Sir Ian was about to pick up the tongs HRH swung her right leg and kicked the tongs the full length of the table from under his nose. A shocked Sir Ian jerked his head upwards, striking the underside of the table with a loud bang and rattling all the glassware and cutlery. I could see a smile spread across Margaret's face, but she didn't miss a beat in the conversation. It was clear that she knew exactly what she had done. Well, I suppose even Royalty has to have some fun. The day drew to a close and we saw the Princess off in her helicopter back to London accompanied by her lady in waiting and Sir Ian and Lady Bowater.

It was later reported to me that on the flight back, Margaret said to Sir Ian, 'You should make that boy a Haberdasher' referring to me. Acting on Royal command, this happened later that year. I received a letter from the Haberdashers' Company inviting me to become an apprentice to the company, the first step to becoming involved with them. Of course, I accepted.

I was duly invited down to Haberdashers' Hall to sign my indentures in the presence of my father. It was a very grand affair. The Livery company's history originates in the middle ages. There have been three Livery halls over the centuries. The first hall was completed in 1458. That original hall was burnt down in the Great Fire of London in 1666, coincidentally the same year that my old school Adams' Grammar School was founded. The current hall is situated in West Smithfield and is a very beautiful building. Before this last move, the hall was in Gresham Street and was an altogether more dour building with lots of heavy dark oak panelling.

We were ushered into a room called the binding parlour, a large rectangular shaped room, the walls of which were bedecked with portraits of past Haberdashers including the founder of our school in Newport, William Adams. The court of Haberdashers were all wearing their blue robes with ermine collars, arranged around a horseshoe shaped table. In the centre of the horseshoe was a small writing desk and chair. On the table were my indentures which I was going to be asked to sign. I was taken to the chair and sat down with my father standing behind me. According to ancient laws of the livery companies, when an apprentice is taken on by the company and signs the agreement, the company purportedly take over responsibility for the youngster and hence the father has to give his permission.

I sat down, and as instructed by dear grandfather never to sign anything without reading the small print, I began to read. It was written in medieval English. After I had been studying it for several minutes, the Master spoke, addressing my father:

> Mr Wells, I think that it is alright for your son to sign the document as it hasn't changed in the last six hundred years, and we have not had any previous problems.

Very sheepishly, I signed the document.

Then came a grand luncheon where I was placed opposite the Master at the high table. The first hurdle for me was the multitude of gleaming silver knives and forks of all shapes and sizes, the like of which I had never seen before. These were accompanied by several wine glasses of varying sizes. Clearly noticing my uncertainty of where to start one of the waiters, dressed in a beautiful red coat with wig and gaiters, quietly whispered in my ear, 'Don't worry, just start from the outside and work your way in.' Worse was to come. The cutlery was indeed solid silver and quite heavy. My nervousness whilst trying to engage the Master in conversation caused me to become somewhat animated. Without my noticing it, the handle of one of the knives had worked its way partially into the sleeve of my jacket. In a nervous twitch I raised my hand to scratch my head and as I did so I saw a silver arc of metal flash through the air towards the Master, who at the time was looking down into his soup. It missed him by inches and with barely a sound, the waiter standing behind him reached out a hand and caught it mid-flight. Tucking it behind his back he gave me a wink and a smile. What a start it would have been to impale the master on the end of a steak knife on my first meeting. After that, the rest of the day passed without further event and Dad and I went home having enjoyed it all enormously.

Apprentices were not meant to be married without the consent of the master and our guardian, who in my case was the loveliest of old gentlemen Roddy Hawes. It also stated that we must not be found in houses of 'ill repute', nor caught gambling. All very sensible. The apprenticeship lasted three years, after which I was admitted into the company as a Freeman. On gaining the Freedom of the company one was also admitted as a Freeman of the City of London. On going to the Guildhall to sign the Great Freedom Book, I noticed that the signature above mine was that of Prince Charles. Clearly I was in some good company.

All too soon, the 'A' level exams came around again, and with offers of places at two medical schools I sat them with a greater degree of optimism. I only had to improve Chemistry and Physics by one grade, having attained a good grade in Biology and an S level in the subject.

At the end of term speech day, I had to make the toast of thanks to the Worshipful Company of Haberdashers and to summarise the events of the term. I had been very apprehensive about this but prepared as well as I could. I still have my notes for that speech, and it makes slightly embarrassing reading more than five decades late. The highlight of the event was being awarded the headmaster's prize for overall best contribution to the school in that year.

The summer holidays began, and this time Mum had made arrangements for me to work in a tyre factory in the nearby town of Knighton. Joy of joys! This time instead of working in the fresh air cleaning cars and de-gunking new ones ready for delivery to their owners, I was trapped inside a dark, dingy, and very smelly building stacking tyres and learning how to change giant tyres on tractors. I hated every minute of it.

Mum was now very limited in what she could do, but still courageously insisted on being installed in a chair in the shop every morning, conversing with the customers and taking the money. Dear Grandad continued to encourage me with the piano and the arts. Granny was the lynchpin of household activities and spent a lot of time with our younger sister, now seven years old. Rosamond was doing well at Dr Williams' school, and I can remember that her worst complaint was having to sit O level Welsh.

Too soon the examination results arrived. I was horrified but not really surprised to find that although my grades had improved, they were still not sufficient to take the offered place in medical school. The conditional place at Westminster was lost. What to do? Once my mother's anger had subsided, her gritty determination that I should succeed kicked in once again, and it was decided that I should have one final shot at gaining a place to do medicine. My paternal grandmother, who had died a month before my birth had left me £350, quite a lot of money in 1968. A place for me at the Davies, Laing and Dick cramming college in Pembroke square, Notting Hill, was booked and off I went in September with three months to improve, but this time on a different examination board.

Just before I left Clun, my grandfather sent to me a lovely letter. It is dated 21 September 1968 and it reads,

> Dear Francis
> Kindly accept the enclosed which may come in handy on your new venture, [a gift of money to help me on my way] I have no doubt about your ability to win through and wish you good luck & good health and may I say be selective about the company you keep and always keep in mind the high principal your Father and Mother have set you,
> With best wishes & good luck
> Love Grandad.

I was, and still am, so moved by this letter that I have kept it with me wherever I have moved. It reveals the moral environment that we were brought up in, and his deeply caring nature, which shone through until the end. His was always a reassuring and cheering voice no matter the difficulties that I faced. He had always been the one quietly there for me.

Term began at the cramming college on Monday 23 September. I had nowhere to stay in London at that time and my aunt and uncle took me into their home in Abbots Langley until I could find somewhere centrally. Joan was the second wife of Uncle Tom, a tax inspector with Her Majesty's Inland Revenue and as such, highly regarded within the family. His first wife had died of breast cancer and David, his son from that marriage, had been a medical student at Guy's hospital and had been an additional inspiration for me to do medicine. I sought his opinion about gaining entry to medical school and which one to choose. His words on selection criteria reveal a significant difference from selection today. He stressed the importance of non-academic qualifications stating that most regarded a sporting ability to be very favourable. This reflected the positive attitude that I received from Guy's and Charing Cross when discussing my membership of both the rugby and hockey clubs. Advising me to avoid St Thomas' with a barge pole, he stated that the choice really didn't matter from the point of view of the quality of training but the effect of that school on later appointments did. A further coincidence in my life was that David had been at Guy's alongside my future mentor and colleague Terence English. I still have in my possession that inspirational letter from David, encouraging me to take up medicine as a career. David became a very successful consultant ear, nose and throat surgeon and his wife Isabel, a consultant anaesthetist. One of his claims to fame was persuading the manufacturers of Biro pens to put a hole in the small cap at the end of the barrel, which originally was a solid piece of black plastic. In his practice he had had to remove these small objects from the airways of children who had removed them with their teeth and then inhaled them. There had been several near-death experiences. The companies adopted the change and perhaps some small lives were spared as a result.

In anticipation of my last-ditch attempt at entry to medical school, in September1968, my parents found lodgings in 123 St George's Square, Westminster. That was a Toc H establishment, a Christian organisation. It offered homely lodgings at very reasonable prices. It also offered a ready fellowship in a vast and strange city. Having grown up in the beautiful but relatively isolating Shropshire hills, and then being constrained within a boarding school environment, my parents rationally thought that supportive surroundings would be essential for my well-being. After all, this was my first time living away from home on my own and proved a most interesting development. I was thrown into a human bouillabaisse of fascinating people from all over the world, experiencing London for their first time. I can still clearly remember walking cautiously into the common room for the first time, very fearful of meeting so many new people. As I entered, I heard music that I had never experienced before. It was Jose Feliciano and the iconic 1968 song, 'Light my Fire'. A young Brazilian student was playing along with his guitar. I was mesmerised and I remember the feeling of excitement at this new world.

I had never been exposed to, nor understood, racism. In our home everyone was regarded as an equal. Therefore, meeting so many exciting people from so many different and exotic places in the world was exhilarating. I made many new friends. This experience was to be repeated a few years later when I went to live in the International Students' house on Regent's Park. Sadly, money was so limited and the work schedule so intense that I had little time for much of a social life.

Toc H was named for Talbot House. The son of Edward Talbot, then Bishop of Winchester, Gilbert Talbot had been killed at Hooge in Belgium in 1915. Toc signified the letter T in the signals alphabet used by the British army in the First World War. Regardless of rank, all soldiers were made welcome for respite and recovery from the horrors of the war. Talbot House was founded in December 1915 as a rest house for soldiers from the frontlines, many suffering from both mental and physical wounds.

Next door to Toc H was one of the Westminster Hospital nurse's homes. For fire practice we were supposed to exit through a connecting passageway into one of their dormitories. To everyone's disappointment that was never necessary.

Whilst the money that I had allowed subsistence at a very basic level, good food was in short supply. Luckily across the Grosvenor Road was a high-class club, Caesar's Palace. Not having the wherewithal to cross the threshold to eat, one day I spotted the chefs outside enjoying a cigarette. I cheekily introduced myself to them. Once they understood my predicament, they kindly left out high quality leftovers for me at the end of the evening. I owe them a great deal.

Although I was financially severely restricted, life was not all constant lectures and book work. London was in full swing and Carnaby Street and the King's Road were the places to be. A note in my diary on 30 November records bumping into John Lennon and Yoko Ono. Recently divorced from Cynthia, Lennon had paid a heavy financial price extricating himself from that marriage and helping Yoko to do the same from her marriage. We teenage students were all shocked at his being in thrall to, as we saw it then, a rather strange, not very attractive Japanese artist best known in England at that time for a movie of naked backsides. Also, for those of us who were fans of The Beatles, the imminent break-up of the band was a common talking point. Strolling up and down the King's Road soaking up the atmosphere was exhilarating for me. I remember the colourful shops such as Biba and all the exotic young people hovering outside.

The course was intense, and realising that this was now my last chance, I applied myself with few distractions. We were an eclectic bunch. One young lady I recall being delivered each day in a chauffeur-driven Rolls Royce, swathed in luxurious furs. She was able to avail herself of lots of male support in the areas she found more difficult. I'm not sure that the outcome for her was very successful.

Once again I applied to five medical schools: Guy's, St Thomas', Westminster, Charing cross and the Royal Free. Remarkably, I was invited to interview at all of them. Things were looking up. The interview at Guy's started on the wrong note. My grandfather had instructed me that first impressions were very important and to be gently confident in my manner. The door to the dean's office was a large heavy oak door with a very large brass knob. Unfortunately, on entering I pushed too hard on the heavy door which was on very light hinges. It swung open wildly, banged against the wall and rebounded with force striking me in the face and causing a considerable nosebleed, before slamming shut with me on the wrong side. I could hear the laughter within and entered more cautiously. The interview went well after that and despite the minor injury I was offered a conditional place, perhaps out of sympathy.

I have no memory of the interview at St Thomas' and was not offered a place there. I was offered an unconditional place at the Royal Free Hospital, but being way out of central London in Hampstead it did not appeal to me. Westminster offered me a conditional place, with an improvement in my grade in chemistry. The interview at Charing Cross, however, also went extremely well. It appeared that all that they were interested in was what position I could play on the rugby pitch. Lock, I replied, and apparently that was what they were looking for as on 7 December 1968, I was offered an unconditional place based on my previous year's A level results. Not only was that a huge relief, but it was also my first choice. I had placed a map of central London on my desk and stuck a pin in the medical school closest to the Royal Opera House, the National Gallery, and the theatre district. It is obvious where my interests really lay. Within days the Guy's offer arrived, conditional upon improvement by one grade in Physics, which I considered to be unlikely. I therefore without further hesitation accepted the offer from the Cross. I have never regretted that decision.

Finally, I had been able to repay my parents' unstinting support of me. Whilst the approach my mother took often seemed harsh, I can now see that she knew her son well and knew what it would take for me to achieve my potential. In return, to underscore what another failure might have looked like, I was sent to work in a chicken factory for the nine months prior to starting at medical school. Chukie Chicken of Craven Arms became the new centre of my life and it was truly awful. The day began with a nine-mile bus ride, picking up the women workers on the way from Clun to Craven Arms. The vast majority of workers there were women. Their high-pitched cackling laughter was irritating in the extreme. The bus was filled with high-pitched chatter, usually declaiming how useless their husbands or children were, accompanied by raucous laughter. On arrival, we were disgorged to the weighing and packing room. I eventually gained promotion to the rank of capon grader. All seemed to be going well and as the young token male, I was taken under the wing, or perhaps I should say the bosom, of these rather large, but charming ladies. They liked to smother me with unwelcome affection. However, it seemed to keep them happy in their work. I was, of course, teased mercilessly. The pushing and touching seemed harmless enough until one rather large lady dropped a fourteen pound deep frozen capon onto my previously broken foot (remember Calpurnia!). Following this trauma I was promoted again, this time to the cold store, auditing stocks of deep-frozen chickens and turkeys. I had really arrived on the scene of the frozen chicken world. The hours were long and tedious, but the manual work kept a degree of fitness and the verbal repartee maintained a degree of mental agility.

I settled into the routine of clocking on, coffee at 11 a.m., an hour for lunch with prepacked sandwiches, and tea in the middle of the afternoon. Finally, we clocked off and boarded the bus back to Clun.

Painfully slowly, the summer drew to a close and I readied myself with great excitement for my next great adventure, Charing Cross Hospital Medical school.

4

Medical School at Last

> I talked of the cheerfulness of Fleet Street, owing to the quick succession of people which we perceive passing through it. Why sir, fleet street has a very animated appearance; but I think the full tide of human existence is at Charing Cross.[1]

This conversation between Samuel Johnson and James Boswell, recorded by Boswell in his biography of the life of Johnson, expressed Johnson's love of an urban environment and noted that even in the mid-eighteenth century Charing Cross was at the heart of 'human existence'. Indeed, Charing Cross hospital is right in the heart of theatre land and close to many world-famous art institutions. I had longed to be able to experience the full richness of the arts and that desire largely drove my choice of medical school. Also, the small number of students in each year suggested an environment that might have a family feel with the opportunity to receive more intense small group teaching. Both of these hopes were fulfilled and life at Charing Cross was immensely rewarding.

The excitement that I felt as the day approached can only be imagined. The traumas of repeated efforts at A levels were behind me, along with the uncertainty of the future. My parents were relieved that I was finally on the way to achieving something meaningful. My applications for county grants were successful, relieving us of modern-day student fees. The first job was to find somewhere to live. Sometime in late August Dad and I set off for London in the trusty Ford. It was one of the few trips that we made together without Mum or other members of the family. In retrospect the apparent confidence with which my father undertook this task without meaningful experience of London was extraordinary. I remember that it was very hot, and we needed to accomplish the job in one day. Little had I appreciated the enormity of finding a suitable and affordable place in the vast suburbs of London. We had followed up an invitation to contact the medical school secretary Christine for help with suggested areas where we might look and we had made something of a shortlist, but I think that we greatly underestimated the task.

We left Clun very early, arriving in the morning rush hour. I remember that we bought an Evening Standard newspaper in Notting Hill Gate at a newsagent that is surprisingly still in business. It was, of course, long before the age of digital communications and we had to rely on our map reading skills using the A–Z of London. We sat in the car scouring the rental pages for quite a while, earmarking several that looked worth visiting. Appointments had to be made by telephone. We found a red phone box on the corner of Kensington High Street that uncannily still exists, although it is heavily vandalised. We set off buoyantly crossing the Thames over Westminster Bridge towards Balham, gaily called 'the gateway to the south' by Peter Sellers in a radio skit called *The Third Division*, written by Dennis Norden and Frank Muir. What we found was hardly a place for the bon vivants. It was my first experience of uninspiring rural living. Of the several properties we visited, one particularly stands out in my mind. It was a small, terraced house in which the couple who owned it had seven students lodging with them. I was offered a put-up bed on the landing behind a curtain. On the other side of the hall, similarly accommodated, was a student from the one of the Royal Schools of Music who was majoring in the trumpet. Living and studying in that environment was going to be impossible and so the search went on. We were shocked to see the conditions that many students were forced to live in.

Finally, as the day was coming to an end, we found a house in Fernthorpe Road, Streatham. The house was owned by a Mr and Mrs Futcher. Mr Futcher was a diminutive cockney carpenter. Mrs Futcher was a Mrs Doubtfire lookalike, a large and loud Glaswegian lady who towered above her husband. She was, however, very warm and welcoming to us. I was offered a pleasant single room with a view of the garden. We were told that there were two other students lodging there, a trainee accountant and a philosophy student. Once we got to know each other, we got on well, but our lives were very separate. Mrs Futcher ran a very tight ship. An excellent cooked breakfast was provided each morning in time for me to catch the train around 7.00 a.m. and to be at Charing Cross Station well in time for lectures. I quickly became used to the commute from Streatham Station, changing at Clapham. At the end of the day there was a wholesome dinner, and then quiet time to work. It was a homely environment in which to begin my life in London.

Occasionally there was tension between our hosts, usually as Mrs Futcher tried her best to keep a neat and tidy house. The worst episode happened during the 1970 Football World Cup. Mr Futcher invited the three of us to join him to watch the Brazilian quarter final against England, the reigning world champions. He had bought a small case of beer which we were sharing when Mrs Futcher, who had been out, returned unexpectedly. The resultant row between our two hosts, although somewhat amusing to us, was very traumatic for Mr Futcher, who felt the full force of his wife's anger. We were expelled to our rooms. Generally, however Mrs Futcher always had our best interests at heart and looked after us well.

Once I had settled into the course, I had little confidence and really did not want to fail again. I was determined to redeem myself scholastically and began to work extremely hard, leaving little time for socialising in the various public houses around the hospital as other more self-confident students did. I do remember occasional discussions late into the night with the philosophy student. In attempt to keep up I had bought Bertrand Russell's seminal text *The History of Western Philosophy*, which I still have. The character that I remember most clearly from it is Bishop Berkeley and his limerick establishing the proof there is a God, and wrote,

> There once was a man who said 'God' must think it exceedingly odd if he finds that this tree continues to be when there's no one about in the quad. Dear Sir, your astonishment's odd. I am always about in the quad. And that's why the tree. Continues to be, since observed by yours faithfully, God.

This proof, whilst entertaining much strenuous debate between us, seemed an utterly fatuous argument of no consequence to life. Needless to say, the accountant agreed with me.

Our first day at medical school began at 10.00 a.m. on 8 October 1969. We assembled in the old main lecture theatre. This was a Paduan style, steeply sloped theatre in a semi-circle. Professor Willie Hamilton, a large Northern Irish embryologist and placentologist, strode into the room and began to boom at us how we were expected to comport ourselves. We were informed that the men must have short hair, the women should have their hair neatly tied back, and that we should all dress professionally. This was 1969 the age of the summer of love, long hair, drugs, free love, and rock 'n' roll, not that we saw much of that. It clearly seemed necessary to remind us of our impact on the public as future doctors. We were told that if we didn't like it, we could leave, take a number 59 bus and not come back. I still remember clearly looking around the room at all of the new faces that were to become lifelong friends. Following this introduction to the world of professional work, we were taken up to the dissecting room to meet our body. We were divided into groups of four, two on each side for our dissection practicals. No one fainted, but there were a lot of apprehensive looks as the pungent smell of formalin invaded our senses. Dissection sets rolled up in green canvas holders were obtained along with the three volumes of dissection manuals that we were going to be expected to work through. I still have them all, and the smell of formalin, even fifty-seven years later, remains strong and just as offensive, with the fat stains on the pages of the books equally as evident. This was our welcome to the world of medicine.

The timetable was going to be intense. The subjects were anatomy, physiology, biochemistry, histology, embryology, pharmacology and statistics. Everyone seemed to be excited to get started.

The hall porter Bill had been there for years. He was a large and friendly man with nine brothers, eight working in a different west end theatre and one in the fruit and vegetable market in Covent Garden, still functioning then, just around the corner from the medical school. The market was in full swing throughout the night and business was concluded by six a.m.. On arrival at medical school, we commonly found a crate of fresh fruit on the steps of the medical school building courtesy of Bill's brother.

Luckily, not many of my new colleagues seemed to be interested in the arts. This left the field open for me. One of Bill's brothers worked at the Royal Albert Hall. He supplied me with a season's tickets for the Promenade concerts the following summer. Another brother gave me my first seats at the Royal Opera House, where I was able to enjoy ballet for the first time. The first one I saw was Kenneth MacMillan's *Romeo and Juliet* with Margot Fonteyn and Rudolph Nureyev in the starring roles. I was starting at the pinnacle of classical ballet. I remember that there were cameras in the auditorium filming the performance. Many years later I operated on a lady who had been in the corps de ballet at Covent Garden and later danced in the New York Ballet. The nurses on the ward had told the patient of my love for ballet and when I saw her after her surgery, she asked me what the first ballet was that I had seen. I described that performance and my excitement at witnessing two of the finest dancers that there had ever been in one of their last years together. She told me that she had known and danced with the pair of them several times. I listened to her stories, absolutely enthralled. She then asked me if I remembered if it had been filmed. I said that it had, and we moved on to discuss other performances. A month or so after her discharge, a package arrived in the post from her. In it was a video recording of the performance and a pair of Margot Fonteyn's ballet shoes, still with stains of her blood within. A beautiful gift from a very thoughtful patient whom I have never forgotten. I treasure those objects. Occasionally I would see Nureyev with his turban like headdress going in and out of the Opera House, which was just around the corner from the medical school. Several other trips to the theatre and to openings of art exhibitions followed. A unique event was the cinema preview of the hit television series, *MASH*. The producers had wanted to secure the approval of some medics and true to form, Bill had secured a few tickets to the preview in Leicester Square. Little did we know the success that it would go on to attain on both the small and the large screen.

Bill's other talent was as a crafty salesman. Sitting at his desk in his hall kiosk, he would attract our attention as we walked by to the common room. Below his desk, hidden from view, was a pile of old textbooks that he had collected from departing students. The average age of the books was eight to ten years. As new students, we weren't aware of the short redundancy times of these books and Bill impressed upon us, falsely of course, how essential they were and that we were so lucky as he only had a few of them, hence, first come first served. A rather more naughty trait of his was tempting us to buy recycled dissection white coats. These side hustles made him a steady income of beer money. A lasting memory that I have of dear old Bill, was on climbing the steps into the medical school one day, seeing him nonchalantly reading the *Beano* comic, sitting on a newly delivered coffin, quite oblivious to the students passing around him.

Whilst the medical school was situated on Chandos Street on the north side of The Strand, the medical school library was housed in the Adelphi, a grand building close to the Embankment. We had to cross The Strand to reach it. The library was on the first floor of that wonderful Art Deco building. There were arresting views out over the Thames embankment and the Festival Hall on the opposite side. Despite its wonderful vista I don't remember many other students being there. One I do remember was Helen, a lovely bright and caring person who worked terribly hard, and with whom I vied for top spot in the examinations. Helen married a quiet but confident fellow student David, who was an excellent semi-professional rugby player, playing for the Wasps first team. They seemed to keep themselves to themselves but were very happy and I liked being around them. I can clearly remember walking through the beds of tulips in the springtime on the Embankment Gardens to the tube station with Helen at the end of intense days of study.

Charing Cross had a small but very colourful intake of students in those days. The newness of everything and the intensity of the experience drew us together rapidly and lifelong friendships were formed. Coming from the social wilderness of south Shropshire caused a significant level of anxiety as to whether I would fit in with fellow students, many of whom I anticipated would have been through public schools. That was not the case, even with a future lord of the realm in our midst we all mucked in together in tight knit groups. Everyone was keen to support a colleague perceived to be struggling in any way.

There was a significant number of very impressive women, both in appearance and intelligence. I'm not sure of the exact proportion of female students, but through the force of their personalities there seemed to be a lot. Cilla McGuire Sampson had come from Roedean, a select private girls' school in Sussex. Her grandfather was Sir Richard Doll, the man who was responsible for statistically linking smoking to lung cancer. Cilla was charming and I must confess to having a crush on her but never the courage to express it, nor the likelihood of success. We were good friends, and I remember helping her quite a lot with her studies. Cilla went on to great things as a child psychiatrist and, with another female colleague, was the first woman to create a women's job-share as a new consultant, allowing her and her counterpart to continue to work and enjoy motherhood.

Just down the street from the medical school entrance, west, towards St Martin's Lane was Bedfordbury Street, on which was situated our adopted local public house The Lemon Tree. Several hours were spent in this establishment. A striking feature was a door in the left-hand wall of the bar area, which opened onto a staircase which descended into the orchestra pit of the London Coliseum. At the beginning of the interval of a performance, most of the orchestra could be seen disgorging from the doorway into the small area in front of the bar. They had pre-ordered their drinks, which were already set up for them.

Behind the bar there were the few trophies that the medical school rugby and hockey teams had won over the years, along with the Charing Cross shield and badges. Sadly, with the move of the hospital to Fulham in 1974–5 all of these memorabilia were removed some years ago. It was the place where our second MB examination results were announced. It was also the place where we rendezvoused prior to rugby matches on a Saturday lunch time. Probably unacceptable today was the practice of the nurses, who followed the team, washing and delivering the clean kit to the team at the pub. On one occasion the shirts arrived late and two of us set off to the ground in Cobham, approximately a forty-five-minute drive in those days.

In an attempt to get there on time we drove at high speed with the roof off his Triumph TR3. Somewhere along the A3 we heard the 'dring, dring' of a police car, not the horrible noise that they produce these days, in hot pursuit. We pulled over, as did the police car behind us. With the usual 'What's going on here then', the policeman introduced himself and informed us that we were well over the speed limit. We got out, apologised, and politely explained that we were on our way to play a rugby match against the Metropolitan police, H division and that we were late. Much to our amazement he said, 'Come on gentlemen, follow me you can't be late for that', and off we went, this time with a police escort. It is difficult to imagine a breach of the law not ending with points on the licence and a fine these days.

Playing rugby against the police was always a bit like the American football match in the movie *MASH*. We were no match for them in size or aggression. It was a day for them to work out their frustrations on what they saw as a bunch of lily-livered medical students. The scores were usually more appropriate for a cricket match and varying degrees of injury were sustained. It was a similar story against Barclays bank. The most memorable pitch to play on was that of the Honourable Artillery Company in the middle of the City of London. This was a beautifully prepared pitch surrounded on all sides by high rise office buildings. Quite an incongruous sight. I can remember an artillery field gun placed at one end of the pitch as though a warning of things to come for the opposition.

We were not a very strong team, but we did have the occasional surprising success. One game that I clearly remember was in the inter-hospitals cup, against St Mary's when the great JPR Williams was playing for them. This wizard of the rugby pitch was one of the toughest players on the international scene, never mind the local club level. His role in the Gareth Edwards try scored for the Barbarians playing against the fearsome New Zealand All Blacks in 1973 remains one of the greatest tries of the century. Even with most of our team attempting to mark him, he ran rings around us, and we ended on the wrong side of a cricket score. Nevertheless, it has always felt a privilege to have been able to be on the field graced with such a legendary player. He went on to become an accident and emergency surgeon and an expert in sports medicine.

Entry to the medical school was off Chandos Place at the top of Agar Street. There was a butcher's shop on the corner opposite the entrance. This was of some comfort with the smells reminding me of home. Above it were the on-call rooms for the junior doctors. Just to the right of the entrance to the medical school was a small café which we frequented. On entering the medical school, one walked up a short flight of quite broad stairs into the entrance hall. To the left was a large noticeboard occupying the whole length of the wall, extending for about 20 feet horizontally and approximately 4 feet in height. It was there that all examination results were posted. The excitement of crowding around to check your results remains with me to this day. Straight ahead was a passageway that went past Bill's porter's lodge and into a common room with a piano against the wall. To the right of Bill's lodge there was an old gate-style elevator which we were not allowed to use, and next to it, the main stairs up to the lecture theatre and some of the laboratories with the anatomy department on the top floor.

On our second day, we began our journey into dissection of our cadavers. Something that I haven't revealed before was the surprise that I felt on seeing the address from which our 'body' had come. He had been the next-door neighbour of the family with whom I had digs in Streatham. An extraordinary coincidence. Naturally, I have never divulged this fact to anyone until now, fifty-three years later.

I think that we were all fairly apprehensive about meeting our donor but most adapted quite quickly. Even though I had been brought up in the butchery business, I was quite overawed by the sight, and the pungent smell of the formaldehyde used to preserve the tissues insinuated itself everywhere: eyes, nose, clothes and hair. After a morning's dissection the pads of one's fingers began to wrinkle and the smell was impossible to wash out. I cannot think why we were not made to wear gloves. It must have been quite unpleasant for those passengers around us on the tube after a session in the dissection room. The utility of laborious dissection is questioned widely today and many, if not most, medical schools have abandoned it, substituting prosected specimens or virtual reality programmes. Good though they are, they do not allow the immediacy of discovering and understanding the true relationships of structures to one another. This is particularly important for those intent upon a career in surgery.

Before we began dissection, we were instructed to show absolute respect towards what had once been a vital human being, and to appreciate the kindness of the stranger that had made their precious donation. Any misdemeanour could result in dismissal. There were two anatomy department technicians, brothers Reg and Fred, who ran the dissection room. Reg was very much the boss but the more diminutive man, whereas Fred was heavier built and significantly taller. Both were proudly cockney. They were responsible for preparing the bodies and for keeping the dissection room and the museum of specimens in the best state possible. Reg, although quite brusque, had a great sense of humour. Fred was somewhat quieter but caring of 'his' students. To the side of the room were large metal tanks with body parts stored inside steeped in the dreaded formalin. Occasionally, they were brought out to show us what the end result ought to look like.

As previously mentioned, the professor of anatomy was William Hamilton, or Willie as we knew him. He was a large Northern Irishman who had an international reputation in embryology and Placentology. He was also professor of anatomy at the Royal Academy of Art, a position once held by the great William Hunter, brother of John. He was Dean of Charing Cross from 1956 to 1962. During that time, he succeeded in obtaining chairs in obstetrics and gynaecology, surgery and medicine for the hospital, all within the space of three years. He could be quite daunting but as one got to know him the true warmth of his character came to the fore. I observed that warmth during the final anatomical viva practical for anatomy. One of our year, an extremely bright student was struggling with the visiting professor from Liverpool and became tongue-tied when asked to name, and to point out the muscles of the sole of the foot. Willie was examining me with a second visiting professor. He knew how bright she was and hearing her hesitation, left my side to go over to her. He gently asked her what structure she was looking at. 'A foot, Professor Hamilton,' came the reply. 'Well done,' he said, 'And which side is that foot?' 'It's a left foot, sir,' and away she went, her anxiety lifted, and she was able to excel with her knowledge to the visiting professor. Not something that could happen today in the professional educationalist led examination structure of best possible answer multiple choice papers. Today examiners are prohibited from speaking to the candidates but merely mark down their findings. I always found that I learnt a great deal in those more open discursive forms of examination, which under the stress of the moment one never forgot.

With his interest and expertise in the placenta, Professor Hamilton was often called to London Zoo to collect interesting placentae. On one occasion, I went with him to collect that of an Elephant. It was a really interesting experience and a chance to be close to the baby Elephant. Such a beautiful animal. Watching the caring way in which the mother kept her close was very moving. I developed a real and lasting affection for those magnificent creatures.

Hamilton was ably assisted by Professor Tony Glenister and his lovely Scottish senior lecturer Jeannie Ross. Professor Glenister was also an embryologist and geneticist. He had served in the Royal Army Medical Corps and had been awarded the military CBE.

A very prominent military man and also a student of Charing Cross in the early 1870s was Sir James Cantlie. He regularly dressed in a kilt, bonnet and Highland cloak, being proud of his Scottish heritage. He became a demonstrator in anatomy and following an episode of typhoid fever and septicaemia contracted in the dissection room he turned to surgery. He spent time in Hong Kong and China, followed by an extensive tour in India, He was largely responsible for setting up the Volunteer Medical Staff Corps that eventually became the Royal Army Medical Corps, an important development that an alumnus of Charing Cross had a major influence upon.

Professor Glenister was a genial man, rather softly spoken, who always had a mischievous glint in his eye, made more interesting by the monocle he often wore and always sported in his top pocket. He followed Hamilton as Dean of the Medical School. They were a powerful duo.

Jeannie was a lovely woman, if somewhat strait laced. A large-bosomed lady with quite prominent teeth she always had a smile and a soft, warm, Scottish encouraging voice. She went from table to table demonstrating structures and explaining difficult concepts. I feel sure that she was the reason that many of us did well in anatomy. She had been married to Dr. McAllister, a rather dry, Victorian looking man who taught us biochemistry.

In complete contrast, there was a rather wonderful character who taught us biochemistry, Jeanie Turnbull. A diminutive red head with great flare, she often used to climb onto the laboratory bench, striding up and down whilst describing chemical reactions and molecular structures. She held our attention for what could be a very dry subject. Attention that was heightened when, on one occasion, in full flow she put her foot into a sink on the desktop and disappeared into the bottles of reagents, thankfully emerging apparently unharmed, other than with hurt pride and an even redder face than usual.

Another lecturer, who held the attention of the ladies, in the group was Dr Max Lab. A rather short but flamboyant South African on whom most of the girls had a crush at one time or another. He taught cardiac physiology well and I still remember those lectures.

For our anatomy dissections, we had to follow Cunningham's dissection manual and at the end of every section we had to pass an oral test, a viva voce, with one of the demonstrators or with Jeannie; fail, and it had to be repeated. This ensured a high standard in the subject. First were the upper and lower limbs, then thorax and abdomen, followed by head, neck and brain.

I struck up a friendship with Barry Jones and Paul Slade early into our time together. Barry and I came from similar relatively humble backgrounds. He was (and still is) an elegant man, quite confident but very pleasant to be around. Hard working, he spent every Saturday at his job in a fashionable clothes store on Oxford Street. He was very kind, inviting me to his parents' house in South London. A keen and good guitarist, many years later he went on to perform at significant venues with his band, as a warmup act in Hyde Park for an assembly of thousands for the 'Moonwalk' in aid of breast cancer. Barry has become one of the world's leading plastic surgeons doing amazing work for children with serious and often life-threatening base of skull problems. Paul's father was an officer in the RAF. He married a lovely ballet dancer, Anne, whilst still a student. I remember being in awe of several of my other colleagues. Andy Stewart had a wonderful sense of humour, and in combination with Barry, Joss Law, Paul Slade, Chris Peach and Nick Ingram made an enviable band of brothers that has stood the test of time and survives as the Balham Boot Boys. The name coming from lodgings they shared together. Several seemed to be able to combine sporting prowess and an easy-going manner with an ability to absorb the work with minimal studying. I was not prepared to take the chance, having made such a mess of my studies at school and overworked considerably. Paul had, and still has, a wonderful sense of dry humour and kept everyone around him very amused. His girlfriend, soon to be his long-time wife, Anne was studying at the Royal Ballet school and eventually danced in the corps du ballet. This seemed to me to be very exotic, and although I knew nothing about the art form, I was very drawn to it. They decided that they wanted to get married, and I think that Paul was somewhat intimidated to share this news with his RAF father. In an attempt to soften the blow, I was invited to dinner with Paul and his parents at which he was to announce his intentions. My memory is of a well-appointed dining room, formally laid out for dinner and a very pleasant evening. All seemed to go very well as far as I could tell and in due course Paul and Anne were married and have had a wonderful life together. Paul became an excellent GP, and a television company made a series of programmes following him through his daily life, including his work on his pig farm.

John Turner, another of the year of students, was a man without fear, and possessed a wonderful sense of humour. One day a group of us were sitting in the Chandos café when he came flying up Agar Street on his bike, which he quickly abandoned and ran inside to hide amongst us. Apparently, he was being chased by the police for dangerous cycling along Piccadilly. He joined the RAF as a student and somehow before long was able to buy a beautiful green Aston Martin. Not long after graduating John switched to a flying career and became one of the very few medics to fly jet fighters. His brave recklessness has survived with him all of his life.

Another bold soul was Tim Riley. Tim joined the army and was one of the medics on the frontline at Goose Green in the Falklands war. He and his colleagues continued to manage wounded British and Argentinian soldiers in a makeshift operating theatre with a 500-lb bomb in the rafters whilst bomb disposal experts sat next to the ordinance to give confidence. I believe that their message was to carry on whilst they were there. 'If you see us run, then do the same'. They completed their shift without event, after which the bomb was diffused. Much to their great credit was the fact that no soldier of whatever country died if they reached their hands. The time-tested practice of control the bleeding, debride the wound and leave it open to heal by second intention was the rule and it worked a charm.

To help with our studies, we had the opportunity to buy a real half-skeleton. I don't know anyone who bought a full one, although they were available. These were obtained from 'abroad', Bill suggested that they were from the Philippines. I still shudder at the thought of families being tempted to sell the bones of their deceased loved ones for money. Bill was the one who delivered mine. I cannot forget the day I took it home on the tube. It was housed in a sturdy cardboard box. On the way home to Streatham, I managed to drop the box in a busy tube carriage. The skull fell out and began to roll along the carriage floor, to the horror of fellow passengers. With the jogging of the train, every time I reached down to grab it, it rolled off in a different direction. Perhaps the commuters on the Circle Line from Charing Cross had seen it all before as few seemed disturbed by the otherwise bizarre sight of a young, short-haired (bizarre enough in 1969) person chasing after an errant skull. I still have that skeleton and with the passage of time am unsure how to deal with it out of respect for the human being it once was. It has been extremely useful throughout my career, however, and I owe a huge debt of gratitude to him (for it is a male skeleton) and his family wherever they may be.

I enjoyed learning anatomy enormously and immersed myself in it. I found that if I read a section in *Gray's Anatomy* and then closed the book and drew the part in detail from memory it really stuck in my mind. A glance at those drawings today rapidly brings back most of the knowledge acquired more than fifty years ago. Though not exactly the modern idea of mind maps, they served that purpose for me. I encourage current students to try that system of learning. I continue to use drawing when recording operative procedures that I was learning, and latterly in the operation notes of patients.

The anatomy, physiology and biochemistry lectures were regular fixtures in the steeply tiered lecture theatre. If late in arrival, there was a small door high up at the back of the theatre, behind the uppermost row of seats that we used to creep in unnoticed, or so we thought. If opened quietly, one could surreptitiously sneak in. Professor Glenister, however, seemed to have a sixth sense and whilst continuing to lecture and to write on the large blackboard would holler out the name of the miscreant, making clear that his or her (usually his) tardiness had been noticed. Years later he revealed the secret of his apparent prescience. He kept his half-moon glasses highly polished and could see reflected image of the offender.

I think that most of us had read the *Doctor in the House* books by Richard Gordon. They were published a generation before our time at medical school, but they still had a strong ring of truth about them. Much hilarity was had throughout the course which seemed to mimic the goings on in Richard Gordon's mind.

At the beginning of 1970 there were a series of coal miners' strikes which led to the three-day week to reduce energy consumption. It was an eerie but quite beautiful sight walking along The Strand in the late winter afternoons with no electric light and what illumination there was provided by candles. There can be a positive side to everything.

Travel from London to south Shropshire was a tedious business with lengthy train journeys interrupted by changes and waiting for connections, then hitching a lift back from Shrewsbury or waiting for my grandfather to pick me up. It would regularly take all day. In 1970 my parents agreed to buy a car for me so that I could get back and forth to London under my own steam. Once again, my dear grandfather stepped in and offered to help. He tried to persuade me that the car to have would be an old Morris Minor. He duly had the local garage bring one up to the square in Clun for me to see. Whilst this would have been the safest and best solution for the job in hand, it was not at all what I had in mind. A small sports car was what I really wanted. One Sunday afternoon driving back to London with Mum and Dad we passed a small garage in Leominster with a bright red Austin Healey Sprite Mk III in the window. This was the ticket. Exactly what I had in mind. To my great surprise, Mum quickly jumped to my support, clearly seeing the appeal of the car, and although Dad had his reservations he bought it for me the following week. This little car was a dream come true. In those days they cost around £750 new. Ours cost a little over £200, as it was a few years old. Nowadays a good example sells for more than £10,000, even though they will be at least fifty years old. When I see them now, it is hard for me to imagine how I travelled so comfortably in mine. Indeed, even harder to imagine was my father, all 6 feet 5 inches of him managing to get in as well. This was the situation we found ourselves in when we became the victims of road rage in Ludlow on our way to the market. The young lout in the other car got out and started shouting and gesticulating at us with the usual vulgar hand signals. The surprise and shock on his face was a joy to behold as two greater than 6-foot men began to emerge from the tiny car and to stride determinedly towards him. We rapidly saw his heels as he leapt back into his car and raced off.

Owning and running a car in central London then was a very viable proposition, as parking was not a problem. At that time in 1970, it was possible to park my little car outside the hospital on Agar Street where there were no restrictions. Also, there were no speed cameras. I quickly learnt the rat runs through Wandsworth and Fulham to get to the hospital from Streatham in the shortest possible time. It was a joy driving through the London streets with the roof down in relatively light traffic at the time in the morning that I left home. By working in the holidays I was able to earn enough to keep it on the road. Using his engineering knowledge gleaned from the REME, Dad taught me how to service the car and how to balance its twin SU carburettors using my stethoscope, saving considerably on service bills.

There were some wonderfully colourful characters in our year of 1969. A good friend Andy Davidson had acquired a lovely sky-blue Triumph Spitfire. The other car owners amongst us were John Williams with another blue car, a Hillman Imp, which I believe he still has. Far more up market was an Aston Martin DB IV, owned by a young man whose father we thought was an arms dealer. A flamboyant and vibrant character, he didn't stay the course and probably went on to much more financially rewarding things.

At the end of each term, we had examinations in all subjects. The results were published on the medical school notice board, and I remember the clamour of everyone leaning forwards to see their results. For the first time since primary school, I achieved some good results and the hard work had put me at, or near, the top of the class in most subjects. In retrospect, I do regret somewhat working so hard, indeed overworking, because it did limit the time that I spent socialising with others. I suspect a factor, other than not wanting to mess up again, was my significant shyness amongst so many outgoing and talented people.

The pre-clinical course lasted eighteen months, with terms like those of secondary school, except longer. It was called the second MB course, as first MB were the subjects of Chemistry, Biology and Physics to A level standard. We had a postgraduate entrant, unusual in those days. Leslie Guinea had worked at the Berlin Opera Company before deciding to switch to medicine. Leslie seemed positively ancient to us being 29 when she joined the group. However, her maturity shone through and she mixed in with us juveniles extremely well. We became close friends, and I found her extremely kind and supportive, as I had what is now referred to as imposter syndrome in spades. Having struggled so much to get into medicine, I found myself with an extremely bright bunch of people who had got in on their first attempt with A level grades that I could only dream of. I remember very clearly thinking as I first crossed the threshold and entered the medical school that now the slate could be wiped clean and I finally had the chance to prove myself. I was absolutely determined not to let the chance slip away. Everything would be new to all of us. It was a level academic playing field.

Looking back on those years it is interesting to note that for a medical school known for producing good solid general practitioners we produced surprisingly many experts in other areas. Almost fifty percent became surgeons of one kind or another, with several consultants in other hospital medicine specialties as well, several of whom developed international reputations. It is a testament to the type of student that the selection procedure produced. Now regarded as outmoded and unfair, it seemed to do the job well in those days.

The London Medical Group

During my first year, I was introduced to an ethical discussion group The London Medical Group (LMG). This had been set up as a forum for the discussion of medical ethics by the Reverend Edward Shotter, or Ted as we came to call him. He was a lovely man, extremely supportive of us students. The president was Lord Amulree, a distinguished gerontologist. Law students and students of the cloth were involved as well as medical students. The speakers were of the highest quality and the standard of debate was quite exhilarating. I had been captain of our debating society at school and always enjoyed the format. Dame Cicely Saunders was a regular speaker and made the passionate case for palliative care, a completely new concept at that time. She founded the earliest hospice and was a wonderful caring and compassionate woman. She always gave freely of her time.

The LMG was the forerunner of the Society for the Study of Medical Ethics, later the Institute of Medical Ethics. *The Journal of Medical Ethics* grew out of it. Ted deliberately never chaired a meeting nor lectured as he was very keen for it not to be seen as an exercise in chaplaincy, so as to maintain the most open interest and discussion. In this he succeeded admirably. I became the secretary of the group in my third year and enjoyed getting to know some of the biggest names in medicine and the law of the time. Lord Amulree, or Basil William Sholto Mackenzie, 2nd Baron Amulree KBE MD FRCP, was a lovely man with a gentle stutter, who regarded his role in teaching very highly. He had a wide circle of friends and knew the artists Pablo Picasso and Graham Sutherland. At first meeting he could be a little intimidating for a butcher's boy from Clun with his monocle and slightly halting, aristocratic voice. He was a passionate advocate for the aged and chronically sick and spoke volubly in their support in the House of Lords. He felt passionately that the hand of the bureaucrat should be kept as far as possible from the care of the sick and elderly. How we could do with his like today. At the time that I knew him he would have been in his early seventies having been born in 1900. His foresight made him a pioneer in the provision of hospital care for the elderly and extended to linking hospital services with care in the home. He never married and lived in a splendid house in Hans Crescent. As secretary of the LMG I was invited to dinner with him at his home. Somewhat nervously I arrived quite early and rang the doorbell. Soon a gartered Butler arrived at the front door and welcomed me in. I remember a short hallway to a staircase which rose to a beautiful living room with an open fire in the hearth. On climbing the stairs, I noticed the quite wonderful series of what I thought were prints of Toulouse Lautrec, Monet, Manet and Van Gogh pictures. Shortly, Lord Amulree descended from an upper room and graciously introduced himself to me.

After the usual pleasantries I blurted out, feeling I was relatively knowledgeable about art and artists, that I admired his wonderful prints on the staircase. He smiled and being the gentleman that he was he gently suggested that I show him the ones that I meant, as he thought that they were originals when he had looked at them earlier that morning. I realised that I had made something of a faux pas. 'Oh, those', he said with a broad smile as I pointed them out to him. 'Yes, they are real paintings collected by the family from the artists.' He immediately diffused my obvious embarrassment by saying, 'I can see that you are interested in art. Allow me to show you some of my favourite things.' We walked through to his study, and he drew out a large portfolio. 'This is one of my favourites,' he said, showing me a pastel drawing of a blurred image of a matador and a passing bull with a flash of red that was the matador's cape. On turning the sheet over was written 'Sholto with best wishes from Picasso'. This was a whole new world for me. The dinner passed delightfully with excellent wine and food.

The time came to leave and Ted, who had joined us, left with me. I offered him a lift home in my trusty Sprite. We set off slowly, but as soon as we reached the junction with Basil Street a Mini, travelling at right angles to my car and far too fast, jumped a stop sign and slammed into the side of it, tearing off most of the front and with it the engine, before ricocheting from us into a row of parked cars on the other side of the street, doing serious damage to at least four of them. Amazingly, we were unhurt despite the fact that my legs were dangling in the open air. I had consumed quite a lot of wine as a result of the nervousness that I felt in the gathering of nobility and following my art faux pas. Ted did not drink alcohol and, with the introduction of the breathalyser in 1967, was concerned that I would lose my driving licence. 'Quickly', he said, 'jump out and I will say that I was driving.' A noble gesture for a man of the cloth. The police arrived and took statements but did not breathalyse either of us and proceeded to book the hapless Mini driver for dangerous driving. My poor little Sprite was carried away on a transporter to be an insurance write-off. I didn't inform my parents that evening as no-one had been hurt and it was very late. But the next morning, I called home at 7.30 from a push-button pay phone outside the London Hospital. My mother answered, and before I could say a word, she said, 'You have had an accident, and it was last night at about 10.30 p.m.' I was flabbergasted; how could she have known? 'I knew,' she said, 'and I knew that you were not hurt.' On discussing it with my father much later he said that this was not an uncommon event with Mum, who seemed to have second sight as it was called then. Luckily as the car was deemed a write-off, but fully insured, I was eventually able to replace it with a younger MK IV Austin Healey Sprite.

My Earliest Experience of Open-Heart Surgery

One day after the first round of lectures, Lesley Guinea, our mature student and ex-opera director, told me that there was an open-heart case going on in the operating theatres under the care of Mr Arthur Makey. Mr Makey had been appointed to develop cardiac surgery at Charing Cross. He was an accomplished thoracic and general surgeon of the old training style. His teaching was encouraging and quite gentle. He never ridiculed anyone, a trait of some of other consultants.

The operating theatre at the old Charing Cross had a viewing gallery from which students and interested doctors could watch the proceedings. It was reached through a small staircase climbing high into the hospital roof space and approached through a small door. Lesley asked me if I would like to go and watch with her. Of course, I jumped at the chance. Looking down on the operative field with the masked and gowned surgeons working quietly on the human heart was breath-taking.

It was a slow procedure, taking much of the day, with a lot of time spent controlling bleeding at the end. However, the patient was successfully removed to the intensive care unit for recovery after nearly eight hours of surgery. Sadly, I was to learn three days later that she had succumbed to it all and had not survived. Cardiac surgery at that time was in its infancy and patients were referred very late in their disease process and as such, faced very high risks. Nevertheless, my enthusiasm was undimmed, and I could not wait to get closer to the action. A cardiologist had been appointed from Leeds to work with Mr Makey. His name was Peter Nixon and he had become established in the profession at a very young age, being only in his thirties at that time. Sadly, he was to fall dramatically from grace in 1997 when he began a libel action against Channel 4 for calling him a charlatan for claiming that hyperventilation was the cause of many serious medical conditions, amongst them serious heart disease. When challenged with the evidence he admitted to false claims in papers that he had written and withdrew his action being then faced with a large bill in costs and the ruination of his reputation.

In stark contrast to that debacle, Makey was a much-loved consultant who led a very distinguished career and held the respect of his patients, colleagues, students and trainees. There is no doubt that he was held back in the development of cardiac surgery by Nixon, who reduced his referrals for surgery believing that patients with coronary artery disease could be best treated by being put to sleep for weeks at a time. Our admiration for Arthur was magnified by the cases that he had to take on as a result of Nixon's obduracy in referral of sensible cases. What should have been a dream team turned out to be a nightmare association. However, in those days training for surgery encompassed the whole of general surgery and Arthur more than made up for this abysmal relationship with a wonderful general practice. He was truly a general surgeon. A list that I remember consisted of a gall bladder removal, some large bowel surgery, a partial lung removal and the extraction of wisdom teeth. This led to excellent teaching material for us students. Many years later, after I had become a consultant cardiothoracic surgeon and received the Hunterian Professorship from the Royal College of Surgeons, I arranged a dinner to follow my lecture and invited those who had figured most in my career. Arthur, of course, was at the top of the guest list. At the end of the evening he thanked me for the invitation. Just as he was turning to leave he said, 'You are probably a better cardiac surgeon than me, but I was a much better thoracic surgeon.' I am sure that he was correct in the latter part of his statement. I sensed from him a feeling of opportunities lost because of the appalling behaviour of Peter Nixon.

Another early experience that had a big influence on my desire to follow a surgical career came when witnessing the last operating list of Norman Tanner. Tanner was the most experienced upper gastrointestinal tract surgeon in the UK at the time and one of the world leaders, such that Frank Lahey, (originator of the Lahey clinic in Boston Massachusetts) who visited him, and watched him operate, commented that the surgery he witnessed at Tanner's hands was the finest display of surgical skill that he had ever witnessed.

His last list was in the old theatres at Charing Cross in 1970. It was a truly general list with, of course, his eponymous procedures, the Tanner Gastrectomy, the Tanner Slide for inguinal hernia repair and, for a finale, an appendicectomy with long instruments carried out through a left diaphragm incision whilst doing a trans-thoracic hiatal hernia repair. The end of the list was met with a prolonged round of applause from the gallery and within the operating theatre. A further famed name on the staff at the time was Norman Plummer, one of the very outstanding physicians of the time. Sadly, our contact was small as he had attachments to several other institutions as was the norm for eminent medical men of the time. Also, he was at the end of his career. However, he was a very fine teacher and again enjoyed a strong international reputation.

The wards were laid out in the Nightingale tradition with six to eight beds on each side of the ward with a good space between them. In the centre was a table at which the nurses sat to make their notes. At the end of the ward were cupboards to store the essential equipment. Some of the wards at the old hospital were adorned with beautiful hand painted tiles which have become invaluable. They were moved to the Victoria and Albert museum for a period of time but now are installed in the new hospital, albeit hard to find.

The wards were usually too hot and the environment was perfect for cockroaches. I remember opening a cupboard one day to find a mass of them spilling out onto the ward floor and scuttling away. At Christmas, the consultant whose patients were on a particular ward would come in with his family to carve the Turkey for the patients, a tradition now long since gone.

Ward rounds were always officious occasions. They were led by the consultant with the ward sister and one or two other nurses by his side. On the opposite side of the bed would be the junior doctors, the registrar, senior registrar, and the housemen or women. And standing at the foot of the bed, the firm of medical students trying to look engaged and knowledgeable. The patients were made to sit upright propped up against their pillows, tightly bound in place by their bed sheets and blankets. Questions would be fired at them and then the junior doctors and the students grilled in front of them. There is a moment in the old *Doctor in the House* Film where the patient in that setting has the temerity to ask a question. James Robertson Justice playing Sir Lancelot Sprat boomed out, 'Shut up man, this has nothing whatever to do with you.' The times have changed now, but back then it was very accurate in its depiction of the hierarchy of the staff and students. Most of us dreaded being called forward to examine the patient and to come up with a possible diagnosis. Being the tallest in the group it was hard for me to hide behind the others and so I got picked out very frequently.

During the eighteen months of second MB, we had university holidays. During the summer break, Paul Slade and I decided to try to get work on a building site, as he had heard that there was good money to be made. After trying a few sites, we struck gold with the redevelopment of Marks and Spencer's main site at the junction of Oxford and Orchard Street. Bovis were doing the developments, and it included reroofing over the Orchard Street pedestrian footpath and refacing the walls in the store amongst other things. I'm not sure about Paul, but my knowledge of anything to do with building was zero. We were put to work as 'go-fors' which turned out to be the most important job of acquiring miniature bottles of alcohol for the real workers from Selfridges across the street. The main contingent of workers were wonderful Geordies who had worked together for a long time. They were very good to us, demanding very little. Much of the time was spent sitting in the roof space wolf-whistling at the passing girls. Now of course completely outlawed, they seemed to enjoy it, and the ladies cast lovely smiles back at them. It was non-threatening and meant in good fun.

On one occasion, the foreman announced that the team, of which we were now very much a part, were going to Brighton for a weekend's work on the branch of M&S there. Pay would be double time on Saturday and triple time on Sunday, with all travel and hotel costs paid. We set off at the end of the working day on Friday. As soon as we arrived, we went to the store and immediately started work. We worked until the early hours completing the job and then retired to bed. The next two days were spent sun-bathing on the beach or drifting through the bars of Brighton. It was a very profitable weekend.

Towards the end of that time, I remember a conversation with one of them. They seemed quite amused by having two medical students in their midst. He turned to me and said with a smile:

> One day when you are a rich and famous doc, you will be gliding down Oxford Street in your chauffeur driven Rolls-Royce with your lady wife by your side, and you will glance over at this store and as you remember these days, a smile will cross your face. Your wife will ask you 'Why are

> you smiling?', but you will gently dismiss the question without confessing to your time with us.

I was a little saddened that he thought that we would disown the memory as we had a wonderful time with them. Indeed, I still think about those wonderful characters every time I pass Selfridges. Travelling to and from Oxford Street and Streatham on the tube, I read *The Iliad* for the first time. The contrast between the daily conversation at work and this journey into the classics was starkly amusing.

Seemingly very quickly, the time passed, and the second MB examinations arrived. In those times the examinations consisted of two written papers for each subject and an oral test in anatomy. We were told that if we were handed a foetal skull or a first rib, we were either up for honours, or it was a chance to raise ourselves up from a borderline fail to a pass. I made sure that I knew those anatomical parts very well. You can imagine my delight when both were put in from of me. After the results had been published on the famous notice board, most of us then removed to the Lemon Tree pub. The manager, who knew us well, shut the doors at closing time in the afternoon, confining us in the bar. The window opening out onto the street was frosted for the lower half. As the drinks flowed, we noticed a very familiar head bobbing up and down towards the entrance followed by a brisk knock at the locked door. Professor Willy Hamilton was outside. The bar man looked at us and shrugged his shoulder asking what to do. Apprehensively, we told him to let him in, wondering what was about to transpire. We were surprised and delighted when he came in and ordered drinks for everyone and simply wanted to join in with the celebrations. Later, I was delighted to hear that I had won some prizes including the Huxley Prize in Physiology.

Intercalated Anatomy B.Sc. (Hons.)

At the end of the term we all left to go home to prepare for our clinical years. Prior to leaving, we acquired our new, non-formalin-stained white coats and stethoscopes. Now it was going to become very interesting and what we were there for. At last, we would meet patients and get on with learning how to become doctors. We said our farewells and left for a well-earned holiday.

I had been at home for about a week when the phone rang. I answered it to find to my great surprise that Professor Glenister was on the line. After the usual pleasantries, he informed me that he thought that I should not proceed with the clinical years, that I should pause to do an honours B.Sc.

in anatomy. This would take another eighteen months. It would consist of course units in anthropology, experimental embryology, primatology and cell biology. Whilst I was flattered and it sounded very interesting, I was keen to get on with the clinical years and politely declined. I thought no more about it until the phone rang again the next day, and this time my grandfather answered it. I heard a brief conversation following which he beckoned me over and with his hand over the mouthpiece, informed me that it was Professor Glenister again, who had asked that I reconsider the offer. With a smile, my grandfather, said that he had accepted on my behalf, and assured him that I would be there at the start of term. The professor was delighted and wanted to discuss the details with me. What could I do but accept gracefully and agree that I would take up the offer. Dear Grandad had led me into a parallel world that I would not have otherwise known. It was the beginning of a fascinating time which became very productive for me as my career developed. I could not have known at that stage how profitable it would be. Clearly, even with no academic experience at all, my grandfather had realised its importance. Once again, I am indebted to him.

Our intercalated degree course included just five students, two from St Thomas', two from The London and me from Charing Cross. One of the Thomas' students Steve Capps and I struck up a close friendship.

The whole course was fascinating, particularly the anthropology unit. Professor Glenister and his counterpart at St Thomas's hospital Michael Day had a close relationship with several of the important names in the subject at the time. One such personality on the world stage was Richard Leakey. There was great excitement when we heard that the great man was coming to lecture and to be with us for a week. Richard, son of the great Louis and Mary Leakey was another pioneer in anthropological research, following his distinguished parents. Although taught by a governess and latterly at Waverley College where he didn't do well, he secured the help of an English teacher and was admitted to St John's College, Cambridge. In his final examinations he asked to be examined in Swahili. Having passed his viva voce in Swahili he was asked to examine a fellow candidate in the same language.

The Leakeys lived and studied in East Africa and made many distinguished discoveries near Olduvai gorge in Tanzania. It became known as Leakey country. The lowest level of this stratified gorge dated back to between 1.7 and 2.1 million years ago. It was here that Homo Habilis, the earliest Hominid remains were found. As well as those primitive members of the Hominidae family were the bones of elephant, giraffes, hyenas and baboons. Along with the bones of these ancient precursors of ours were found elementary stone tools and evidence of a refining diet. Mary Leakey produced unequivocal evidence to show that there was tool making throughout these levels. The most common were pebble choppers, a cobblestone that had been chipped, or flaked to use the jargon, to make cutting edges. Jane Goodall and Diane Fossey were protégés of Louis. They developed their own important careers, working with chimpanzees and gorillas. We were treated to lectures by Jane Goodall, John Napier and Michael Day, Professor of Anatomy and Anthropology at St Thomas' hospital. Another wonderful lecturer was J. Z. Young, from University College London. His book *The Life of the Vertebrates* remains a classic.

Richard Leakey brought the small female skull of the famous Australopithecus aforensis, known as Lucy, for us to see. This skull is now locked away in the anthropology museum in Addis Ababa in Ethiopia where I was privileged to see her once again, this time through the glass of the exhibition cabinet. Learning about the importance of the Galapagos islands in the understanding of evolution as seen through the eyes of Charles Darwin and learning the thirty-two differences between the new- and old-world monkeys were but two of the joys of the course. Frequent trips behind the scenes at the Natural History Museum and free passes to London Zoo to watch the gibbons brachiate, were some of the privileges that the course afforded us.

In cell biology we were introduced to the wonders of the ultra-microscopic world seen through an early electron microscope. Learning how to do freeze-fracturing of tissues and then to scan the revealed surface seemed magical to me at that time. Professor Lynne Reid, travelled from Harvard, where she was to become professor of pathology and pathologist-in-chief at the Children's Hospital in Boston to give us one week of her time. At the time she had been appointed the Dean of the Cardio-thoracic Institute in London, somewhere that was to become my own Alma Mater in future years. Her work on the detailed structure of the lungs was seminal. Seeing for the first time the ultrastructure of the lungs was magical.

For the different course units, we moved between the anatomy departments of The London, St Thomas', Charing Cross hospitals and University College.

I had moved from my 'digs' in Streatham to the International Students' House, affectionately known as ISH, on Regent's Park at the instigation of Tim Riley who had heard about a new extension opening on the south side of the park. This beautiful building was part of the John Nash (1752–1835) development around the park. Nash was responsible for the layout of much of Regency London. Most of the very beautiful buildings in London, including Clarence house, the Terraces on Regent's Park, Marble Arch and the Staterooms in Buckingham Palace were his work. The main International Students' House building is on Portland place. Latterly the Terrace on the south side of the park was acquired in 1968 and developed for student accommodation. Tim and I applied and, perhaps because of our generally respectable appearance in the age of long hair and flower power, we were accepted. The deal was that for around £5 per week we had full board on the agreement that we would spend at least four hours per week with the foreign students, helping them to feel at home and showing them around London as necessary. For an extra one pound per week, I had the privilege of parking my little sports car in their underground car park. There was also free parking on the outer circle of the park at that time. I was given a room on the first floor overlooking the terrace opposite the back of the Royal Academy of Music. Directly opposite my room were practice rooms in the Academy. For a period of time the great jazz musician Johnny Dankworth taught there, and he could be heard practicing with his wife Cleo Lane. In the summer months, with the windows open, we were treated to their practice concerts. Some of us would gather together in my room with a beer and enjoy the music.

Looking after the foreign students was a joy and we made so many good friends with occasional exciting opportunities. I remember driving two beautiful Brazilian girls around London. Dressed all in white against their brown sun-kissed skin, sitting on the back of my little sports car with soft top down, they made a head-turning sight. I became particularly fond of the students from Africa and South America. They were charming, polite and very hard-working.

Not long after we arrived, in 1972 the Queen mother came to officially open the building. Tim and I were chosen to greet her in the downstairs common room. When she arrived with her entourage, she was absolutely charming but admitted to being rather thirsty. Without thinking, we asked her if she would like a cup of tea, to which she immediately said 'that would be rather nice.' The only source readily to hand was a dispensing machine and so I put the money in and brought her a plastic cup of tea whilst Tim, being much more socially adept than me, held her in conversation. She insisted that we join her and so we did. We all sat down oblivious to the others in the room. With the tea being so hot it took a while to drink. The Queen Mother, however, was very relaxed and chatted away asking us what we were studying. She found the medical course interesting and quizzed us in some depth. The Royal family had significant links to the Charing Cross hospital, and she was delighted to hear that was where we were studying. Finally, after about twenty minutes she moved on, encouraged to do so by her lady in waiting. I was surprised when, after her death in 2002, in a review of her life her lady in waiting retold the story on the BBC. Apparently we made her late for her next engagement. Keeping Royalty waiting might have lost us our heads in centuries gone by.

During the summer holiday of 1973, Steve Capps and I decided to drive to stay with his friend, or it might have been his cousin, in an apartment in Calpe near Alicante. He and his girlfriend were working for a package holiday company and they invited us to stay with them. After planning our route, we set off in my Austin Healey Sprite. A distance of over 1,300 miles lay ahead. We planned to do it in two days. The route down took us through the centre of France and we reached Perpignan very late at night. We decided to bed down in our sleeping bags on the side of the road and to get up very early the next morning to complete the journey. After a rather poor night on the tarmac in a layby on the side of a mountain we set off to complete the journey. The little car ran faultlessly. Steven was not insured to drive and so that fell to me. Finally, fairly tired and quite sunburnt from driving in the open air, we arrived, and met our hosts for the next ten days. The girlfriend was a flamboyant bohemian type who greeted us at the door in her birthday suit. Surprising though this was to me, she seemed quite unphased by it. A further shock to my boarding school, country bumpkin breeding was waking in the night to find her sitting on the toilet, door open, facing me, again quite naked emptying her bladder. Clearly this was going to be an interesting stay.

One morning, I awoke to find her standing fully naked on the balcony of the next room overlooking a building site. When I looked towards the building site, I noticed a workman who had spotted her whilst pushing a wheelbarrow full of sand. Clearly intoxicated by the site he hadn't noticed that he was approaching the edge of the incomplete second floor and before I or anyone else could shout to warn him, over the edge he went. Luckily for him he landed in a pile of sand and was able to stagger to his feet dazed but with no apparent serious damage. Our host simply turned away and returned inside as though nothing had happened.

The other feature I remember was a notice stuck to the wall inside the elevator that warned you not to enter with bare feet, 'for fear of electrocution'.

The time came to return home, and we decided to drive a different route and to pass through Saragossa. Being an age without digital on demand media and not being able to read Spanish we were unaware that Saragossa was in the grip of a Cholera epidemic. The first that we knew of it as we approached the town, were signs of skull and cross bones with severe warnings in Spanish, which of course, we were unable to read. Acknowledging that something sinister was going on, we decided not to make the planned stop there for lunch and continued to our border crossing at San Sebastian.

On the route up to Bordeaux the fan belt broke miles from a town or village. We resorted to trying to flag down passing cars. Eventually a young woman stopped, taking pity on us. We showed her the problem and she declared that she could not help us. Quick as a flash we said 'Well, do you think you could remove your stockings, which we could then use as a temporary replacement for the fan belt?' Initially a bit taken aback, she agreed and shed the said undergarments while we turned our backs. In exchange we gave her a bottle of wine that we happened to have in the car and parted. I had read that this was a short-term solution for the problem and so it proved. It lasted long enough for us to reach a garage in the next town where a replacement belt was jury-rigged by the lovely moustachioed garage owner. The remainder of the journey was remarkably uneventful, and we arrived back in London well satisfied with ourselves having experienced more of the world than perhaps we had expected.

The time that I spent working for the degree was very relaxing compared with the intensity of the medical course. There was much more down time, although the lectures seemed to be more densely packed into the week than current student timetables.

The final examination for the Bachelor of Science degree was split into the usual combination of written essay papers, viva voces and practical examinations. The very last examination was practical anthropology which we were told didn't count for very many marks. Steve Capps had managed to negotiate tickets to the Jesus College May Ball in Cambridge the night before and so all of us, bar one, decided to go. We arrived in Cambridge in our best penguin suits and dresses and had a wonderful time, staying up for the obligatory survivors' breakfast on the River Cam in a punt. Suddenly someone remembered what we were supposed to be doing that morning, and in a bit of a panic, the four of us raced back, crammed into my Sprite, to The London Hospital where the anthropology practical was taking place. We arrived thirty minutes late, but were allowed in. Margaret, the lone student who had not gone with us was already well on with her answers.

Finally, it was all over and we could relax. Several days later we were instructed to go to the Blind Beggar pub on the Mile end road where we would be informed of our results by the Professor Johnson, our anatomy professor. We assembled and ordered our drinks. After a while he came in and very simply stated, 'well, you have all passed. The swat got the first, the rest of you got upper seconds.' That was a little unkind to Margaret, but her diligence had paid off.

A final summer holiday ensued before we returned to our respective medical schools and the clinical course. I was approached by Dr Norman Robinson, Lecturer in Anatomy at The London and asked if I had plans for the summer. Dreading the possibility of another summer in the chicken factory, I replied that I didn't. He asked me if I would like to do a research project with him on Neuroanatomy. I was very happy to become involved, especially as it was paid employment. I had joined the Brain Research Association (B.R.A.) as I was extremely interested in brain function. The project was to try to establish whether Gamma Amino-Butyric Acid (G.A.B.A.) was a neurotransmitter in the adult rat brain and to establish its distribution and localisation. It was funded by the Friedrichs' Ataxia Group and the Action for the Crippled Child Fund. The experiments required removing the brain from anaesthetised adult Sprague Dawley rats. The work was detailed and required a great deal of care to protect the animals from discomfort or pain. It taught me detailed staining techniques and the practical use of the microscope and data recording. Also, the surgical techniques, although relatively limited, needed to be carried out with great care and precision. In conclusion we were able to show to a reasonable degree of satisfaction that GABA was very likely to be an inhibitory neurotransmitter and add information on its localisation in the adult rat brain. This resulted in a paper in the *Journal of Anatomy* in 1973, my first publication.[2] That was accompanied by a letter in Nature. It was a very satisfactory use of the summer months that gave me a very good start for my CV.

Early that Summer we were invited to the Royal Albert Hall to receive our degrees. The Queen Mother was the chancellor of the university at that time and our tea break at ISH was in my mind as she conferred my degree upon me. Other than the excitement of mounting the stage, what I remember is the boredom of sitting through what seemed to be thousands of pharmacists receiving theirs. Mum and Dad had come down to London to support me in this, but I remember what a struggle it was for Mum as there was no available parking nearby and she would not have a disabled sticker in the car; they had to walk slowly for a considerable distance to get there. She was quite exhausted as a result. We found a hotel on Kensington Gore for lunch and immediately afterwards they had to head back on the long drive to Clun. Dad must have been utterly exhausted but was up at 5.00 a.m. the next day despite it all to get on with the shop work. His moral and physical strength I can only admire and never hope to emulate.

With the end of the summer, the clinical years loomed ahead and with them the excitement of learning how to be proper doctors.

Charing Cross Hospital: A History

Charing Cross Hospital Medical School, though it is perhaps not as well-known as Guy's, St Thomas', King's, St George's and others, has a noble history. It was founded by Benjamin Golding. He was born in 1793, the youngest of sixteen children, in St Osyth, a small seaside village in Essex, beyond the Colne valley. Half of his siblings died in childhood, perhaps the stimulus for him to study medicine. It is reported that the young Benjamin was impressed by the kind works of the grand priory in St Osyth. For centuries the Monks supported the poor and the sick of the area. His father was well to do, owning several houses and businesses, including as my father did, a butcher's business with slaughterhouse, lending a note of resonance with my own start in life.

At the time there was no formal medical training in London. Professional skills and knowledge were acquired through pupil apprenticeships to recognised physicians or surgeons, rather like pupillage for trainee barristers today. For example, John Hunter began his career working as an assistant to his brother William in his anatomy school in central London. Edinburgh was ahead of English hospitals and training was well established there by the middle of the eighteenth century. Benjamin enrolled at the university of Edinburgh in 1811. After only two years he moved back to London having received his M.D. from the University of St Andrews where degrees could be issued by testimonial alone. He registered at St Thomas' hospital in the same year. It is notable that Benjamin wrote the first major history of that hospital, indicating his interest in medical training and the administration of health care in general, something that perhaps he is not known well enough for.[3] He lived close to Leicester Square, where John Hunter had lived and where his collection of anatomical and pathological specimens, along with his comparative anatomy collection, had been housed before being moved to the Royal College of Surgeons in 1799. Perhaps, knowledge of this collection was also a spur to his ambitions. As a medical student he had the vision of creating a hospital for the poor in the then squalid streets around Charing Cross. Within a couple of years, in 1815, Benjamin had opened his own house to the poor, as the area around him was impoverished and the housing meagre at best. Disease was rife. He would see patients at his house in the morning before going to St Thomas' in the afternoon to continue his studies. These are Golding's own words about his first conception of the hospital in 1815,

> I consider that a young medical man, whose time is but partly occupied, cannot be employed more beneficially, either to himself or others, than in

> adding to his practical knowledge, and in extending, by every means in his power, his opportunities of seeing diseases in their multifarious forms and complications; and that, to attain this object, and at the same time to render himself useful to others, he cannot do better than to devote some hours daily, for the first few years of his professional life, to the seeing, and prescribing for, gratuitously, those sick persons who require his aid but who are too poor to remunerate him. With these views I opened my house in the year 1815 to such poor persons as desired gratuitous advice and prescribed daily for all such applicants from eight o'clock in the morning until one in the afternoon; and this practice I continued for several years. Residing at that time in Leicester place, and afterwards in St Martin's Lane, in the neighbourhood where sickness and poverty so constantly abound among its dense population.[4]

In his own words, he stated seeing in excess of 20,000 poor people.

In 1823, with public support, he raised sufficient funds to open what was called the West London Infirmary, situated just behind the Haymarket Theatre. In 1825 he received his MRCS (Member of the Royal College of Surgeons) and LRCP (Licentiate of the Royal College of Physicians). He continued his treatment centre for several years. This endeavour grew into his plans for a much larger institution which led to his concept for the Charing Cross Hospital, named so in 1827. The hospital was formally opened in 1834. The then Princess Victoria consented to the principal ward for women being called the Victoria Ward. The Medical College was opened in the following year 1835. The opening lecture was given by Dr William Shearman, the Senior Physician. It was followed by lectures on anatomy and physiology, botany. chemistry, Materia Medica, midwifery (Dr Golding), morbid anatomy and surgery on successive days. Interestingly, in this age of anti-vaccers, one of the stated important objects and intentions of the charity was to disseminate the benefits of vaccination by gratuitously employing that salutary preventative of Variolous Infection to all poor persons and children who apply for the same.

There was no distinction in who would be treated. Foreigners as well as locals were welcome. None were charged and the doctors gave their services for free. Money was raised for the upkeep, drugs and to pay the domestic staff. A committee of local ladies was set up to provide flowers, books and linen. The first patron of the hospital was a son of King George III, the Duke of York. As the demand grew, larger premises were required and a property was found in Villiers Street. To keep patients moving through the beds, they were discharged as soon as the most distressing symptoms had abated, a forerunner of modern-day NHS early discharge policies. The discharged patients would receive gratuitous attendance in their own home until perfect health had been restored. This approach has a ring of modernity about it, as under-resourced NHS beds are oversubscribed and the concept of virtual wards have evolved. Early discharge is not a new phenomenon.

The plan for a medical school was in place from the very beginning and was begun as soon as the move to Villiers Street had been accomplished. The medical school course lasted six years, although postgraduate students were admitted for shorter periods. The path remains the same today, with the postgraduate course taking four years. Rather like the welcome we were to receive on our first day as medical students, those of the day were warned, 'Students are expected to be answerable for their conduct to the committee and are liable, if irregular, idle or dissolute, to censure and dismissal.' As described earlier, the opening remarks by Professor William Hamilton to us new students in 1969 on day one in lecture one reiterated those sentiments.

As this is being written, the government has announced its intention to begin apprenticeships in medicine whereby the student will provide work for the NHS at the same time as trying to train to be a doctor. Interestingly, this concept is not new and existed in those early days at Charing Cross. Four apprentices were taken on each year in the dispensary and became responsible to the chief dispenser and were required to perform minor procedures such as cupping, bleeding, teeth extraction, lancing of abscesses and the like, for a much-reduced educational fee.

The demands on the new Charing Cross grew rapidly and considerably and after lobbying for a new hospital, including that against the plan to rebuild Westminster hospital near the proposed site, the hospital committee were given the go-ahead, albeit with insufficient funding. Decimus Burton was awarded the contract to design and build it. The design was completed in 1830. The foundation stone was laid on 15 September 1831 by the Duke of Sussex, brother of King William IV.

Troubled years lay ahead, and Golding and his committee had to see off competition from King's and University College to maintain their independence. The most heated rivalry was with King's College in The Strand, which had no attached hospital. Their management made repeated attempts to affiliate with the new and rapidly growing Charing Cross hospital but all failed. Eventually they built their own hospital in Denmark Hill. This explains the continued undergraduate pre-clinical course in The Strand. Golding and his team were successful, however, and the future of the hospital secured.

Two famous names in British history were early students at 'The Cross', Dr David Livingstone and later Dr Thomas Huxley. Livingstone was born in 1813 in the mill town of Blantyre. Despite an unpropitious start in life, he became one of the most popular British heroes of the late nineteenth century. He was the second of seven children. At the age of ten he was put to work in a local cotton mill to support his poor family. He was to work there until the age of twenty-six. His father heavily influenced him in the Christian tradition of benevolence and caring. His Sunday school teacher was a further important influence and as a result of these influences he became interested in the potential of missionary work. His missionary zeal is conveyed in his words, 'In the glow of love that Christianity inspired, I resolved to devote my life to the alleviation of human suffering.' He studied hard every minute he could, even learning Latin with a primer in front of him whilst working the spinning jennies and mules in the mill. These were very noisy machines and must have yielded an exhausting environment. His desire to become a medical missionary grew. In pursuit of that ambition, in 1836 he began studies in Anderson's University in Glasgow. He was entirely self-taught. He moved to London to enrol in the London Missionary Society. At first, he was regarded as a rather rustic country bumpkin who needed the rough edges to be removed. Following an episode of emotional tongue-tie when attempting a sermon, he was advised to focus on his medical studies and that is when the move to Charing Cross occurred. He transferred to Charing Cross in 1839. On completing the course, he returned to Glasgow for his final medical examinations. He wanted to travel to China, but his desire to do this was frustrated by the Opium Wars and so he went to Africa in 1840. Other than for two short episodes he wasn't to return to England until his funeral in Westminster Abbey.

He became an explorer and a passionate advocate for the abolition of slavery, abhorring it in all its forms. He wrote that,

> ...the strangest disease I have seen in this country, seems to be broken-heartedness, and it attacks free-men who have been captured and made slaves.

Livingstone's fame abounded. He had become a fabled explorer, besieged in the street by adoring fans. Among his achievements were the discovery of the Victoria Falls and crossing the Kalahari Desert. The most evocative memory which endures to this day, however, is the apocryphal remark of Henry Morton Stanley on finding him, 'Dr. Livingstone, I presume.' Livingstone had seemingly been lost for four years on a search for the source of the River Nile. This quest was of mythical proportions. According to Herodotus writing in 460 BCE many attempts had been made to find the source of the Nile, but none succeeded. An eighteenth century French author wrote that 'it is not for mere mortals to discover the Nile feeble at its source'. Most explorers before him had been British and many had perished in the attempt. There was an enduring pride amongst the academic and military classes in the British achievements in exploration and discovery. Arising from this, Sir Roderick Murchison, a Scottish geologist who had served as the Director-General of the British Geological Society had asked Livingstone to take on this daunting task. He left England in 1865 planning a journey time of approximately two years. He suffered badly with multiple diseases and malnutrition and was isolated in what is now Tanzania. As the two years expired and contact with Livingstone was lost, concerns were raised. Efforts were made to find him, but none succeeded until the efforts of the now infamous Stanley.

Henry Morton Stanley was a British journalist, working as a reporter on the New York Herald. As Stanley had fought in the American Civil War, the editor had thought that he was American and it would be a great coup for an American to succeed where the British had failed in finding Livingstone. Clearly not being fully in touch with his staff he hadn't known that Stanley was not American. Nor did he know that Stanley was hardly a born explorer and viewed the venture with scepticism and fear. However, he accepted the proposition and set off in 1871. In the process he was ravaged by dysentery, starvation, and malaria, developing cerebral malaria which caused dementia. On making some recovery from this he contracted smallpox. Many of his porters died as did his two white companions. The travails of both Stanley and Livingstone were legion, and it was a miracle that they both survived long enough for them to meet and the immortal words to be uttered. Stanley returned to civilisation a hero, but Livingstone stayed on his quest but died in Zambia eighteen months after his discovery by Stanley. He was buried in Westminster Abbey with Stanley a pall bearer. Stanley died of a stroke in 1904 in London. He was denied his burial in Westminster Abbey close to his friend Livingstone as later he began to promote the slave trade, undermining his credibility.

Another student who matured into a great scientist was Thomas Huxley. Born in Ealing in 1825, the son of a schoolteacher, he entered Charing Cross as a free scholar. One of the signatories of his application was John Henry Newman, later cardinal Newman. Thomas' brother James had apprenticed in pharmacy and had been appointed dispenser at Gloucester Asylum. He had been so well regarded that a post had been kept open for him at Charing Cross. In a supportive note to his application, Cardinal Newman expressed his belief that these two young men would hereafter reflect credit on any institution from which they may receive their education. How true those words became. It was an exception for two members of the same family to be taken in as free scholars, but it was an exception which was made for them. Thomas began his studies at 'The Cross' in 1842, aged just seventeen. He studied hard and was heavily influenced by T. Wharton Jones, the lecturer in physiology. Wharton Jones made several significant discoveries, including describing the granular nature of neutrophil leucocytes and described in detail the mammalian oocyte. They got on very well and it was Wharton Jones who encouraged Huxley to publish his first paper. In it he described for the first time the inner root sheath of hair cells, still known as Huxley's Layer.

On completion of his studies Huxley was encouraged to apply for a post as a ship's doctor by a respected colleague, Joseph Frayer. Frayer won almost all possible prizes. He was later knighted. Huxley was appointed to Royal Navy Haslar, which had an extensive museum of specimens from all over the world. Sir John Richardson, a renowned explorer and naturalist was head of Haslar. He noticed Huxley and became very impressed by his diligence and capabilities. A cruise was heading off on a survey of exploration in the Torres straits between northern Australia and New Guinea. The captain was looking for a ship's surgeon and Huxley seized the opportunity. They sailed in December 1866 and so began a remarkable career which brought about a revolution in zoological knowledge. At the age of twenty-five, Huxley was made a Fellow of the Royal Society. In time he was to become president of that august institution. He maintained his loyalty to Charing Cross and often expressed his gratitude for the education that he had received there. He became a great supporter of Charles Darwin's theory of evolution, being referred to as Darwin's Bulldog

On his death and in his honour, Charing Cross Medical School established the Huxley Lectureship, its stated aim being on recent advances in science in their bearing on medicine and Surgery. It was delivered biannually. Among them were many of the greatest names in medicine at that time: Rudolf Virchow, Professor of Pathology in Berlin, 1898, The Right Hon. Lord Lister, for what was to be his last public lecture in 1900, Professor Pavlov of St Petersburg, 1906, and Professor Simon Flexner, Director of the Rockefeller Institute in New York, 1912. All paid their respects

By 1850, Charing Cross Hospital was in a strong financial position. In 1868, 19,000 patients were treated. The first trained nurses were taken on in 1866. Until then the nursing staff had been recruited from the domestic team and were in general a scruffy bunch of reprobates, often stealing from patients and demanding money from them. They were described as illiterate, ignorant of manners and often in the grip of excessive alcohol intake. It was clear that something would have to be done. However, this move towards formal training and better selection was not without its detractors. The doctors reacted with hostility fearing that they may begin to undermine their position, a concern that has re-emerged today with specialist nursing and physician's assistant roles in the modern NHS. The pupil nurses were stratified into three grades. The probationers had to be eighteen years old and able to read and to write but were of servant class. Their training lasted for three years, following which they were referred to as nurses. The group above them were educated women and could be referred to as nurses from their first day. Their course took five years, and they became certified nurses if successful. Both of these first two groups were expected to live in the establishment. The third group were fully trained and called Sisters. They were taken from a superior social class and could either live in or at home with their families. There were five nurses for forty-eight male and female beds, with three for the twenty children's cots. Charing Cross took these nurses from an Anglican order of the Sisters of Mercy, known as St John's House. Some donors objected to the use of women from this order as they claimed that it was undermining the protestant order of their beliefs. It was in 1854 that Florence Nightingale took thirty-eight volunteer nurses out to the Ottoman Empire to help the sick and wounded soldiers in the Crimean War.

William Golding continued to fight with vigour for the expansion of the hospital until his retirement in September of 1862. He lived for only a further eight months to the age of sixty-nine. His contribution had been enormous and it is undoubtedly true that without him Charing Cross Hospital would not have come into existence.

By the late 1870s students were travelling from many corners of the globe including India, Egypt, South Africa, and South America to study at Charing Cross. As the education demands grew, the need for a formal medical school building became ever more clear. In 1878 fundraising began. The Duke of Bedford, whose name is recognised in the designation of Bedford Street in that area, owned much of the property around Chandos Place. He was the first to subscribe and to lease a plot on which the medical school was eventually built. Ultimately the funds were raised quite quickly but there were ongoing disputes between local residents and the hospital committee about the eventual height of the building. All of these problems were overcome however and by 1 October 1881 the school was finished.

One of the complaints from the students at that time had been that the dissection room had to be shared with the mortuary in the basement of the hospital. There was no refrigeration to slow down putrefaction and the smell was terrible. Finally, to overcome this problem a tunnel was constructed beneath Agar Street and its junction with Chandos Place for the bodies to be transferred to the new anatomy department on the top floor of the medical school. It wasn't an easy excavation because of sewer, gas and water pipes in the way. As a result, it was only 3 feet in height but adequate for the job.

More than a century and a half later it, was to serve as an escape route for a few of my own colleagues during our time at the school. Towards the end of second MB, at the time of my twenty-first birthday, a few of us decided to play a prank on the passing pedestrians and to dress up. Two had hired Gorilla outfits from one of the several theatrical costumiers on New Row, off St Martin's Lane, behind the medical school. Four others put on white coats and pretended to be their handlers. The gorillas pretended to escape from the medical school and to run down The Strand causing mayhem. One of them, Charles Townsend Rose (later to become a hereditary peer) climbed a lamp post and was happily regaling the passers-by. They then took off for Trafalgar Square, grabbing a bunch of bananas from the habitual fruit seller on the corner of its south entrance. Rushing on they managed to mount one of Landseer's Lions close by, and proceed to eat the bananas with the four handlers pretending to try to capture them. Then Charles spotted a rather lovely young lady and decided to imitate King Kong. He jumped down and whisked her off her feet, only to find that her parents were close behind her. There then followed a Buster Keaton type chase, with our gorillas followed in hot pursuit by the parents of the hapless girl calling for police help, followed by us white coated students and a policeman with truncheon drawn bringing up the rear. Back on The Strand, next to the Lyons Corner House, was an Army careers office. With some quick thinking we all dashed in there, and as the surprised WRAC officer looked up, Charles asked if we could sign on as guerrillas. The poor lass nearly fainted but we were able to make our escape through a back door and run back to the accident and emergency entrance of the hospital, with the gorillas removing their costumes as they ran. The final part of the escape was made on the trolley through the tunnel to the medical school. We should express our thanks to the nineteenth century hospital committee for their far-sightedness in constructing our escape route.

'The Cross' went through many episodes of financial difficulty and, as today, there were periods when wards were closed. There were several famous beneficiaries, amongst them was Sarah Bernhardt the famous French actress. Her Royal Command Performance in 1912 in front of the King and Queen, at the Coliseum, raising £3,750 for the hospital, equivalent to £500,000 today. She also visited the hospital and talked to a number of patients, making her own donation on leaving.

In the Boer War, a group of seven Charing Cross nurses in long blue capes, long skirts and small hats, travelled to the South African theatre of war to provide care for the sick and wounded in hospitals near the front, as did several of the doctors and many of the students, rendering the hospital short of staff. Convalescence for returning wounded soldiers was provided at a house in Surrey bought for the purpose by Passmore Evans, a great supporter of Charing Cross.

The day following the declaration of war in 1914, Maud Hopton, a ward sister at Charing Cross signed a war office contract agreeing to serve with the military nursing service at home or abroad for a period of a year and prepared to embark for No. 2 General Hospital. This was based in Le Havre and took many frontline injured soldiers. When they could travel, they were transported back to Charing Cross, where 300 beds were made over to the battle wounded. Support for the work that the hospital was doing for injured servicemen continued to be recognised by the royal household. Once a week a wagonette would arrive from Buckingham Palace and take some of the recovering injured soldiers out for a drive. A further contribution to the war effort by the hospital was the making of sphagnum moss dressings. This remarkable plant can absorb twenty times its own weight in fluid and has antibacterial properties. In remembrance of this, one of the wards was named Moss Ward.

The war and competition with King's medical school dramatically reduced the number of students at 'The Cross'. As today, recruits from abroad were encouraged to make up the difference. Students came from India, Egypt, South Africa and Spain and other parts of Europe not directly caught up in the war.

An ever-present pressure for the hospital was a lack of sufficient space. The triangular site just off The Strand didn't allow outward expansion. After the First World War several developments were made possible by the hugely energetic efforts of Philip Inman, later Lord Inman, first appointed as secretary and superintendent in 1921. This most remarkable young man, continuing in the mould of the hospital's founder, William Golding, led years of fundraising at home and abroad, travelling to the United States several times. Just as the need for space was forever increasing, so it was for funds. Inman proved to be the perfect person for the job. Being in the heart of theatre land, much help came from actors, dancers and many others in the world of the arts. Notable amongst them was Gerald du Maurier who, once informed about Charing Cross by Inman, became a lifelong supporter. Another famous name, the impresario Lord Lonsdale also became a passionate supporter of the hospital. There were extensive allies amongst the royals; Princess Louise became the president of the hospital.

During the Second World War as the Nazi bombs rained down on London, most of the beds had to be moved out of the centre of the city, with the main base in Ashridge, a large country house. Norman C. Lake became the senior surgeon there. (A prized possession of mine is the Norman C. Lake prize in surgery which I was awarded at my final examinations.) As the blitz progressed the hospital was hit by an incendiary bomb, but damage was relatively slight. As a result of this threat, everyone was accommodated in the basement along with the patients.

Prior to the war, plans had been put in place to rebuild the hospital on a nearby site. Many properties had been bought in anticipation of this. However, it became clear after the war that this would not work as the government planned to move many of the local inhabitants out of the centre. A large plot of land at Northwick Park was purchased, with great enthusiasm as a secondary plan. However, with the inception of the National Health Service and the abolition of voluntary hospitals, notice was given by the University of London that it would be outside of their purview and henceforth could not be a recognised University of London medical school.

Plans were then switched to Fulham and the development of that site. Initially this came into a lot of criticism by local residents, councillors, and local doctors, but once the benefits had been realised and the opportunity of such a new development was grasped, it was then accepted enthusiastically. There was a lot of sadness at the closure of the old hospital, which had given such great service in the centre of London.

In fact, the emotions expressed were not new and are reflected in a poem written in 1647 at the pulling down of the original Charing Cross monument, from which the hospital took its name. The name Charing, meaning riverbend, was derived from a hamlet that had occupied the area in medieval times. The cross referred to an Eleanor Cross, once marking the site of an important road junction at those times. A chain of crosses had been commissioned by King Edward I stretching from Lincoln to that site between 1291 and 1295, as a memorial to his wife Eleanor of Castile. It had stood there from 1294 until 1647. It was destroyed by Oliver Cromwell's men and after the fall of The Protectorate a bronze equestrian statue of Charles I had been placed on the same site as the original cross. Now there is a reproduction of that cross outside Charing Cross station.

Here are two verses from more than 300 years earlier titled 'A Puritanical Ballad' that was meant to commemorate that event,

The Downfall of Charing Cross
Undone, undone the lawyers are,
They wander about the towne,
Nor can find the way to Westminster,
Now Charing cross is downe;
At the end of the Strand they make a stand,

Swearing they are at a loss
And Chaffing say, that's not the way
They must go by Charing Cross.

Me thinks the Common Council should
Of it taken pity,
'cause, good old Cross, it always stood
So firmly in the city.
Since Crosses you so much disdain
Faith, if I were as you,
For fear the King should rule again
I'll pull down Tyburn too.

As the site in Fulham was being cleared and the new hospital built, life had to continue at the old Charing Cross. I was saddened to have to leave the original site at the heart of London and the centre of the arts and theatre land, where I had chosen for my medical training. However, I am happy that I was able to spend the first years of my training at that wonderful hospital and medical school and in such a glamorous location, the exact antipathy of my origins.

The Clinical Years

Having spent the previous two years studying for the intercalated B.Sc., my original colleagues had moved on and were well into their clinical training. I joined the students of the year below who had failed their 2nd M.B. examination the first time and were resitting. It was like starting all over again making new friends because, although we were a small medical school, each year was quite self-contained, other than on the sports field, playing for the hospital teams. Most of the group that I joined were now eighteen months to three years younger than me as a result of my delayed start. However, I soon settled in and made some new lifelong friends.

Unlike today's training, we were grouped together into what were called firms. We would be attached to one or two consultants in a specialty, the senior registrar, registrar, senior house officer and houseman. The housemen, male or female, were referred to as housedogs because of the drudgery of much of the work. Newly graduated everyone had to satisfactorily complete that year prior to being registered with the General Medical Council (G.M.C.). There were six students attached to each firm, who then rotated together around the specialties for the next three years.

The building of the new hospital on the Fulham site was well under way. From the aerial view it was in the form of a large cross, reprising the origin of the name taken from the original.

My new year of students was the last to undertake our first round of medicine and surgery firms at the old hospital. The first firm was with two remarkable surgeons: Arthur Makey, the cardiothoracic surgeon and John Pendower, a superb general abdominal surgeon. Two more different personalities of surgeons would be difficult to find. Makey, tall, elegant and softly spoken and Pendower, short, stocky and very dynamic. Both immaculately dressed. Mr Pendower would arrive at the hospital in his open top MGB sports car with the roof down, come rain or shine. Dressed in a duffle-coat and bobble hat, his initial appearance would fool everyone, as when he got out of the car, he removed them and donned a morning suit jacket, with red carnation already in the buttonhole and morning suit trousers already in place. He would then fix the tonneau cover over the driver's seat and stride briskly into the hospital ward to make rounds. He had a highly ordered and quick mind. His teaching was staccato and to the point. Pharmacology was summed up by the sentence, 'An adequate dose for an adequate time, if it doesn't work change the treatment.' Taking a patient's history was summarised as, 'What is the patient complaining of, the history of the present complaint, past medical history, general health, bowels, waterworks, allergies and current medication'. All done in quick time.

In the operating room he was just as direct with swift and accurate movements, no time wasted. Despite this apparent machine-like approach, he was caring and humorous. I was to experience his deeply caring nature later as his houseman.

Makey was more considered and ponderous but equally as effective. I never saw him flustered even in the worst situations in the operating room. The cardiac cases that were referred to him, were often at the end-stage of disease, partly because of Peter Nixon, the new cardiologist's attitude, and partly as a result of the novel nature of cardiac surgery in those early days. They were extremely challenging. No matter, he patiently worked his way through the many obstacles. His fingers were long and spider-like (arachnodactyly) and moved with a mesmerising delicacy. Both men drew great loyalty from their students and their junior staff. The breadth of surgery that we witnessed on that firm was enormous. The professorial firm on the other hand, was with an obturate man Harding Rains. His firm was far less dynamic, and anaemic compared with theirs. This made the Pendower/Makey firm the most sought after. The comparison stimulated the often-quoted phrase about surgeons, 'Those who can operate do, those who can't become academics.'

Ward rounds were conducted with the whole entourage of consultant, junior doctors, students, and the ward sister. Patients sat to attention whilst their case was presented by the houseman or the students who were then grilled on the physical signs and the management of each case. Having to examine the poor patient in front of such an audience was nerve-wracking and often produced a ripple of stifled laughter by the group if our technique was lacking, which it frequently was. This may sound disrespectful to the patient, but it always seemed to be done in such a way that the patient was able to join in the fun. Occasionally he or she would whisper to us where we were going wrong. 'Not there doc, over'[h]ere', as he guided your hand to the appropriate spot. One of the tricks to assess how bad any genito-urinary bleeding (haematuria) might be was to hold up a freshly passed urinary sample and look through it to see if we could see the buildings across the street a technique illustrated in texts from as long ago as the fourteenth century.

Time was spent on the wards, in lectures and in the outpatient and casualty departments. Much of it was structured and we were expected to attend all of the firm's ward rounds where variable amounts of teaching went on. A&E and attendance at the outpatient clinics was more observational, but we were asked to examine patients in front of the consultant and to discuss our findings. This could be quite stressful but also amusing. The very first patient I was asked to examine was a young woman of about twenty-four who had presented with a lump in her breast. She was frightened, but not half as much as I was at the prospect. Happily, it turned out to be what is referred to as a breast mouse, a fibroadenoma, whose chief physical principals are that they are quite hard and highly mobile in the breast tissue, hence the name. Our first rectal examinations were equally as embarrassing for both parties, but as we were constantly told, 'If you don't put your finger in, you will put your foot in it.' In the modern wokist world, rectal, vaginal and breast examinations are taught on plastic models. Such is progress but it really can't properly prepare the young doctor for the realities of life in the clinic.

The operating theatres were on the top floor of the hospital and had large windows which could be opened to allow a flow of fresh air; we had a similar feature at the old Papworth Hospital. It didn't seem to have any impact on the frequency of wound infections, which I remember as being very low. When a biopsy was taken to assess the nature of a lesion during an operation, the specimen would be sent for rapid analysis. It would be run down to the ground floor, through the hospital and across William IVth Street to the pathology laboratory, which was situated in what had once been the old Edwardian restaurant Gatti's. Beautiful crystal chandeliers were still in place reflecting the style of a lost age. The biopsy material was snap frozen in liquid nitrogen, then sections were cut of the fresh material and stained. The windows in both buildings would be thrown open for the result to be shouted across. Professor Sloper was the pathologist at that time, and he would shout across the street above the heads of the Londoners passing by, 'Caaarcinoooma', or not as the case may have been. All of this seemed quite normal at the time. Prof. Sloper had the distinction of his great-great grandfather being one of the very first students probably along with William Golding in the opening era of the hospital.

This was such an exciting time, and I think that the charisma of those excellent surgeons had everything to do with the fact that half my peer group of the original year became surgeons themselves.

The surgical firm was followed by our first medical firm with a wonderfully flamboyant and hilarious physician Dr Bruce Fowler, whose son was in our cohort. Bruce was a tall and well-built man with a slight stoop, protruding front teeth and very large, greying sideburns in otherwise reddish hair. He had a permanent grin and almost everything he said was delivered with a chuckle or loud guffaw. His son became just like him. An endocrinologist of serious repute, he was well-known for his description of the retarded relaxation of the knee jerk in myxoedema, or underactive thyroid. His sense of humour was ever present in his lectures. His publications tended to contain humour also. As an example, here he is describing pain in the anus or proctalgia fugax.

> Doctors appear to be particularly prone to this condition, which usually occurs at night. The patient complains that he feels as if a red-hot poker has been momentarily inserted up the back passage. A writer in a learned medical journal makes the suggestion that ice should be inserted into the rectum to relieve the pain. One can only suppose the refrigerator is kept beside the bed, with a compartment for making ice easily detached, and the shape of the cubes suitably modified for their unusual destination, ready to be inserted by the sleepy doctor in the moment or so that the pain is present.

On sunny days he would suddenly declaim, 'White coats on boys and girls, follow me', and we would rush off, following behind him like Konrad Lorenz's ducks (imprinting works wonders with medical students). Off we would go out of the hospital, along The Strand, across Trafalgar Square and on into St James's Park where we would sit under a tree amongst the tourists and government officials going about their business, whilst Brucey, (our nickname for him) would hold forth on a lecture about the thyroid gland. Wonderful days, indeed, halcyon, never to be forgotten. All this is lost in the modern world in the name of safety and appropriate behaviour, whatever that is.

Being able to attend lectures, ward rounds and clinics, and then to stroll to the National Gallery or the Royal Academy for some cerebral refreshment was a gift from the heavens. Surrounded by the arts in all of their glory, a wonderful earthy part of the greatest city on earth, and human beings in all their splendour was unsurpassable. And all of this with no student fees and a local authority grant. We were indeed blessed..

Although everything was done in a very formal way on the wards, there was a great deal of fun to be had as well. As mentioned already, on Christmas Day, the consultants would still come in with their families to carve the turkey delivered to the ward for the poor unfortunate patients trapped there over the festive season. Sadly, this died out quickly on the move to Fulham. Parties in the nurses home were riotous affairs, but curiously for the time I have no memory of any drugs being distributed or used, which was surprising considering what was going on in the outside world.

All too soon, however, it was time to move over to the new hospital in Fulham. Built in the shape of a cross, it was shiny and new, but it never had the charisma of the old 'Cross'. Opened by the Queen in May 1973, the move was staged between the old and the new hospital. The night before the opening we had the hospital rugby club dinner and at the end of the evening, someone decided to remove a chicken and try to fry it under the X-ray machines in the radiography department. Yes, rather too much alcohol had been imbibed. One of our number was a trainee radiographer and she agreed to help with the machines. My memory doesn't serve me well about what happened next, but what I do remember is the anger of the Dean and Head of Radiology Dr Reynolds, who was to show the Queen around his department, when he found the viewing room full of radiographs of our hapless chicken, now defrosting on the x ray table. Someone else also had the idea of removing some bed sheets, sewing them together and painting a For Sale sign on them and replacing the hospital flag with it, to greet the Queen on her arrival. Thankfully everyone's energy ran out before this was accomplished.

Our firm's first move from The Strand was to the West London Hospital at Hammersmith, for Obstetrics and Gynaecology. Dame Josephine Barnes was the head of the gynaecology department and a wonderful woman. As mentioned earlier she would hold history of medicine tutorials for those who were interested. The Chiswick Maternity Home was where we saw and witnessed and assisted at the delivery (or 'catching' as now must be said), of the babies. We had to log at least twenty of them in our attachment. The midwives loved to call us in the middle of the night from our on-call rooms. I have to say that I really enjoyed it, and the experience was to come in very helpful later when on an A&E job after qualification. More of that later. It was during that attachment, one sunny Saturday afternoon that I and the senior house officer Martin were attending a lady who was very slow to progress beyond the second stage of labour. Being granted permission to leave for a break by the senior midwife we went down to the bank of the River Thames where Martin knew that the hospital owned a small boat. We found it easily enough and pushed it into the water. I jumped in and Martin jumped in after me with a Party Seven can of beer. Unfortunately, in our haste we forgot to put the oars into the boat. We could see them left on the shore. We quickly drifted away from the bank, but initially we weren't worried as there was an outboard motor. However, the situation became more serious when we found that we were unable to start it. We drifted out to the centre of the river and then with the ebbing tide we floated off towards the direction of Putney Bridge. There was nothing we could do about it. Luckily, after about ten minutes we were approached by a police launch. The officers had noticed our white coats which we were still wearing and heard our yells for help. After explaining the problem to the officers on board, they kindly towed us back to the point of embarkation. After expressing our profound thanks, we rushed back to the labour ward, leaving the now confiscated beer. Apparently it is illegal to be in control of a boat whilst under the influence. Another example of police tolerance of inept medical students at that time. Back on the unit we were relieved to find that the lady had progressed little since our departure and discussion was underway regarding induction of labour. Later that evening she delivered a beautiful baby girl. The hospital was closed in 1975 as the birth rate in the area had fallen dramatically.

During the first year I had continued to live in Regent's Park. It was so luxurious for a student to emerge from the beautiful Nash buildings onto the park. To be able to climb into my little Austin Healey Sprite and to drive out onto the Marylebone Road and follow the overpass to Hammersmith and Fulham against the incoming traffic each day, was very satisfying, knowing the drudgery of road commutes into central London. Most journeys were taken with the roof down, and the music blaring out of my eight-track stereo tape player, usually Barry White, Percy Sledge, or the Beatles.

Tim Riley, who was also living in I.S.H., suggested that we join the Playboy Club because on a Saturday night for £5 you could buy dinner, as much as you could carry, with multiple returns. The innocence of us medical students shone through and the Bunny girls would look after us so well with generous free drinks. Occasionally if we had some spare cash, we would visit the tables. Not exactly the last of the 'big-time' spenders we would gamble a few pounds. One evening feeling very rash I placed my £5 on a red number. It came up and the winnings kept us in Playboy Saturday night meals for many weeks.

Several of my friends from the original year, had moved into a flat in Balham and when the time came to move out of the International Students' House, they invited me to join them. They were a great bunch, with an amazing sense of humour. Being the only student from the original year, and then having to join the following year's students, and a sub-group at that, it gave me a slight feeling of schizophrenia, being not fully embedded in one year or the other. I felt somewhat outside each group at first and as a result I struggled to feel confident. As a consequence, I decided to move out of the Balham house, having found a tiny room in Hampstead. I had accepted the offer of the room unseen. I piled my few belongings into the Sprite and set off for Hampstead. I had been seduced by the reputation of Hampstead Village and the proximity to the Heath. On arrival I was shocked to find that I could hardly stand up in the room and there were huge heating pipes running down the wall next to the small single bed. There was no room for a desk and the only chair was rickety and tiny. I didn't even unpack the car but headed back to where I had come from. In a day or two I heard that there was a good room available next to the hospital. It was in the Charing Cross student residence called Brandenburg House, just across the road from the hospital. Somewhat relieved, I moved in there. The original group in Balham became very close knit. Now I do regret leaving them and feel silly not having more confidence to stay. Whilst boisterous and great fun, they were, and remain, very nice people. They continue to meet annually as the Balham Boot Boys.

From my days in the sixth form at Adams' Grammar School in Newport, I had a girlfriend Christine. She had a lovely and warm personality. We had met at a sixth form dance between the Girls' High School and ours. Perforce, it had become a long-distance relationship. Even in the months spent at Chuckie Chicken much of the time it was a telephone and written letter relationship, but she was very loyal and we met when we could. When I first went to London, Christine was working in the National Provincial Bank in Newport. Once I had begun my course she transferred to the head office in the City of London. When she first arrived in the city she was working as a cashier and I would go over on the Circle Line to meet her for lunch. I had very strong feelings for her and the relationship lasted for four years. We enjoyed a lot together. A particular pleasant memory was our first trip to Stonehenge. In those days it was permissible to park quite close and to walk amongst the stones. It was quite magical with almost no-one else present. When Christine moved to London, initially she was living with a relative of her mother in South Woodford, a long journey on the Central Line. From there she moved to Beckenham in Kent, an equally difficult place to reach from central London. Christine was having to share a room with another girl who was pleasant but a little strange in her behaviour. If I stayed over for the night, I had to hide under the covers as she stripped for bed. She seemed to like the three of us sleeping in the same room. Eventually, Christine moved to West Hampstead. However, once I began the clinical training, meeting became more difficult, and the relationship came to an end.

The second year of clinical studies was comprised of a series of shorter attachments to the smaller specialties. Obstetrics and gynaecology was followed by a couple of weeks in sexually transmitted diseases (STDs) with a Dr. Fluker. He was a tall, angular man with feline features and half-moon glasses. The diseases were categorised alphabetically, syphilis, the star of the show, being A1, and chlamydia, a lesser being, was C or D. Gloating in the middle was the ever-popular gonorrhoea, an important B1. A cry would go up from behind the cubicle curtain, 'A1, over here', and we would rush over to the poor unfortunate victim to cast an eye over the chancre on full display. With the summer of love not far past and the contraceptive pill freely available, unprotected sex was rampant and so were those nasty little bugs. Once diagnosed, syphilis and gonorrhoea were easily treated, the problem lay in the shyness of the victims to present themselves for help. The nasty ones were chlamydia that could lurk silently in the female genital tract without symptoms, wreaking havoc on the girl's reproductive health and producing chronic pelvic inflammatory disease, a terribly painful and debilitating condition. Before the advent of HIV, perhaps the nastiest was herpes simplex as there was no treatment for that at the time and it became a lifelong burden for the patient. Several cases of secondary and tertiary syphilis were also on show.

Although Charing Cross was regarded as a lesser-known London medical school, compared with Guy's, St Thomas', Kings, and St Mary's, for example, we had a star-studded cast of physicians who were true pioneers in their respective fields. In paediatrics we had Dr. Hugh Jolly, who was probably the best-known medical personality in the United Kingdom. He was the British version of the American television children's guru, Dr. Spock. Hugh Jolly pioneered many aspects of child health and development. He could be regularly heard on the radio, imparting gems of information for worried parents on subjects as wide as vaccination through parenting. A flamboyant and large man with the most dynamic personality he would dominate a room whenever he entered. At that time in the early 1970s Dyslexia was, for most people, an unknown entity and indeed scorned as a concept by many, preferring to suborn afflicted children with the wholly objectionable term 'educationally sub-normal'. Jolly knew that I was interested in this area and raised the funding and the support to set up a study to compare children with this abhorrent label with a group that were being helped in the newly set-up Helen Arkell Dyslexia centre housed on Parsons Green in West London. A patron at that time was Susan Hampshire, who suffered severely from what had been recognised by the team there as Dyslexia. Using state of the art psychological tests of the time, I was able to show a significant difference in performance between children with lower educational abilities and the Dyslexic child who overall scored far higher on all aspects of cognitive testing. We also began to differentiate the numerate dyslexics from the verbal. During the study Miss Hampshire allowed herself to be tested and of course scored very highly. Learning parts for her acting career was a real trial for her and the script would have to be read to acquire the lines. These results clearly showed that Dyslexia was a neuro-cognitive impairment that often afflicted highly performing children and adults. Another self-declared severe dyslexic is Sir Jackie Stewart, multiple Formula 1 world champion. He has vividly described how the condition severely disrupted his school life. Being asked to read aloud in class all that he could see was a jumbled maze of words. Called lazy and stupid by teachers, he was humiliated in front of his class. He describes the pain of it in his biography, *Winning Is Not Enough*. Now it is fully recognised and expert help is on hand for those who suffer from it. For a few pseudo-intellectuals it has almost become a rite of passage to claim they are Dyslexic. I was pleased to be able to make a small early contribution to its understanding.

Another specialty that I enjoyed was Ophthalmology. Mr Eric Arnott was an innovative ophthalmic surgeon who pioneered phacoemulsification in the treatment of cataracts. For a considerable period he was alone in the world outside the United States in developing this treatment. A true innovator, he also went on to develop the earliest foldable, implantable lenses. He was a competition level swimmer, swimming a mile every morning before work in the hospital pool. He kept this up all his life. I went with him on several occasions, but of course could not keep up with him. He even completed the formidable Alcatraz to San Francisco mainland swim, something that few achieved. He was a delightful and charismatic man. Through him I very nearly pursued a career in ophthalmology. One of our number, Paul Kinnear, went on to do just that. I noticed that practically all the eye surgeons that I knew liked to play organ music whilst operating and Paul was no exception. An ophthalmologist that I operated on recently went so far as to record his own recital and gave it to me to play during his operation.

The specialty that we now know as oncology, was hardly known or recognised in the 1960s and was really introduced by Professor Ken Bagshaw, another Charing Cross star. He was the first to develop chemotherapy for Choriocarcinoma, a trophoblastic disease which was almost universally fatal. He rapidly became aware of the need for a separate unit because of the risk of infection in this group of patients who became immunosuppressed with the chemotherapy. The word amongst us students was that you had to be really supersmart to do oncology.

Neurology starred Dr Clifford Rose. Yet another flamboyant consultant who made a huge contribution to his specialty and was respected worldwide. He set up the Centre for the Study of Migraine and Headache, given the eponymous name of the Princess Margaret Centre for the Study of Migraine. He also carried out pioneering research into Motor Neurone Disease. At lunchtime on a Wednesday, he would often demonstrate a neurological condition with a patient brought into the lecture theatre to illustrate the illness. Computerised Tomography and Magnetic Resonance scanners had yet to be invented and introduced into the clinical setting. Hence diagnosis was by history and physical examination. His demonstration of physical signs was theatrical and completely memorable. His flamboyant dress sense of dark chalk stripe three piece suit and very colourful tie made lasting impressions on everyone present.

Another almost daily lunchtime activity was a visit to the post mortem room to see a case demonstrated by the pathologist. Standing on tiered steps behind railings, munching our sandwiches, we would watch whilst the diseased organs were removed and displayed. For some that was a bit too much. This practice implanted in me the importance of always seeing the evidence first hand, whether that be down the microscope, in radiology, or the path lab.

There is a dread in the back of some students' minds that they may faint at the sight of something particularly distressing. The only time that I fainted on the course was during an operation on the lachrymal glands around the eye. I can remember the E.N.T. surgeon picking away at the bone around the ethmoid sinus. The sound reverberating hollowly through the sinus was too much for me and the next thing I knew was coming back to my senses lying on the ground having being pulled away from the table by a nurse and the anaesthetist whilst the operation continued.

Dr. Randall in the psychiatry department was a pioneer in transgender medicine and worked with the senior Charing Cross urologist Mr Peter Phillips, who became the first surgeon in the UK to develop transgender surgery. Previously patients had to travel to Casablanca, Morocco, for the surgery. Randall had an old Rolls Royce motor car, about which he used to regale us with stories. One such tale was having his hub caps stollen on a trip to the French Riviera. He dealt with the patients in a caring and thoughtful way, guiding us through the minefield that was transgender management back then.

A hangover from the old Charing Cross days was the provision of orthopaedic services to the Royal Ballet. Mr Strachan had been their surgeon for several years and did regular clinics for the dancers from the Opera House. The injuries were often horrendous as witness to the severe physical strain that the dancers placed themselves under. Attending those sessions as often as I could brought me a better understanding of the stressful and intense world of classical dance. This increased my admiration for them as they pursued excellence.

Early in my second year, whilst doing my A&E attachment I met a beautiful and warm trainee nurse. After an initial hesitant approach, and much to my surprise she agreed to meet for a drink after work. Her hesitancy was because she was dating an army officer, who at that time was serving outside the country. We got on very well from our first meeting and quickly became very close, albeit with a pause whilst she resolved her relationship with the soldier. I had recently moved to the hospital residence Brandenburg House. Anne had moved into a well-appointed apartment south of the river, close to Hammersmith Bridge, next to the Harrod's depository. For a couple of students, we had a luxurious lifestyle in that penthouse apartment, with wonderful views across the river. I had never felt quite so happy in my personal life before and it appeared to be mutual. We had limited funds but managed to enjoy a lot of things together. My first visit to Cambridge was with her. I remember driving through the fields ablaze as the farmers burnt off the stubble from the harvest in the autumn. With the blessing of her parents, we had planned to marry before I graduated. Unfortunately, probably because of my serial failures to get into medical school, my parents, mother in particular, were absolutely against the idea. Perhaps correctly, my mother feared that with my poor performance at school and all the traumas that were experienced by the family in my multiple attempts to gain a place at medical school, such a profound distraction would cause me to fail to qualify. I came under considerable pressure to break off the engagement and to abandon the idea. After considerable and painful thought, this pressure was not something that I felt I could resist. My parents had sacrificed so much for me to achieve my goal. To my shame, and latterly, much regret, I brought the relationship to an end. I suspect that my life would have taken a different path had I not made that decision, and probably a much happier one. As well as the real joy in the relationship, I was very fond of her parents and would discuss world events and general philosophy with her wonderful father long into the evenings. He was the chief Methodist minister for the RAF, based at the NATO command centre at Northwood. He was a big, red-haired man with a very powerful voice and a ready laugh, which made our conversations hilarious as well as interesting. His having seen so much more of the world, I have no doubt that my contributions to our discussions must have been relatively trivial, but he engaged with me with gusto. I missed him so much latterly.

In our final year, the major firms were in the professorial units of medicine and surgery. The two professors of medicine that we were allocated to were Professors Hugh de Wardener and Abe Guz. Hugh de Wardener was a renal physiologist and excellent physician. His was an extraordinary life. He came from an aristocratic French family who had fled Austria during the French revolution. His forebears had migrated to the USA, and his father had moved to Paris as a commodity broker. There he met Hugh's mother, a singer, also American. When they divorced, Hugh was sent to an English boarding school, initially with no knowledge of English. He trained at St Thomas' hospital. Following graduation, his house physician job was in Scunthorpe, but within a week of arriving there his consultant died, and Hugh was left to look after the adults and children that had been under their care. With outbreak of war, he joined the British army and was drafted to Singapore just a few weeks before it fell to the Japanese. He was seized as a prisoner of war and found himself on the Burma railway, immortalised in books and the movie *Bridge on the River Kwai* starring Alec Guinness. He was held captive in those nightmare conditions for the next three years. Being a scientist and caring doctor, he continued with his calling and carried out astounding work. He successfully treated prisoners of war with Diphtheria using antiserum made from the blood of other patients. He also deduced that Wernicke's Encephalopathy was because of a dietary insufficiency of thiamine. He was able to confirm this with autopsy work. He persuaded the Japanese guards to allow the prisoners to have Marmite, which contains multiple B vitamins. He took specimens of blood from the prisoners of war that he looked after and stored them and his notes in a sealed drum in the grave of one of the prisoners. These were exhumed after the war and published in *The Lancet* in 1947. He suffered severe malnutrition himself, contracting diphtheria, malaria and with it jaundice and tuberculosis. Not only was his work a tribute to his indomitable spirit and inner strength, but so was his very survival, when so many succumbed to disease and ill-treatment.

On return to clinical practice, he became intensely fascinated by renal function and malfunction and made very important contributions to the development of renal dialysis, which at that time was in its infancy. For most in those days renal failure was a death sentence. Sadly, his war experiences caught up with him, and Hugh died with severe peripheral neuropathy. I suspect that few, if any of us, were aware of his amazing history and astounding contributions in his early medical career. His book, simply titled *The Kidney* was a seminal text. I bought a copy when working for him and he wrote this inscription, 'Hoping you get as much fun out of the kidney as I do – and wishing you much luck Hugh de Wardener 29.1.74.'

His colleague Professor Abraham Guz was a completely different animal. Both men were brilliant, but Abe, as we affectionately called him, was a difficult man who had the foible of chewing the end of his tie constantly, causing it to fray. He was the first to recognise that there was a short acting substance within the blood that could cause coronary artery dilatation. This turned out to be nitric oxide, which is used extensively now in the setting of the cardiac catheter labs., and in the coronary intensive care units. He became very interested in the control of respiration, and carried out many experiments on the Vagus nerve, blocking transmission through it in conscious and anaesthetised humans and animals. He followed Hugh de Wardener as the head of clinical research unit at Charing Cross. He developed one of the world's first sleep laboratories. He carried his scientific discipline into his clinical work, and as housemen we were expected to repeat all blood tests three times to ensure the correct analysis. It surprised me how variable the results could be. We were taught rigour and discipline on those wards, something seriously lacking across all aspects of health care provision in modern times. A disciplinary approach is now classified as harassment or even worse, bullying. Telling poorly performing individuals to shape up or ship out is now completely unacceptable, expectations have become so low in the modern NHS because of extremely poor staff recruitment and retention. The very poor working environment has given rise to the acceptance of poor performance. Few in management appear to understand this and spend their time blaming everyone around them, the consultants in particular. It is salutary to see that standards are frequently higher in the American and several European systems as a result of stronger maintenance of discipline, made possible by better working conditions and pay, so that individuals want to maintain their employment.

Surgery is an art form and requires strong technical skills as well as an excellent knowledge of anatomy. There are many big names in the surgical world, but they are not always the best technical surgeons. The old saying, 'Those who can, operate, and those that can't teach', is often true. The first statement in E. H. Gombrich's book, *The Story of Art* (published by Phaidon), is that there really is no such thing as Art. There are only artists. The same can be said of surgery. There is no such thing as surgery; there are only surgeons and they all have varying degrees of experience and technical excellence. It is the elephant in the room in all presentations on surgical results. Some of the most well-known surgeons that I assisted were not the ones that you would want to operate on you or your family. One of the surgeons with the finest of technical skills was a senior registrar when I was in training called Gary Coombs. He had beautiful hand control and great economy of movement. I remember feeling at the time I worked with him that if I could be known for nothing else than my surgical prowess, that would be enough. Not only was his surgery technically brilliant, but, defying all stories about the handwriting of doctors, his writing was just as beautiful as his surgery; flowing, calligraphic script, evenly executed, and a joy to read. Another such surgeon was Al Pacifico, more of whom later. The reduction in training time has been quite counter-productive to producing fine surgeons and maintaining standards.

Towards the middle of the final year, we had to spend time in general practice. Earlier in the year we had to register our preference with the medical school secretary Christine Jackman. Christine was a lovely lady and had been very supportive of me. Her office was in Brandenburg House where I had my room. She had a list of GPs who accepted medical students. They were all alumni of Charing Cross. Most of them were within the confines of London, but there were a few attachments in the countryside. Christine alerted me to a practice in Bideford, a lovely and historic port town on the estuary of the River Torridge on the north coast of Devon. The GP was Dr Alan Riley. A wonderfully kind and caring man who was loved by his patients. He lived with his new partner Liz, an equally lovely and caring person. I arrived at a difficult time for them both. Alan's marriage had just fallen apart, and he and Liz had formed an incredibly strong bond. They lived in a beautiful house in Appledore, just a few miles away. Liz's two boys were living with them, but sadly Alan's children had been made inaccessible to him by his egregious wife. This remains the case and is a source of deep sadness for him. I was supposed to spend two weeks with them; however, I had such an enjoyable time that I stayed on for two more. Alan had table football and every evening on returning home we would play, and every evening Alan's frustration would mount as I repeatedly beat him, but it was all very good natured, and the howls of laughter and complaint of cheating could be heard from a considerable distance.

Each day was so enjoyable that I was seriously considering becoming a GP We began by seeing patients in the practice before lunch. The afternoons were spent on home visits. The doctor was always welcome. It reminded me so much of my days delivering meat to the farmhouses in the Clun countryside. Just calling out, 'Doctor', before opening the door and entering to the same welcoming faces.

It was a glorious early summer and we had some extremely enjoyable trips around and about Devon. One of the most memorable was a boat trip to Lundy Island. On the way back we were entertained by a traditional jazz band; drinking beer on the open deck of the boat as the sun set behind us on our way home was a truly memorable experience.

One of the most memorable people that I met there was a gentleman called Mr Eccles. He made beautiful ship's chronometers. His creations were highly sought after. He was following in the footsteps of John Harrison, who built revolutionary timepieces in the eighteenth century and was eventually awarded the prize for solving the problem of measuring longitude. Whilst latitude had been appreciated and measured accurately for centuries by the position of the sun and the stars, many ships and lives were lost as a result of ignorance of longitude. Longitude is a shifting concept and there was no defined governance that could be uniformly applied to locate it accurately. A longitude committee had been set up in 1714 to attempt to solve this problem. It took many years' work to develop a clock that could withstand the ships' movements at sea in all weathers, but eventually Harrison managed to achieve it. He won the prize after some significant disagreements but was awarded the Copley Gold medal in 1749, a prize shared by a select number of the greatest names in history, Benjamin Franklin, Captain Cooke and Einstein to name a few.[5] Although Mr Eccles seemed quite old to me in my arrogance of youth, we met several times and spent many hours talking. At the end of my time in Devon, Liz and Alan arranged a leaving dinner with the wonderful Mr Eccles. I kept in touch with him for several years afterwards.

Alan and Liz ran a sex therapy clinic on Wednesday evenings. During this time, I was expected to work in my room so as not to interrupt the proceedings. On one occasion I was allowed to sit on the stairs to listen to the counselling session. I learnt a great deal that evening that my inexperienced world never knew existed. I will leave it up to the mind of the reader to imagine some of the topics of discussion, but the first step of the evening was to roll out the rubber mat and to get out the sex toys, all very new and exotic to me.

My time in Devon was coming to a close but there was time for one more episode of excitement. I had woken up in the middle of the night with a strange sensation that I was not alone. Sure enough, I could make out the faint ghostly image of a white-haired gentleman at the foot of my bed. As my focus returned, I could see him staring very intently at me, then slowly the apparition dissolved and was gone. Getting back to sleep was impossible. That morning on joining Liz and Alan for breakfast they asked why I looked so strangely tired. At first, I didn't say anything as it sounded so ridiculous. But then Liz said to Alan, I think that Francis has seen our ghost. That caused me to describe what I had seen. Neither were surprised as apparently he had been seen many times. The previous owner of the house had shot himself in the garden under the window of the room that I was in and several guests had experienced the same thing. Liz's mother was something of a clairvoyant and had experienced such a presentiment several times. She was also the one to predict the ultimate failure of my first marriage.

During my extended stay I was beginning to miss the cut and thrust of hospital medicine, surgery in particular, so Alan made arrangements for me to spend some days with one of the general surgeons in Barnstable and Exeter hospitals.

During my last day in Devon, I had been in Exeter observing surgery. I left a little late but wanted to buy a present for my hosts and so changed very quickly into my outdoor clothes. I arrived back in Appledore with little time to spare. Liz came to the door and burst out laughing, pointing at my groin when she saw me. I looked down and to my horror found that the tail of my white shirt was protruding from my unzipped fly. I hurriedly and embarrassedly adjusted my dress. A leaving dinner with friends including Mr Eccles had been arranged for that evening. During the dinner, and following several glasses of wine, Alan asked me if I would go to his study to retrieve a document for Mr Eccles. Searching on his desk for the piece of paper I saw an unfinished letter still in his typewriter. I noticed my name clearly stated on the letter and couldn't resist looking. What I saw horrified me. Alan had written with fulsome praise of my time with him, but had added a caveat at the end declaring a worrying trend that he had noted and thought that he should report to the dean of the medical school. He stated that he noticed that I had a tendency to expose myself in public and he found this concerning. I returned to the dining room very sheepishly, desperately wanting to proclaim my innocence but of course could say nothing as

I ought not to have snooped on the correspondence written in confidence. Having left me to sweat it out for a while, and seeing my worsening anxiety, they all broke out in hysterical laughter as, clearly, they were all in on the plot. Despite my relief, it took me a few minutes to recover my composure.

We had shared some wonderful experiences, and it was very hard to leave, but the final run of clinical teaching beckoned and could be resisted no longer. I often think back to those times of laughter and learning. Alan is a superb doctor and was a wonderful teacher of the classical kind. He had encyclopaedic knowledge allied to a most empathic nature with a wonderful sense of history. Liz is the most loving and homely person and made my stay with them my home also. I felt real sadness at leaving what had become a second home for me in that lovely part of the country and with such wonderful people. We have remained friends ever since.

My memories of the final months are hazy, made so by intense work in preparation for the final examinations. A very clear memory, however, is meeting Helen Stubbs, who became my wife two years later. As I have explained I had broken off my engagement under pressure from my parents. Following this I had met Helen at a party thrown by a nurse called Marina Midgely. She had the distinction of being a member of the Tolstoy family through her mother's side. At the party I met a vivacious young airline stewardess from Cheshire. As we began to talk it became clear that we had had similar upbringings, she a farmer's daughter in Cheshire and me a butcher's son in Shropshire, neighbouring counties. We began to see each other and a romance blossomed. It was a difficult time for me as I was entering the run into the final exams; if successful this would be followed by the intense working environment of house jobs. Despite this we developed a sound relationship and eventually married in the summer of 1977. My parents seemed happier for me to be with a farmer's daughter from an area of the country where we had family relations. Helen's parents were very nice to me, and I began to feel that I had a warm inviting home to which I could retreat with her whenever we were able. This played a very big part in my attraction and subsequent proposal of marriage.

All too soon the examinations arrived. Again, being out of kilter with the main body of students for the year I had to sit the exams in the autumn rather than the summer months. In preparation and as practice for the 'real thing', most of us sat what were called the Conjoint Examinations. These were the Licentiate Examinations of the Royal College of Physicians and Surgeons. If passed, they allowed for the practice of medicine but were seen to be inferior to the degrees of M.B. (Batchelor of Medicine), B.S. (Batchelor of Surgery), awarded by the University of London. Part of the Conjoint

Examination was undertaken in Queen's Square opposite the Hospital for Nervous Diseases. In the surgery clinical exam there was a patient with a rather untidy above the knee amputation that was being shown to candidates who were expected to take a history and to explain the clinical situation. That particular patient had severe peripheral vascular disease and had lost his leg as a result of poor blood supply. At the end of the day, he had clearly become bored with proceedings and had decided to play a prank on the next student to be confronted by him. There was great hilarity when one of our group came rushing out of the exam hall and ran up to several of us sitting waiting on the grass in the centre of the square, shouting, 'Who got the shark bite, who got the shark bite?' We hardly had the heart to tell him of his error. The examiner must have seen the funny side of it as he passed the examination.

We were also invited to sit some prize examinations. I sat several of them, winning proxime accessit in the Norman C. Lake Prize for Surgery and prizes in E.N.T. and Ophthalmology. Whilst seeming somewhat unimportant at the time, they did serve to swell my CV very meaningfully.

Finals proper began inauspiciously on Monday 13 October 1975. Written exams were held during the first week, with the clinical exams in the second and third weeks. The results were announced on Wednesday 5 November. In anticipation of any bad news a completion of finals party was held the night before in Brandenburg House. Much alcohol was consumed. Thankfully I found that I had passed and more than that, had been awarded the Golding Gold Medal, proxime accessit for the year. A very pleasant if unexpected reward for all the hard work.

A special mention should go to a Dr Choudhuri who gave me individual tutoring in therapeutics, a weak spot of mine. He was extremely patient with me and an excellent teacher of what I regarded as an extremely boring subject. Drug actions and interactions could not ignite any excitement in me. I held to John Pendower's mantra, 'If unsure always look it up.'

Despite the coming of the exams, I noticed from my diaries that I managed to continue to enjoy musical culture with visits to the Royal Albert Hall for Britten and Elgar and a wonderful concert in the Royal Festival Hall with Leonard Bernstein's version of Voltaire's *Candide*.

Later, in 1986 I think it was, Bernstein was conducting a performance himself at the Barbican, and we were lucky enough to get very good, near front row seats. I discovered that he was giving a pre-performance talk with some of the orchestra present in the mid-afternoon and so went along. It was a gem of an experience. Bernstein really engaged with us and gave many tips on what to look out for, particularly a passage when Pangloss was singing. Sure enough, in the actual performance, as the moment approached, he turned to the audience and winked and smiled mouthing, 'Watch this.'

Having completed the exams, we had several weeks to fill before taking up our house jobs. The first thing was to check which jobs we had secured. I was very fortunate and managed to have both of my first choices accepted. This meant that I was to start with six months surgery with Mr Makey and John Pendower, and the second six months with Tiny Maini, (now, an extremely well deserved Professor, Sir Ravindra Maini FRS) and Dr J. T. Scott. I was delighted at the prospect.

In the meantime, I signed up for a short locum in surgery at the Mile End Hospital in East London. That was an eye-opening experience. On the first day I arrived early on the Monday morning and reported to the operating room as instructed. On entering I was greeted by the surgeon who had a huge look of relief on his face. I soon discovered why when he told me that the last two locums had just not shown up for work during the previous week. Immediately we got on well and I had an excellent, if brief, experience of true district general hospital surgery. I had been shown how to do an appendicectomy as a student and was promptly let loose on the general public and accomplished several of them whilst there. Also, the consultant was generous with his time taking me through inguinal hernia repair and other beginner surgical procedures. It also led to some well needed cash in my pocket for the first time since the Oxford Street building site experience three years earlier.

We were so fortunate in those days to have no student fees to pay and to have quite a generous local county council grant from our home county, in my case the Salop County Council, for which I shall always be grateful. The cost of living was so different then and one could live well on a few hundred per annum. Instead of graduating with many tens of thousands of pounds debt, taking years to pay off, if ever, my total debt on beginning my first house job was £2,300, an effective debt today of about £18,000, a very different scenario to that which most students face today.

Finally, I returned to Clun for what would be my last Christmas with family for many years. It was a very brief stay as I had to be on duty on the surgical ward at 9.00 a.m. on New Year's Day. For the next nine years I either found myself on call or moving from one job to another over the Christmas period.

5

Now the Real Pain Begins – Pre-registration House Jobs

> Just as iron rusts from disuse and stagnant water putrefies, or when cold turns to ice, so our intellect wastes unless it is kept in use.[1]

I had been relishing the beginning of life as a 'proper doctor' on a surgical firm. Now I could get my teeth into learning surgical practice and hopefully get some real surgery under my belt. The truth dawned very quickly. I was on what was referred to as a one-in-two rota, every other night and every other weekend on call, which also included a normal full day's work in between. This is where the 100-plus hours per week came from. The day began with a ward round of all patients at 6.30 or 7.00 a.m., depending on how many there were to see. In those days consultant surgeons would operate at least two, and often three full days per week.

As we were working for two consultants, we were in theatre practically every day, unless asked to take part in an outpatient clinic. We also carried the on-call bleep throughout the time that we were on duty. This meant that we could be, and often were, called to casualty for surgical emergencies, and to the wards regularly for every imaginable event, from writing up drugs to GPs' discharge letters, putting up intravenous infusions for blood and other fluid transfusions, insertion of chest drains, oh, and regular cardiac arrest calls. At the end of every day there would be a post-surgery ward round usually with the senior registrar and after that settling down to write up all of the requests for radiography, blood tests etcetera. Then we could begin the important process of a late evening of clerking in the new patients for surgery and taking their consent. If there were relatives present, we would usually involve them in the process and answer any questions they might have. Looking back on it, it was common at first to feel somewhat out of our depth through sheer lack of experience. What questions and how many we would pose to the registrars or consultants, if they were around, depended very much on their characters. I often found myself waking patients after midnight to take their history and consent for that day's morning surgical list. As far as I remember no one, other than the occasional patient, complained as it was seen as a rite of passage that had to be accepted if a surgical career was to be pursued.

Life in surgery was not for the fainthearted as we were regularly reminded, and women were discouraged, only the hardy few fought through the ranks. On one occasion, when second assistant in a case, I found myself falling asleep at the table having been pulling on a retractor for what seemed like several hours. I was saved from falling to the floor by the accidental hooking of my gown onto an intravenous pole at the head of the patient. A brisk tap on my knuckles by the consultant swiftly brought me back to life, although how much use I was is very debatable.

There was an unending tolerance by patients of the system. Today, as patients' expectations rise, the public patience is wearing thin and tolerance within the NHS is being eroded. Government propaganda from serial political parties in power has distorted the truth about the NHS since its inception. The truth of the quality of service and the world ranking of our NHS, has been repeatedly and falsely claimed to be the very best. This has resulted in the population at large accepting almost any inconvenience as 'The poor staff are so overworked.' The latter statement is frequently true, but it comes about through lack of good forward planning and appropriate funding. This approach has seen the service quality steadily diminish over the years with unacceptable waiting times, and lower numbers of doctors and nurses for the population than most other comparable developed countries. This poor service has led to some of the worst outcomes for cancer management in the European Union and the USA.

Of course, healthcare free at the point of delivery is a completely laudable goal, and would lead to the best system if adequately managed and funded. Neither of these requirements has or could ever be met by the remote control of government officialdom, more interested in party politics than meaningful long-term policies and their own survival than the service provided. The NHS has been among the largest employers run from a central government in Europe outside of the Russian Federation and sadly suffers from most of the problems that collective government run organisations do in the communist bloc. It has become a massive, remote-controlled juggernaut, whose controllers are far removed from the action and asleep at the wheel with their desire for personal power driving their agendas. As suggested recently by Tony Blair, ex-Labour Prime Minister, 'There is a risk that politics is for the weird and the wealthy.'[2] This is borne out by the high percentage of politicians enjoying private health cover. The management of public services in the UK, independent of the colour of the political party, would suggest that it is a more accurate statement than they would like to accept. If it is to remain a state-run organisation what is needed, in my opinion, is an all-party commission with a ten-to-fifteen-year rolling plan, to develop and maintain a state-of-the-art health service that the tax paying public deserve. A similar proposition has recently been floated by the current health secretary the Rt. Honourable Wes Streeting MP. It remains to be seen whether this will ever materialise. As one of the six wealthiest nations on earth, with such high levels of taxation, the population paying that tax deserves it.

We all had to live in the hospital for the first year. This was the pre-registration year, now superseded by foundation years one and two. The idea was to start to build the experience of real-life patient management. We were fortunate that the staff accommodation at the new Charing Cross Hospital was of quite a high standard. There were three high rise blocks, one for the on-call medical staff and another two for the nurses. Each apartment had three separate rooms, with a common bathroom and kitchen. I shared an apartment with two good friends Andy Davidson and Stewart Flemming. Stewart was a bit of a fitness fanatic and would coax me out to run with him along the Thames Embankment for a couple of miles, and back again and then to run up the ten flights of stairs to the top of the building. Not my favourite occupation. Stewart went on to be an accomplished plastic surgeon. Andy was more like-minded with me regarding strenuous exercise and would prefer a cigar and a good glass of wine with some black olives rather than a brisk run along the Thames embankment. He and his wife Susan O'Connell became well-liked GPs in Essex.

We only had two-weeks holiday somewhere during the twelve months of our house jobs. Surgical training was such a macho business that serious contenders rarely took all of their leave during those six months. It was in this period particularly that surgery was regarded by some, but by no means all, of the senior surgeons as being too demanding for women such that there was not just a glass ceiling, but what at times felt like a reinforced concrete barrier for them. I am delighted to report that one of the best, if not the very best, trainer that I had was a wonderful woman Miss Marie South, but more of that later.

Despite the demands of the job and the endless hours in the hospital, I have to confess to loving every minute of it. It was challenging and exciting at the same time. The practical nature of surgery appealed to me. Reconstructing, or restructuring the anatomy of the body, using your hands, eyes, and mind to alleviate suffering has great rewards, both in the short- and long-term. I have always enjoyed using my hands in art and music and elements of surgery cross over into those aspects of humanity. Excellence in surgery requires a profound knowledge of anatomy, well-practiced surgical technique, a delicacy of touch, and at all times, a respect for the person who has placed their life and well-being in your hands. A more important and profound responsibility in the moment is hard to imagine.

I have been reflecting on what the appeal of surgery has been for me. To rise each day with a purpose in mind and to retire each night with a sense of something important completed well, gives life a meaning and satisfaction. I have no time for those who enquire after 'the meaning of life' in an abstract sense. Life is an existential fact. Our existence is material and tangible. It is up to each of us to bring meaning to our lives. Life itself is a quirk of the universe. We have to seize upon its reality and make each day count for all around us. What matters is what we do with the time that we have. It can be frittered away unproductively, it can be used with malevolence towards others, or it can be used constructively. To give of your best for each and every person who enters your life in clinical practice or simply in your daily life, brings meaning to an otherwise abstract existence. Surgery allows this. We tend to be somewhat short-termist people. The satisfactory completion of a treatment episode for a patient before moving on to another fits our personalities. Each day can end with immense satisfaction, or extreme tragedy. It can be Shakesperean in challenging emotions. However, a truly empathic personality adds considerably to becoming an excellent surgeon and carer.

The nature of the job means that we are confronted by tragedy and trauma, and things do not always go as one would hope. Surgery is one human being doing their best for another, through the process of accurate diagnosis, appropriate treatment choice and accurate wielding of the knife and other instruments. The very nature of humanness is our fallibility. Some conditions are beyond satisfactory surgical help and even with the advanced nature of imaging preoperatively, this may only be discovered in the process of the operation. In addition, accidents do happen, and in our period of training, the excessive hours that we were expected to work did lead to some otherwise preventable problems for patients. In the middle of my surgical attachment, after four continuous days and nights work, in a state of exhaustion I was called to the accident and emergency department to attend an elderly gentleman who had been brought in with acute abdominal pain, distension and bowel obstruction. History, examination and investigations revealed large bowel obstruction with a tumour. Urgent surgery was necessary. In preparation for surgery, I had placed an intravenous line for fluid replacement. I needed to give an initial dose of appropriate antibiotics and to replace lost potassium. The Casualty department was busy, and the sister demanded that the patient go to the ward before going to the operating theatre to make space for other patients. Despite my protestations, she insisted that I give the drugs on the ward. Another of the nursing staff drew up the drugs, labelled the syringes, and placed them in a tray and sent it to the ward with the patient. Tragically, as I was to discover, the nurse had labelled the syringes the wrong way around. Each was filled with a colourless solution. The only distinction was the label placed by the nurse. I had not been able to check myself as this was done because of the pressure from the casualty Sister.

Now even more exhausted, not helped by the aggression in casualty and the endless lack of sleep, once on the ward, I started to give the drugs intravenously. One syringe contained potassium and was to be injected into a litre bag of saline, diluting it appropriately. The other syringe contained the antibiotics. As I gave what had been labelled as the antibiotic, the patient began to cry out in pain as the infusion passed up through the vein in his arm. Potassium is intensely irritant when infused undiluted directly into a vein. I instantly realised that I was not giving antibiotics but a large bolus dose of Potassium! Perhaps the reader can imagine the profound shock and anxiety which overcame me instantly. Most often this is a fatal error. Almost immediately the patient suffered a cardiac arrest. Realising what had happened I began cardiac massage and called urgently for glucose and insulin, the treatment for potassium overdose. Frantically I worked to restore a cardiac output and thankfully was successful. As soon as we had a stable situation, I called the consultant who would be in charge of the case, Mr Pendower. His reaction was typically caring. He ordered me off duty and to go to my room and to sleep and not to return until contacted by him. He would deal with the problem from then on. In utter exhaustion, I made my way to my room inconsolably distraught and collapsed onto the bed. After some time, I fell into a very disturbed sleep.

Early the following morning, there was a knock at the door of my room. It was John Pendower come to talk, and true to the man, to support me. He was completely understanding of the situation and concerned to know how I was. Once he knew that I was recovering my emotions, he instructed me to take the rest of the day off and only to come back when I felt ready. Thankfully the patient survived and later when recovered I met with him and his family to explain what had happened. As so often is the case when speaking transparently and honestly, they were so generous in their support and kindness. His lovely wife went so far as to place her arms around my shoulders in commiseration. Truly the kindness of strangers. However, this event scarred me for the rest of my years in medicine and I have never forgotten the look of horror and agony on his face as I administered the drug. I have never again administered drugs that I have not drawn up and checked myself from phial to syringe and to the patient. Lessons can be very hard won in our profession.

Both surgeons had an enormously varied practice. One list that Arthur Makey worked through, began with a closed mitral valvotomy where the narrowed mitral valve is opened through an incision in the lateral chest wall. This was followed by a lung resection for cancer, a hiatal hernia repair through the chest, a nephrectomy and as a finale the removal of wisdom teeth. John Pendower tended to stay within the confines of the abdomen, his forte being large bowel surgery. He would also deal with other general surgical problems such as removal of the thyroid gland, hernia repairs and varicose vein stripping, to name but a few. Surgical training was truly general back then. Working for those two men led to a huge experience in many areas of surgery, something that simply doesn't happen these days. And before the criticism is thrown that the standards must have been lower because of the generality of practice, the training was so long and detailed that their experience was vast and as a consequence they were truly general surgeons who could turn their hands to almost anything. They knew tissue planes intimately and their delicacy of handling respected the tissues, minimising the trauma for the patients. Today we are being forced into training proceduralists rather than true surgeons with a large experience.

Very early into the job I was taught how to do appendicectomies, inguinal and femoral hernia repairs, and simple vascular anastomoses. These are surgical procedures that nowadays are not learnt until much further into a surgical training. On our firm we had a wonderfully colourful registrar Gary Coombes and senior registrar Graham Barrett. Both were naturally gifted and eager to teach. They had great patience in supervising us. They created an ideal learning environment.

John Pendower also worked at Croydon Hospital, and it was a real treat to go there with him to sit in his clinic. His previously mentioned economy of words and efficiency of examination remains engrained in my own practice. He had always had an interest in the law and whilst I was working for him, he completed his bar examinations. Eventually, he became Dean of Charing Cross and Westminster Medical Schools. He had a wonderful sense of humour and when the combined medical schools were being rebadged, he vetoed the plan to call it the 'Westminster and Charing Cross Medical School', as he was not going to lead any institution with the initials WC! His pompom hats and morning suits were legendary. He was the finest of tutors and a wonderful example of who and what a surgeon should be. The only other surgeon, so highly skilled that I have had the good fortune to work with was Albert (Al) Pacifico in Alabama. We called him Al Terrifico, so impressive was his skill, but more of that later. Working for such men only fired my enthusiasm for the specialty more.

The nurses at that time were always neatly turned out with their smart uniforms and clean white aprons. They tended to come from respectable families and in the modern world would very likely have become doctors themselves. This is not to run down the profound importance of excellence in nursing. The patients and we doctors were the benefactors of such discipline and caring skills. Ward discipline was strictly maintained by the ward sisters, overseen by the real matron. Sloppy appearance and lateness were simply not acceptable. I'd like to highlight two aspects of their uniform. First, a silver buckle on their waist belt. This was often a present from their parents on becoming State Registered Nurses (SRNs) and something of which they were immensely proud. The second was a bronze cross made from the bronze of a captured cannon from the Crimean War, which they wore with the military ribbon.

Matron was always a highly experienced nurse who was gifted immense powers in the administration of the hospital. The creation of the 'modern matrons' by Tony Blair's government really undermined the true status of what and whom a matron should be. The title has been purloined and degraded by the politicians with no understanding of what it really meant. No one crossed the hospital matron, certainly not the consultants, many of whom were seen as visitors as they also had attachments at other institutions. A legendary matron at The Cross was Miss Cochrane, perhaps the most famous of matrons. Her demeanour portrayed the discipline that she demanded. A rather large lady always immaculately turned out in her pressed uniform and white starched cap, she set the example for all those under to follow.

On Wednesdays, Arthur Makey often did a heart operation. These were mostly heart valve cases but there were occasional coronary patients as well. Numbers of these were limited because of the attitude of Peter Nixon, already discussed, and the procedure was still in its infancy. As the numbers were small and infrequent, the whole team needed to progress slowly, and the results were often poor. However, the experience of working with a team trying to establish the practice of open-heart surgery was invaluable.

The planning for every cardiac case was extensive. For each one we had to bring in blood donors as the blood loss was often considerable. On duty one Saturday evening, I received a telephone call from a doctor claiming to be a cardiology registrar at Harefield Hospital. This was unusual, but not implausible as it is a stand-alone cardiac unit in north London. He claimed that they had a patient with an acute aortic dissection, a life-threatening diagnosis where the aorta, the main arterial pipeline of the body, has split its wall. The threat is of aortic wall rupture and sudden death through exsanguination. In a rather strange Glaswegian accent, he stated that they couldn't deal with the patient at that time, because the surgeons there were already operating, and would we take him as soon as possible. Perhaps the name Dr. McTavish should have rung an alarm bell but being so keen to do the job well, I made the call to the ward sister to request a bed and registered the patient with the theatre staff and the intensive care unit. I rang Harefield back and accepted the patient. I then began the round of calling everyone in, including the multiple blood donors. This took almost an hour. At the end of it, I was settling for a last cup of tea before the onslaught began. As I sat down the phone rang with a very anxious sounding Andy Davidson on the other end. I tried to explain that I didn't really have time to chat then as I had an emergency case coming in. He declared loudly that that was what he wanted to talk to me about. The Harefield doctor was Andy, and he had been trying to get back through to me for the last hour, but my phone was continually engaged! I was furious as I then had to phone everyone and cancel all the arrangements that I had previously made.

Around lunchtime on 21 January 1976 I was in the operating theatre near the top of the building. Each theatre had large windows looking out over west London. Suddenly the theatre was vibrating to a loud noise from outside. Quite low in the sky was the beautiful sight of the supersonic aircraft, Concorde. We were witnessing its first passenger flight from the UK. Built by British Aircraft Corporation and Aerospatiale, it was and remains a wonder of modern technology. The first flights took off simultaneously from Paris and London. It had the capacity to fly at supersonic speeds for longer than any other aircraft, then and now. It also beat the Russians and the Americans in production, despite the espionage tricks of the Russian agents who stole many of the blueprints during development. The Russian Tupolev version, insultingly called Concordski flew a test flight first before Concorde but crashed at the Paris Air Show in 1973, killing all six crew and seven people on the ground, most of whom were children. That ended their programme.

Helen, my fiancée, was working for British Airways ground staff at the time and helped to board that first group of passengers. Little did she know that we watched this amazing, if somewhat noisy aircraft, circle the area of the hospital before flying off from London. With the theatres on the fourteenth floor of the hospital we had a wonderful view. That evening Helen excitedly reported her experience boarding the passengers and was surprised to hear that we had heard it first and then seen it over the hospital. Just over two decades later I was able to experience a flight on that supersonic missile. My daughter Joanna witnessed its final flight to Filton in Wiltshire as it flew over the Clifton Suspension Bridge in Bristol. She was in a crowd of people on the cliff above the Avon Gorge witnessing its passing.

The six months on the surgical firm passed in a blur of work and sleepless nights but was exhilarating and energising and reinforced my desire to become a surgeon. There was a real sense of family within the surgical team which was cemented by the welcoming and supportive nature of the nursing staff. Very sadly, today there is a real concern, backed up by formal review, of bullying of junior medical staff by some nursing staff. In thinking about this, the progressive undermining of medical staff by management has struck me, many of whom these days are senior nursing staff who appear to have been infected by this reduction in respect across the board for doctors and what it takes to achieve a degree in medicine, and the responsibility that all carry on their shoulders. At the same time the advent of the so-called 'modern matron' has devalued the dignity and respect of that post. The discipline of nursing staff on the ward has also been seriously undermined by the effect of significant staff shortages. At that time, in the 1960s and 1970s, both the nurses and the junior doctors were subject to strict disciplinary control and each professional group held the other in the respect that was deserved. Discipline has become a dirty word. It appears that as soon as nursing staff are in any way disciplined they tend to leave and often follow this up with a complaint of bullying and harassment. This is quite unlike the attitude to doctors of all levels of seniority who appear to be regarded as dispensable and easily replaced without regard to their knowledge and experience. Can this ever be reversed? I doubt it and it is a sad fact, as this seriously affects patient care and the satisfaction levels of staff.

The discipline extended to our knowledge of the patients and their details. We were expected to be able to recite their history in detail, know the drugs that they were taking and all of their blood results and other tests without looking them up. It became a matter of pride to ensure that everything was up to date and complete. It was not possible just to make things up, as at the same time the ward sister would have the notes open and could check up on us.

The preparation for these daily ward rounds would extend late into the evening or very early the next morning. Today it is common for the junior staff and indeed the nursing staff to know very little about the patients in their care. It is usually the consultant who knows most about the patient and needs to inform those who should know the detail for each one. This sloppy attitude has infected so much of medicine and is just another reason for increased litigation by patients failed by the system. The introduction of the European working time directive limiting junior doctor's hours requires detailed and accurate hand over between the staff. Too often this is poorly done by both nurses and doctors and leads to a lot of wastage and harm. In some departments the failure to recruit adequate levels of staff, necessarily commensurate with the reduced hours, has resulted in unacceptable waiting times for investigations to be reported. It is common for CT and MRI scan reports to take several weeks. All of this adds to delay in diagnosis and treatment. At that time we would go to the various departments to seek out the results first hand. It also meant that we could look at the pathology slides through the microscope under the supervision of the pathologist adding significantly to our knowledge and bringing the disease alive.

At the end of the six months in surgery I moved overnight into the medical job. This was with Dr J. T. Scott and Dr. Tiny Maini, whose firm I had enjoyed immensely during my student days. Both had a wonderful sense of humour and were very kind and caring men. The lesson that sticks in my mind was imparted by Dr Scott on day one and it went like this,

> Wells, be sure to finish the patient history before the wheelchair stops, because once the patient begins to remove their clothes you will be there all afternoon.

He also stated that I should not think about getting married without his permission as the workload was not commensurate with a satisfactory married life. Can anyone imagine saying that to a twenty-five year old these days, good advice though it was?

There was another salutary lesson that I learnt when a student on their firm. On leaving the old hospital, I was confronted with an *Evening News* billboard announcing that a cure for rheumatoid arthritis had been found. This of course proved to be baseless, and the lesson was not to believe medical announcements in the press. As I have come to realise most, if not all, of them are about trying to raise extra research funding and are embellishments of the truth. This can be heard on a regular basis on radio programmes as well as in the press. The journalists do not seem to have understood that they act as wonderful advertising for fund raising and rarely do they seem to follow up on the claims that they transmit. In many cases this raises hopes falsely for suffering people.

Moving from the excitement and frantic activity of the surgical unit, the rheumatology ward seemed very passive to me. The on-call nights, although less busy, were a source of a little more excitement. We were 'on take' to use the jargon, for all of acute medicine. With properly functioning general practitioners, the referrals that we received were mostly genuine medical emergencies. Through the lack of availability of access to a GP there are many who attend A & E who could easily have been dealt with in general practice. Although specialist rheumatologists had a responsibility for medical emergencies when 'on take', once a putative diagnosis had been made the patients were then triaged to the appropriate medical sub-specialty. The ward rounds were much more lengthy and made up many of the hours in the day.

During the latter part of that attachment, I arranged to see our professor of surgery Professor Harding Rains to discuss a surgical training. I had spoken to him at the end of my training before I began house jobs. Sadly, he remained stubbornly unhelpful, telling me that at twenty-six I was too old to contemplate a career in surgery. And so I made my own plans. At that time there were few run-through training programmes as there are now. We had to chase every job ourselves. This resulted in moving every six months for the first several years. Helen, whom I married in 1977, was very tolerant of this, although it was completely outside her life experience prior to meeting me.

Back in my room following the deflating meeting with Harding Rains, I can remember sitting down with a blank sheet of paper to map out what were, by reputation, the best jobs in the country in surgical training. I arranged them in such a way that each job placed me in the best position for the next one. It worked. A training programme that normally took up to fifteen years and sometimes longer, I achieved in nine, some of it by good fortune but more of that later.

It is strange how some events stick in the mind but this one came at a salutary time. Very late one evening during my house jobs, I remember running into Barry Jones, a friend from my original year. He was by then a senior house officer in surgery and intent on a career in plastic surgery. I asked him how he was finding things at that stage of his training. He oozed excitement and energy, reinvigorating my enthusiasm for a surgical career. Medicine or general practice were not for me.

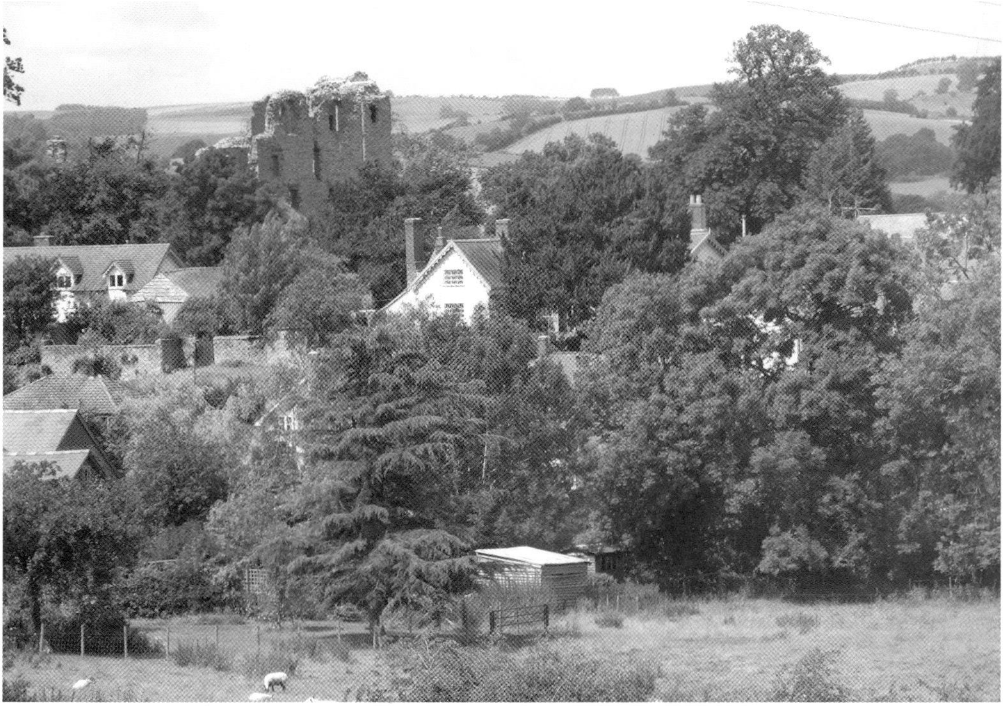

A view across Clun with the Norman Castle on the hill. (*Author's collection*)

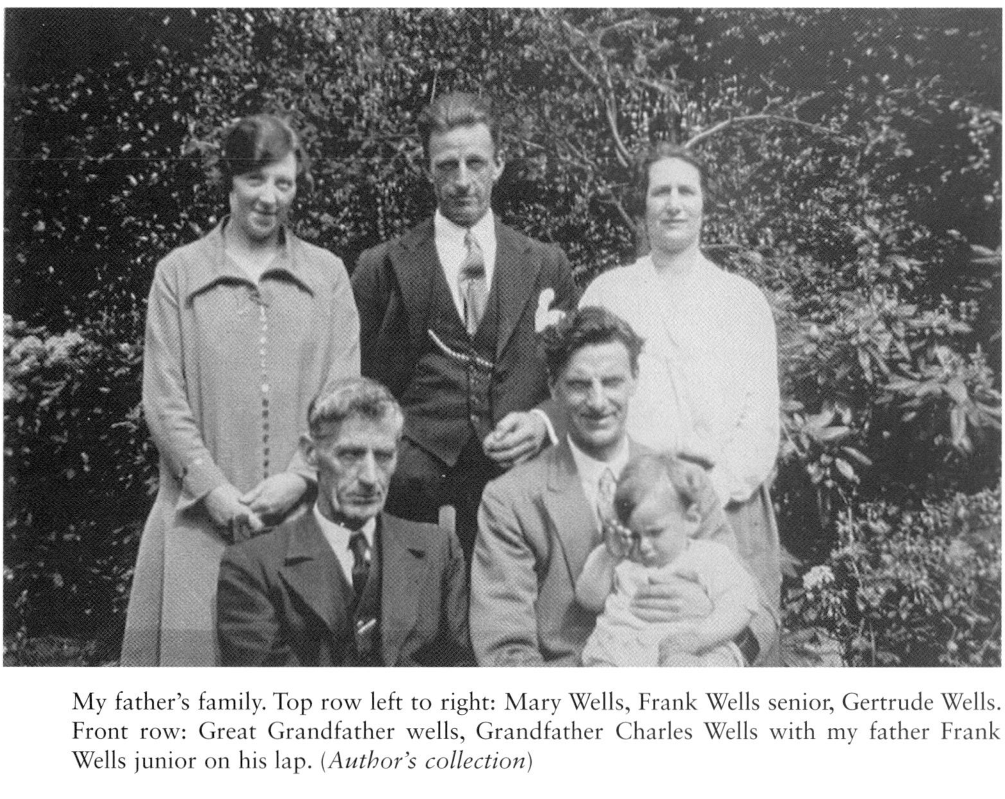

My father's family. Top row left to right: Mary Wells, Frank Wells senior, Gertrude Wells. Front row: Great Grandfather wells, Grandfather Charles Wells with my father Frank Wells junior on his lap. (*Author's collection*)

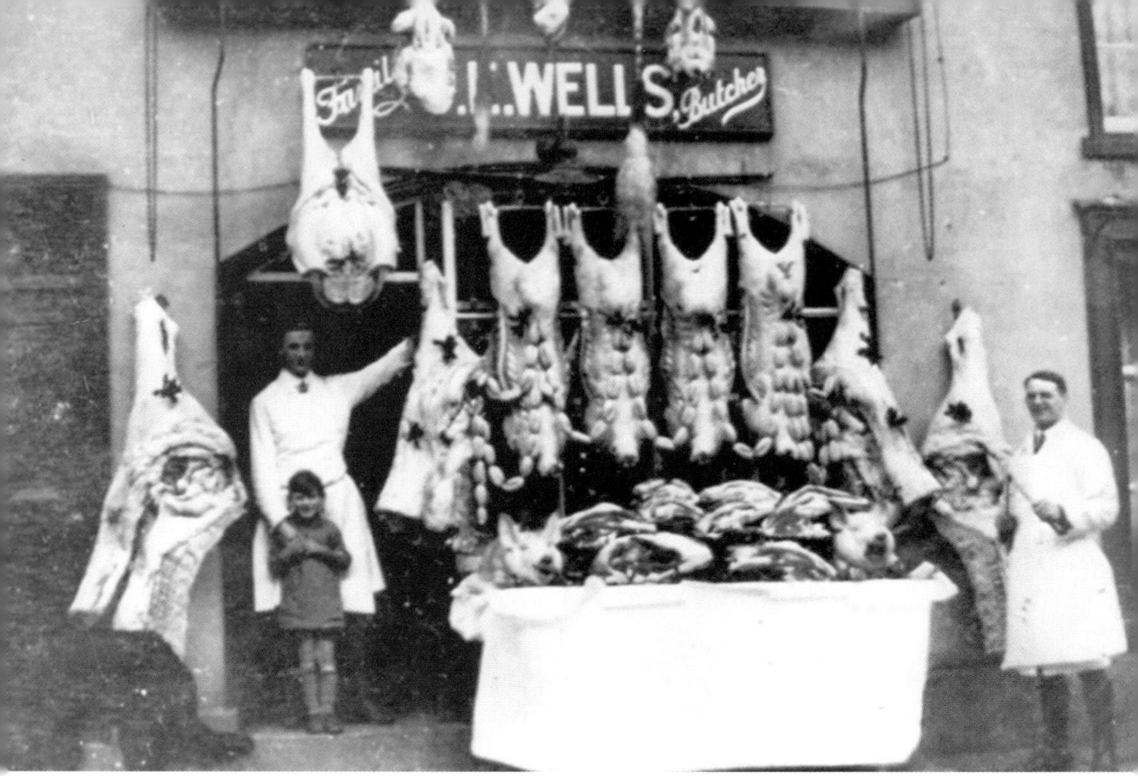

The Shop in Clun, c. 1932. My father aged approximately five years old standing in front of his father Charles Wells, with my great uncle Charlie Griffiths to the right of the picture. Tuesday was market day and the shop was dressed like this every week for many years. (*Author's collection*)

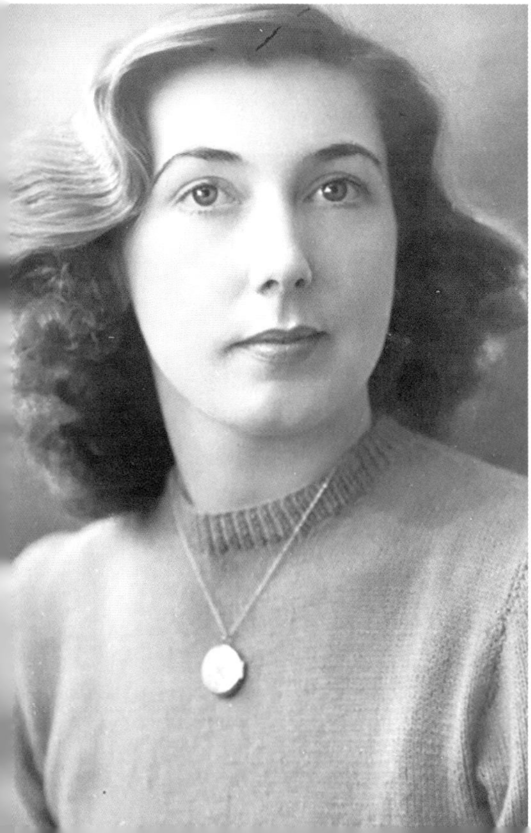

My mother Violet Wells at the time of her marriage to my father. (*Author's collection*)

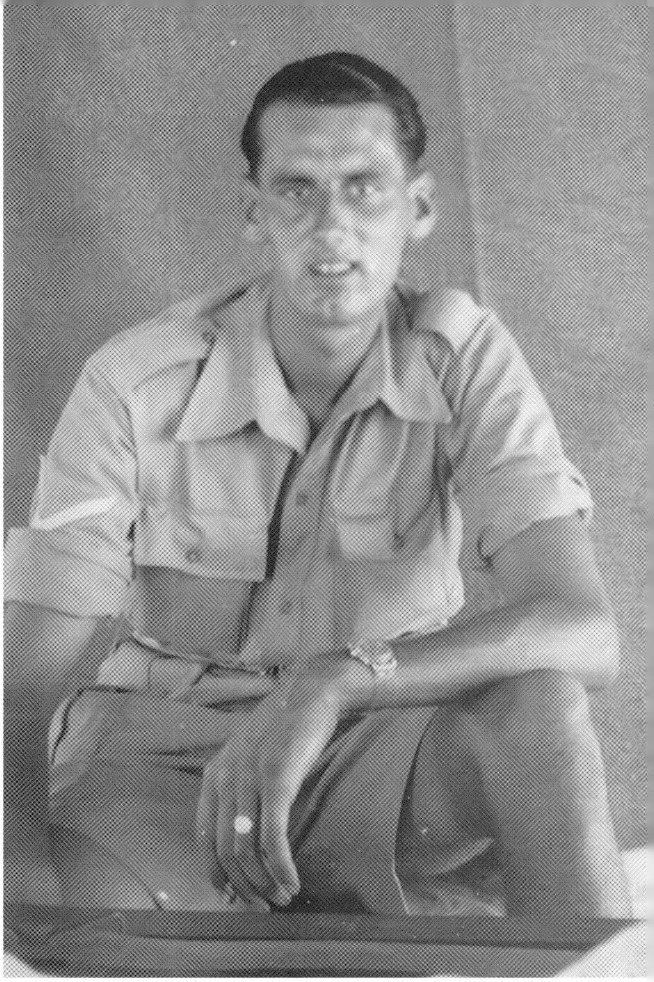

Right: My father Frank Wells in Palestine with the Royal Electrical and Mechanical Engineers. (*Author's collection*)

Below: My mother with her class of pupils at Clun Primary School. (*Author's collection*)

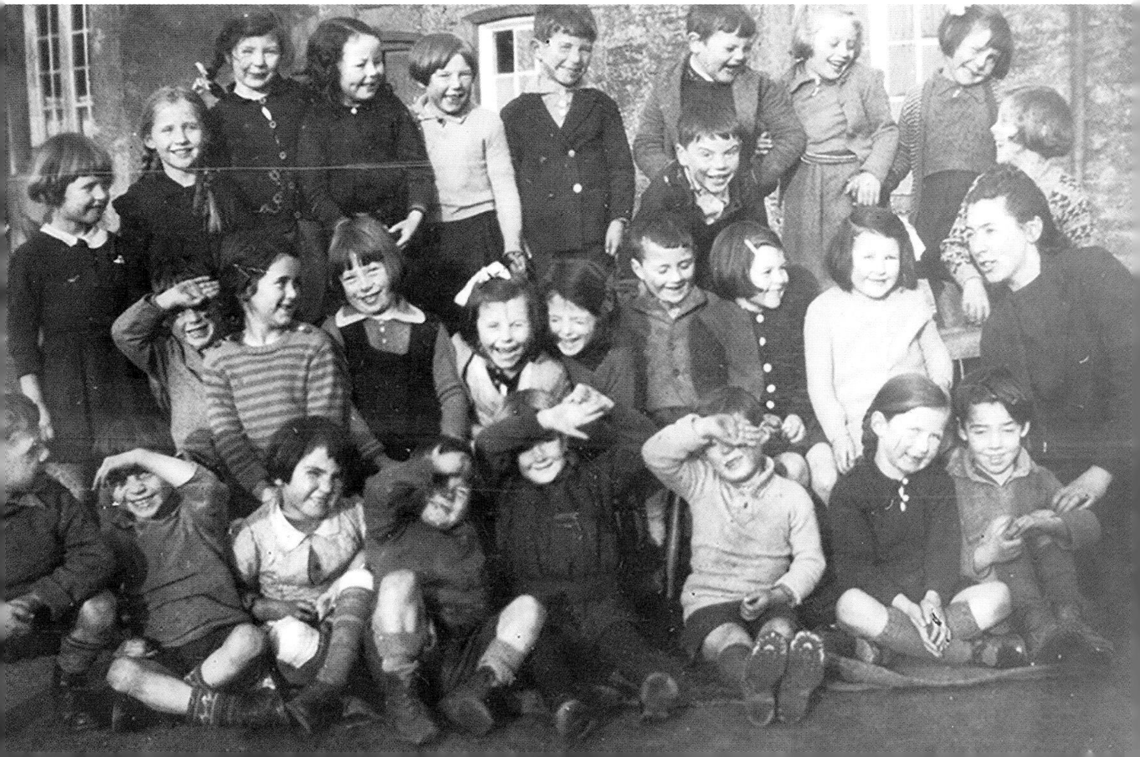

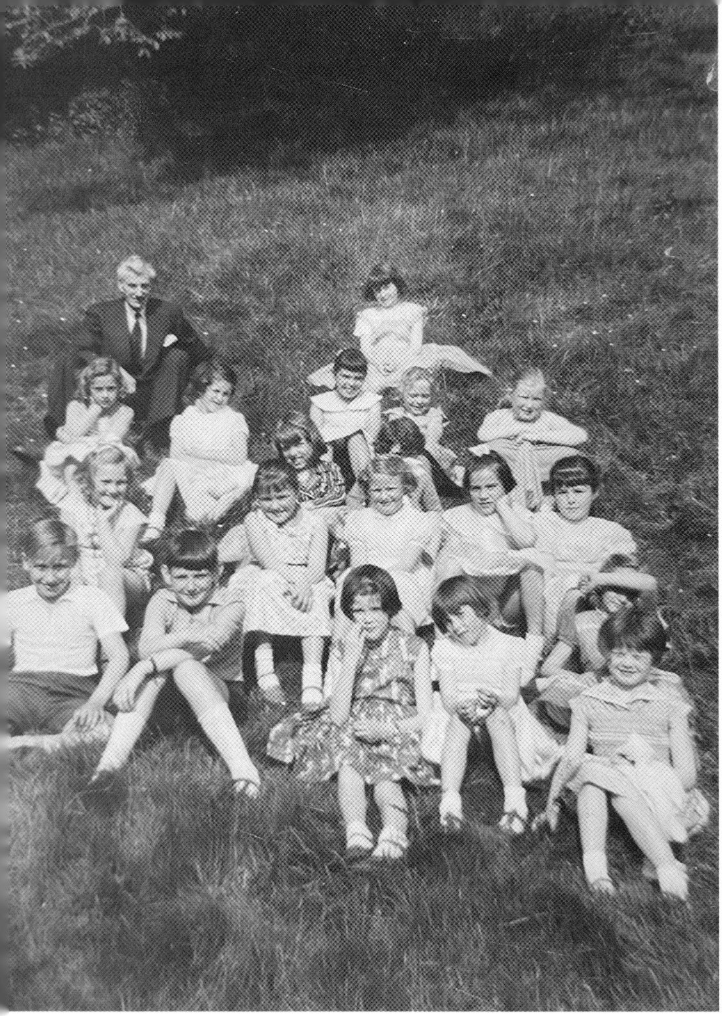

Right: A typical birthday party with games in the old castle grounds. My grandfather organised the entertainment. The author is second from the left in the front row. (*Author's collection*)

Below: An early family outing to Trafalgar Square with Rosamond and Dad, c. 1956.

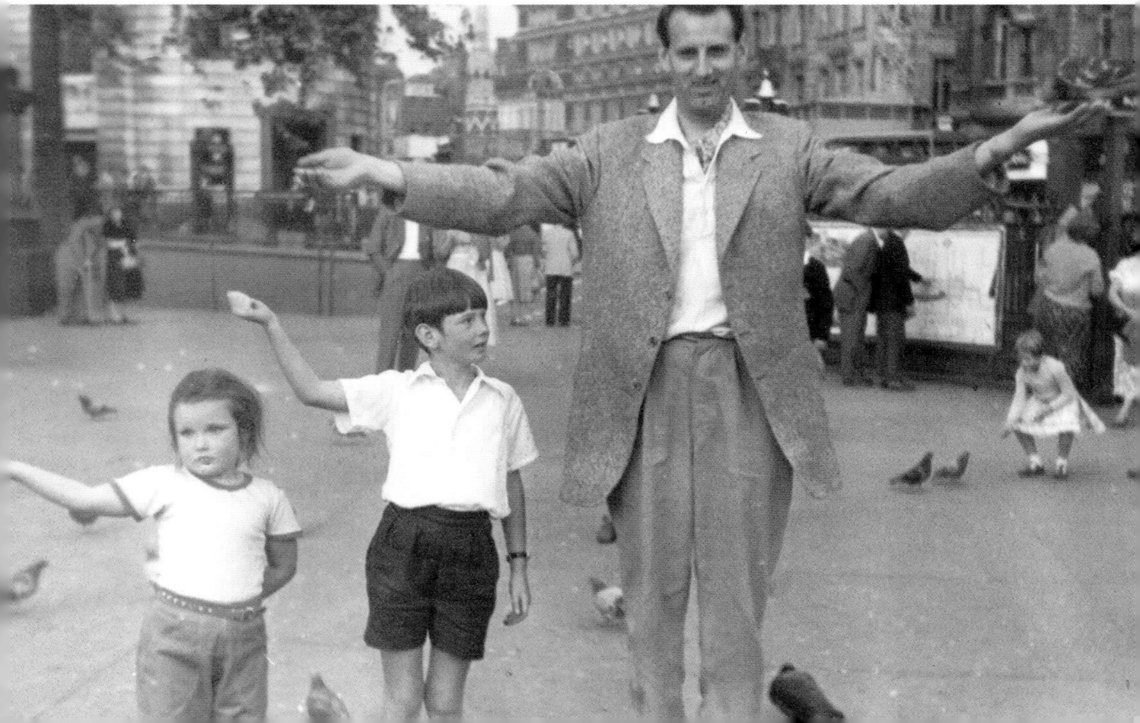

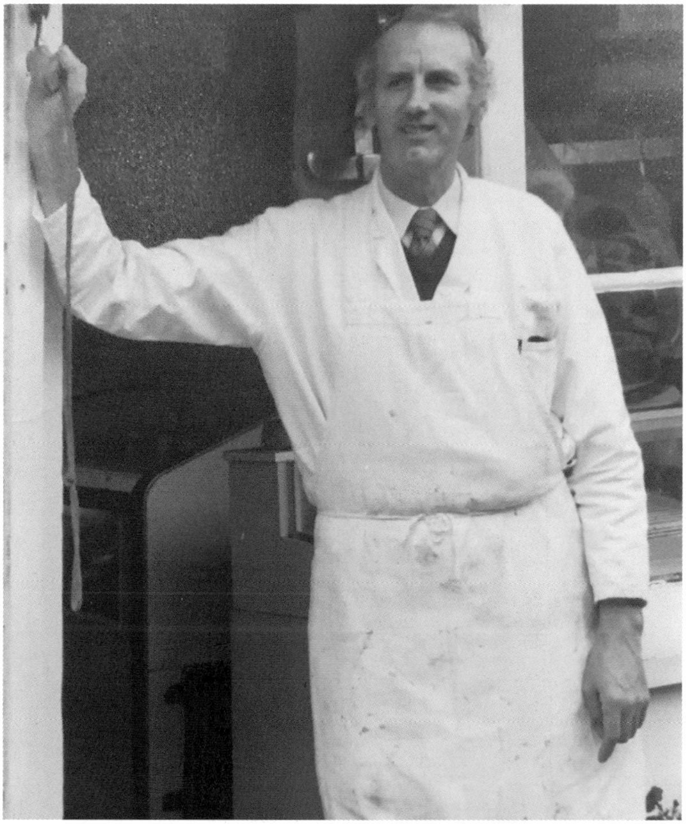

Right: My father outside the shop. (*Author's collection*)

Below: The shop in the square in Clun. (*Author's collection*)

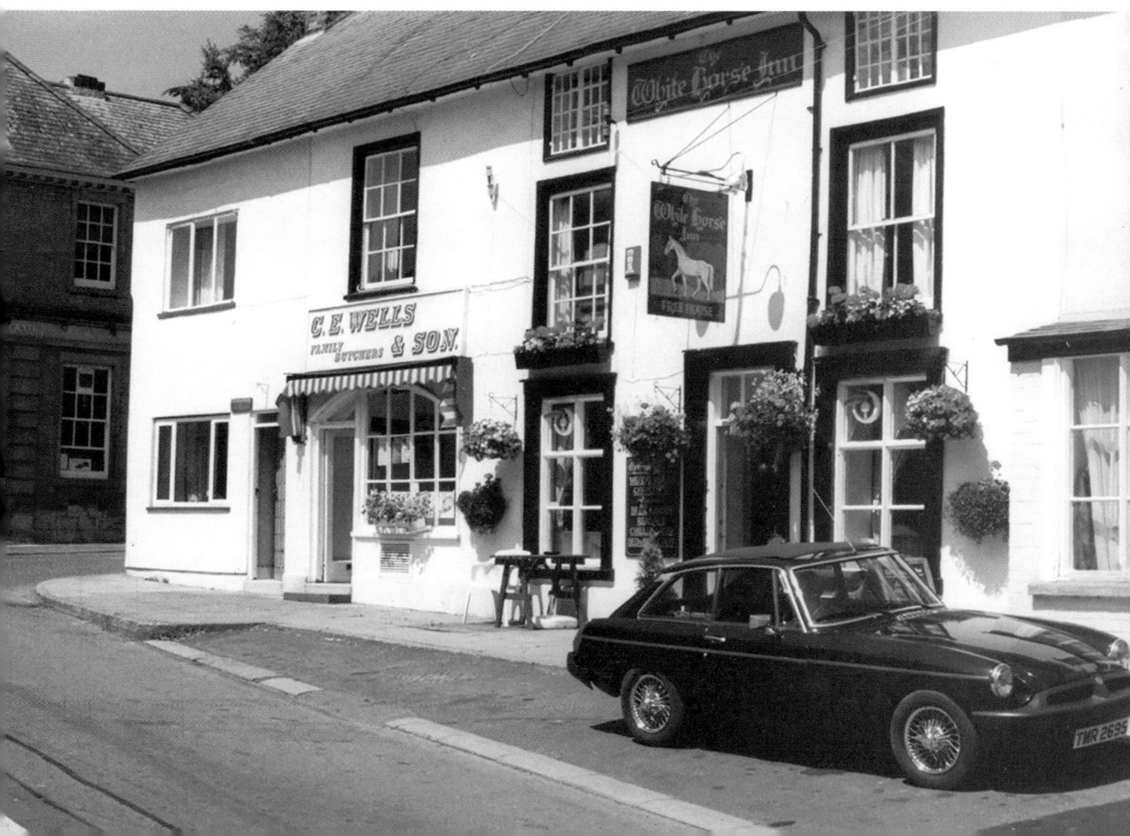

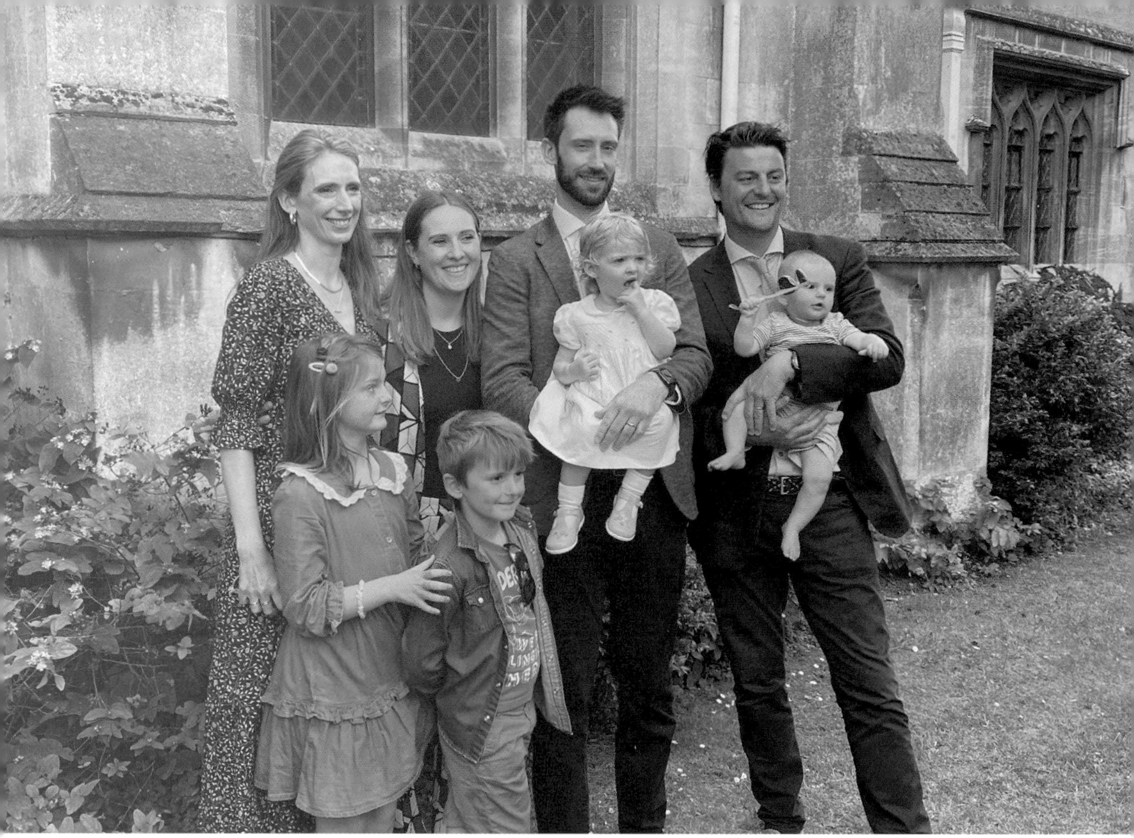

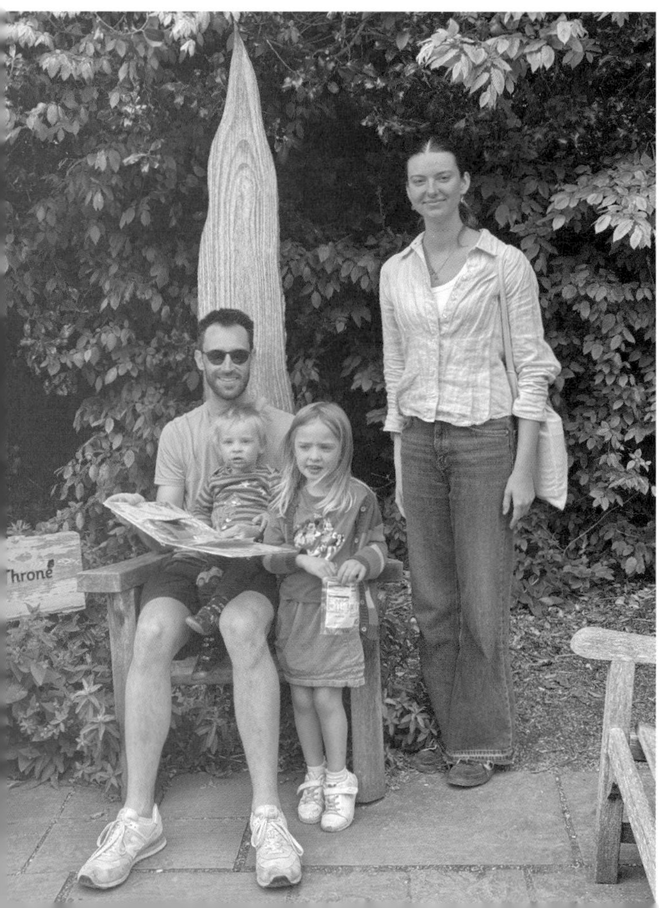

Above: The family at the christening of Florence Winter Wells, here in the arms of her father. My son Nicholas, my daughter Joanna, and Millie, Nicholas's wife, are to his right, with James, my son-in-law, with their new addition, Wilfred, in his arms. Emily and Archie stand in front. (*Author's collection*)

left: Nicholas with his son Arthur and his daughter Florence and my daughter Olivia. (*Author's collection*)

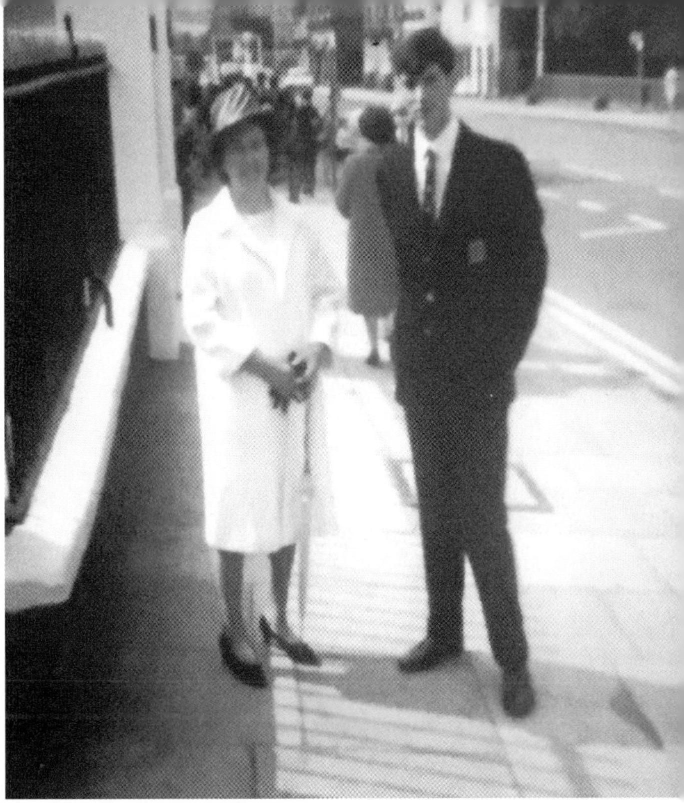

The author as head boy at Adams' School with my mother, 1967. (*Author's collection*)

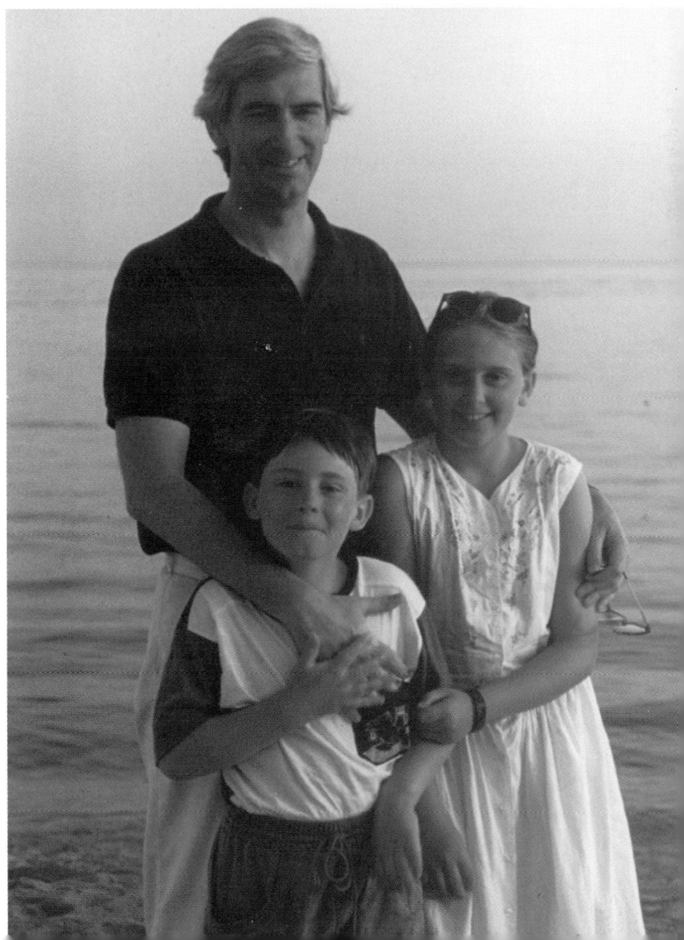

The author with son Nicholas and daughter Joanna. (*Author's collection*)

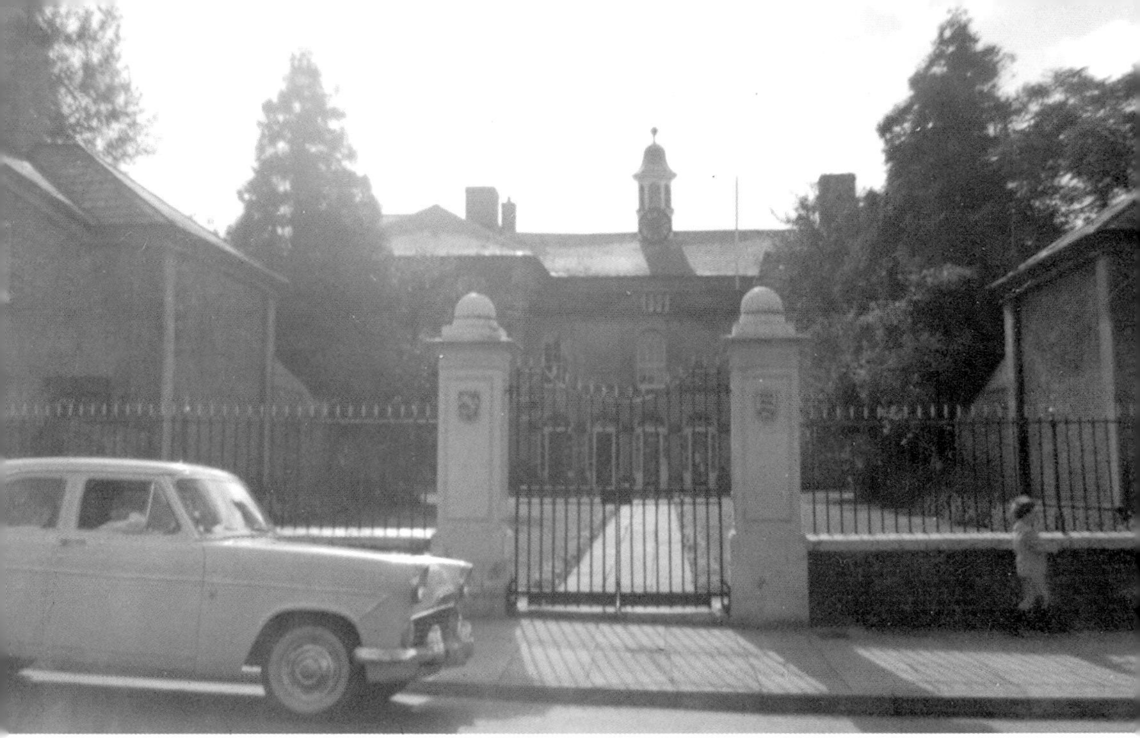

Adams' Grammar School, Newport, Shropshire, taken contemporaneously with my attendance. The alms-houses can be seen either side of the main entrance. (*Author's collection*)

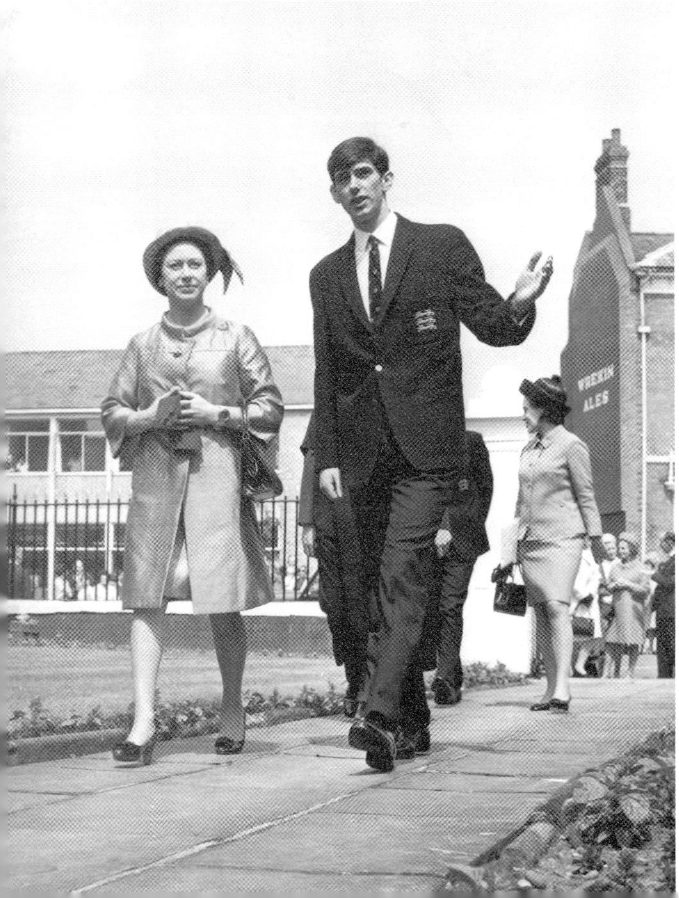

The author with Her Royal Highness Princess Margaret on the occasion of her visiting the school having been made the first lady appointed to the Haberdashers' Company. (*Author's collection*)

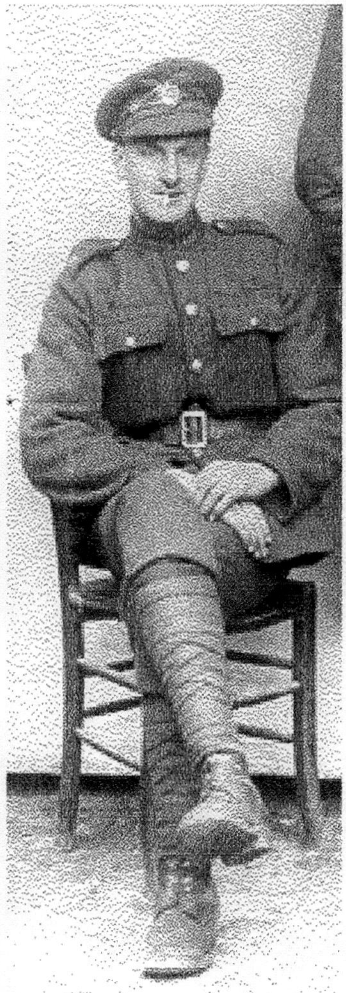

Charles Wells in c. 1915

Right: My grandfather Charles Wells on the Western Front in 1915. (*Author's collection*)

Below: Grandfather in charge of one of the trains used to haul ammunition and big guns to the front. He is dressed in the white overalls in the driver's cabin. (*Author's collection*)

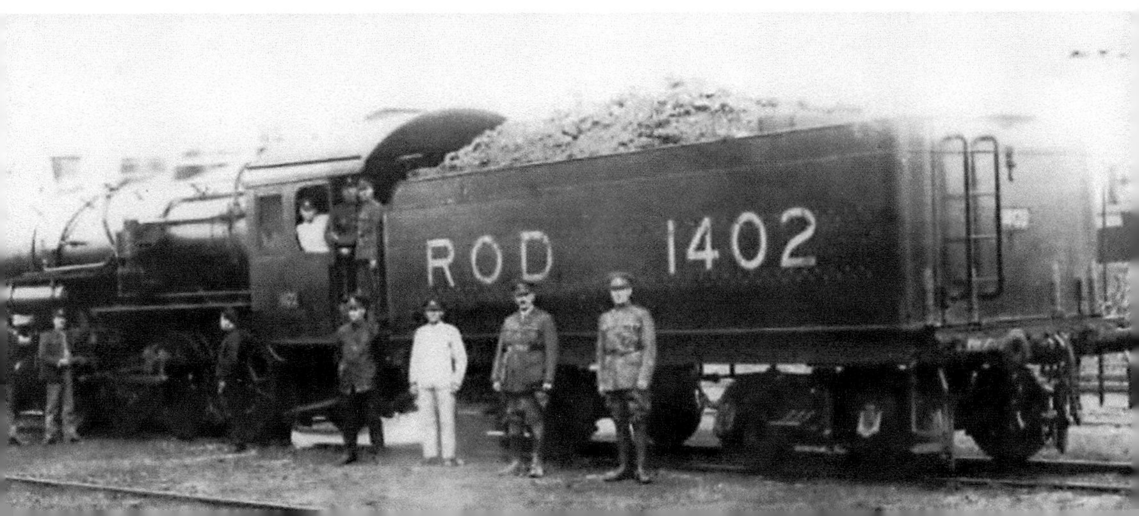

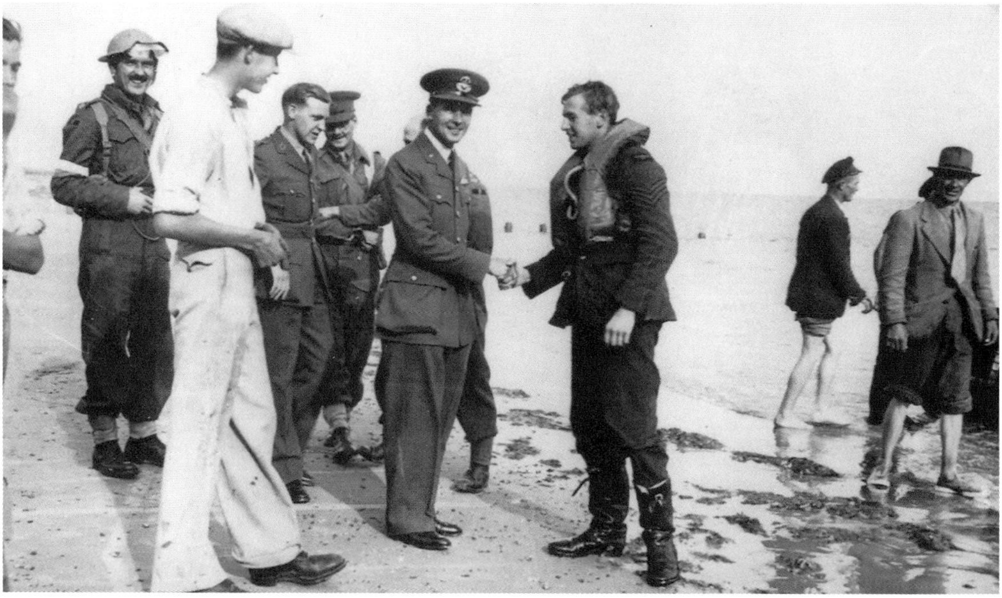

Above: Flying Officer Cyril Babbage having just been rescued from the channel and brought ashore in Bognor Regis after being shot down in his Spitfire engaging a German ace. (*Author's collection*)

Below: My father in his workshop in Garian, northern Libya. The famous 'Lady of Garian' can be seen on the wall behind him painted by the American serviceman Clifford Saber, a volunteer ambulance driver with the 8th Army. (*Author's collection*)

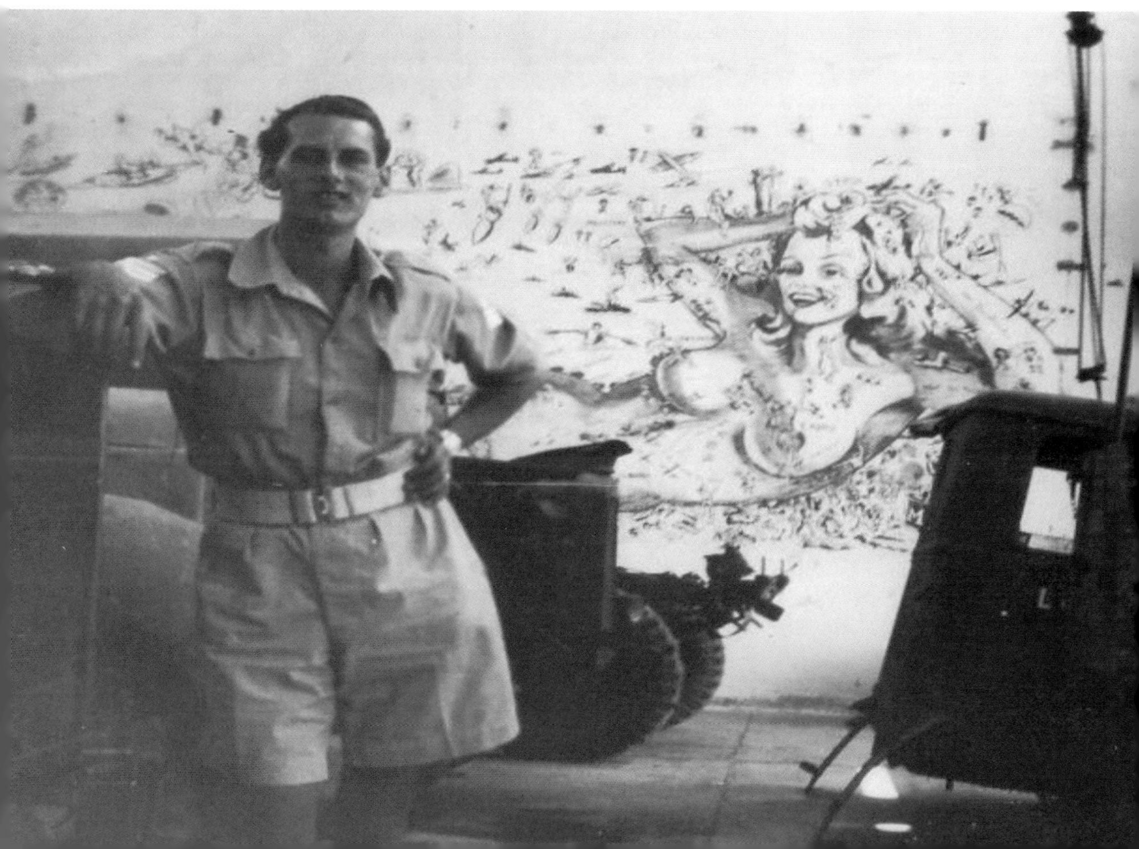

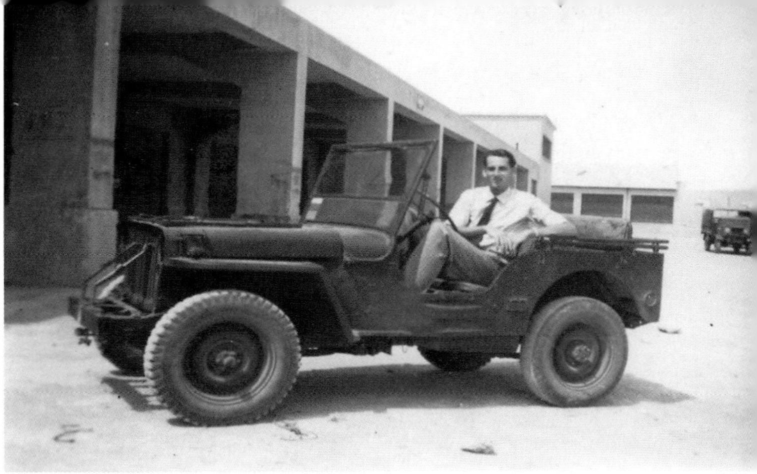

My father in his Willis jeep after a patrol in Palestine, 1947. (*Author's collection*)

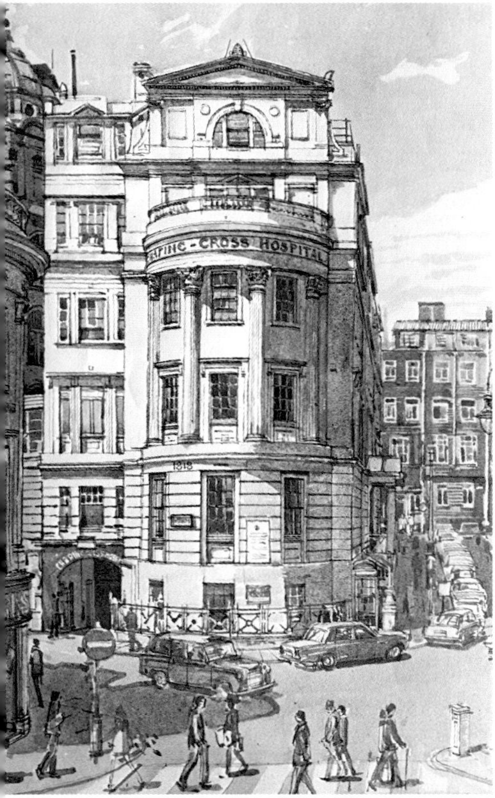

Charing Cross Hospital, just off The Strand in London. (*Print by Dennis Flanders*)

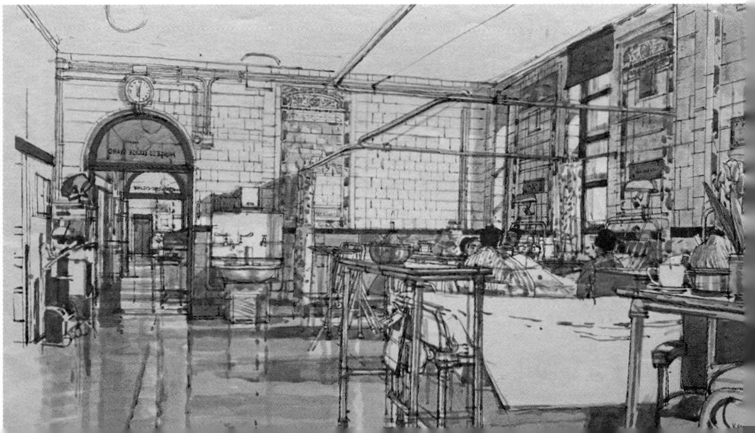

Princess ward in the old Charing Cross Hospital. Note the tiles on the wall above the patients. (*Print by Dennis Flanders*)

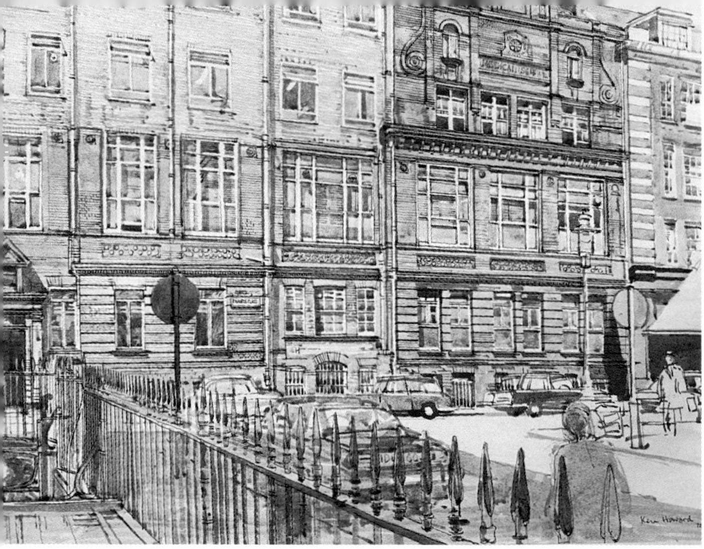

Charing Cross Hospital Medical School, University of London. Since demolished and replaced by offices. (*Print by Dennis Flanders*)

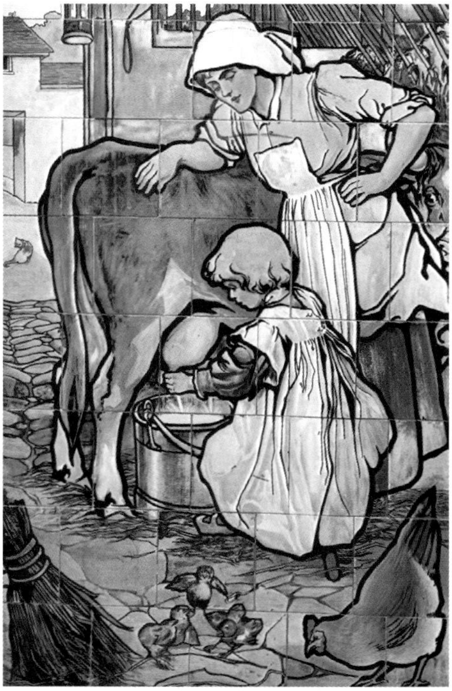

An example of the beautiful hand-coloured tiles that adorned the walls of the wards in the hospital. Now exhibited on the wall of the new hospital with some remaining in the old hospital, now the headquarters of the Central London Metropolitan Police. (*Author's collection*)

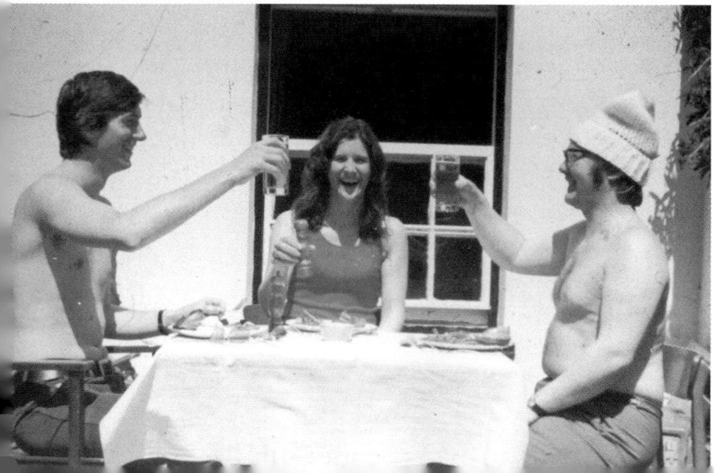

The author enjoying a sunny lunch in Appledore, Devon, with Liz and Alan Riley during my General Practice experience as a medical student. (*Author's collection*)

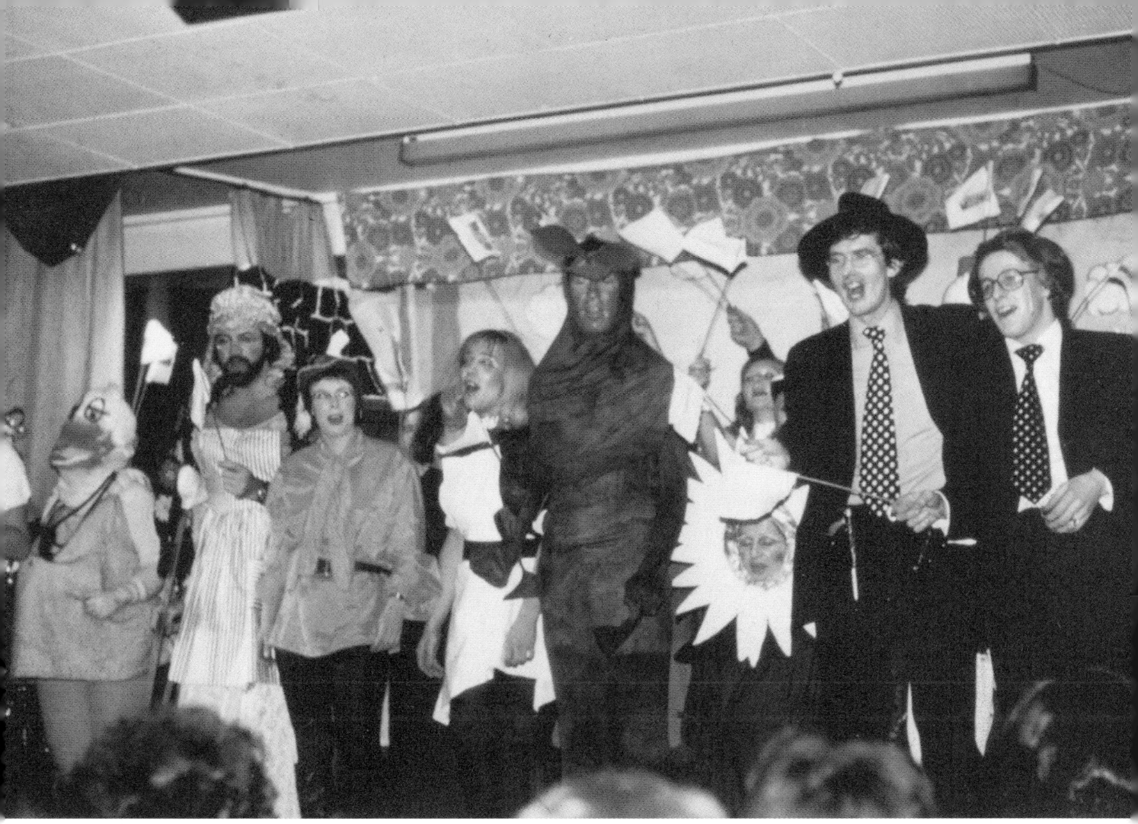

Above: The author in full song in the Christmas show at Winchester County hospital, 1978. (*Author's collection*)

Below: The author with David Dunn, vascular and general surgeon at Addenbrooke's hospital on my first foreign trip to present academic work that we had done together in Garmisch-Partenkirchen, spring 1980. (*Author's collection*)

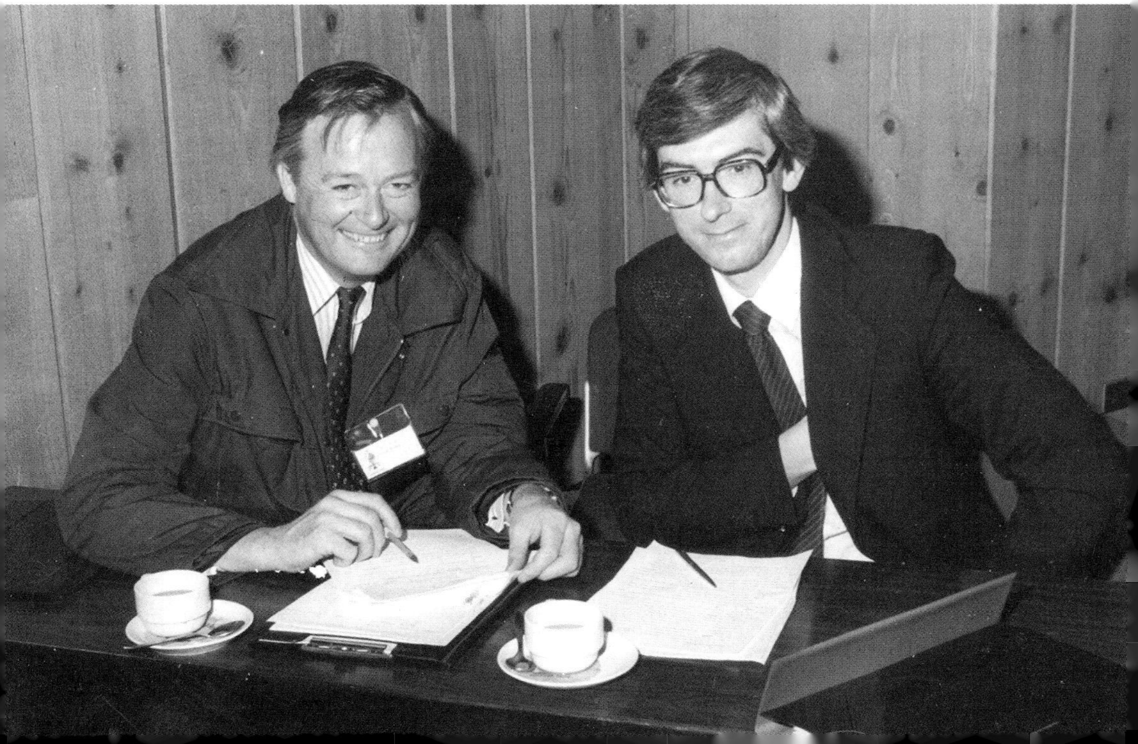

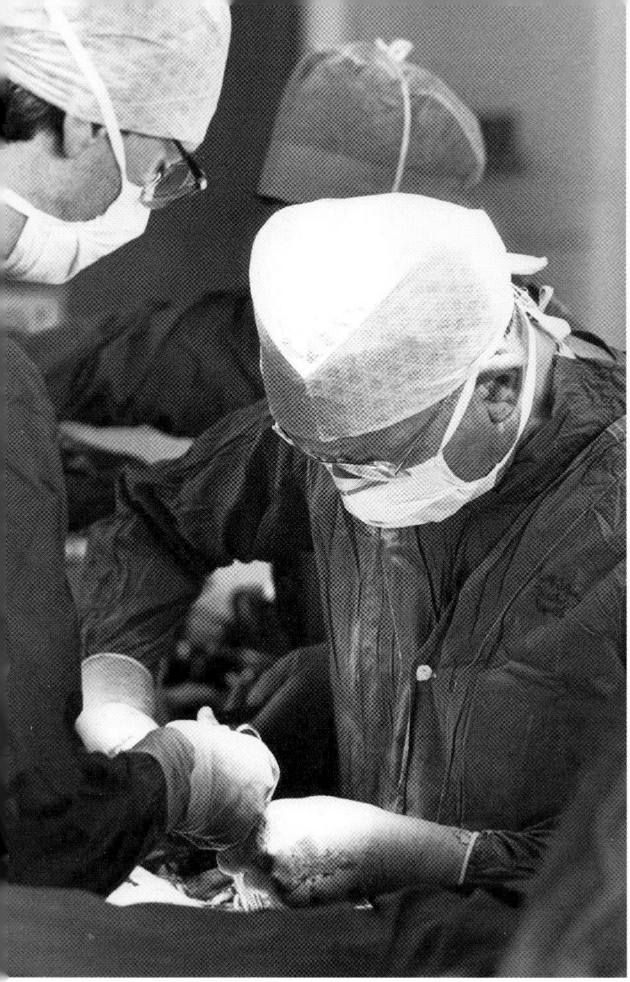

Left: The author as surgical registrar assisting Mr Ben Milstein, consultant cardiothoracic surgeon, at Papworth Hospital in 1981. (*Author's collection*)

Below: At Papworth Hospital as surgical registrar. From left to right, Chris McGregor, senior registrar, the author, Mr. John Wallwork, consultant cardiac surgeon and Mr Ben Milstein. (*Author's collection*)

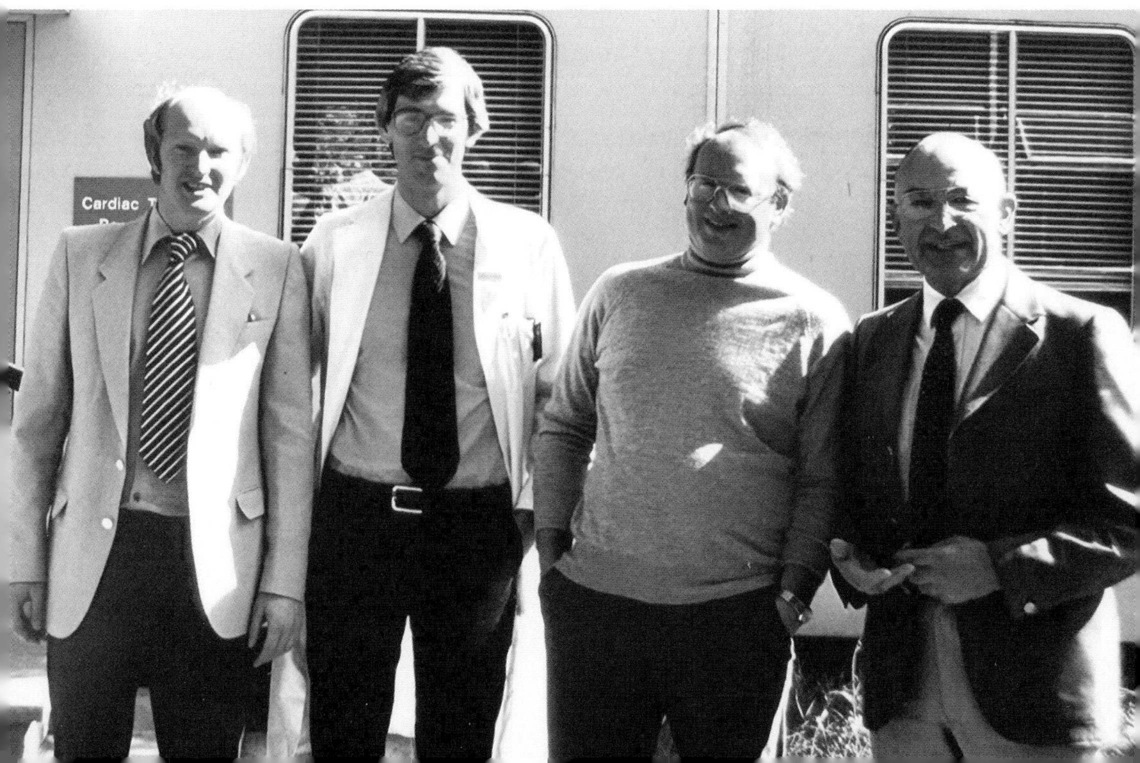

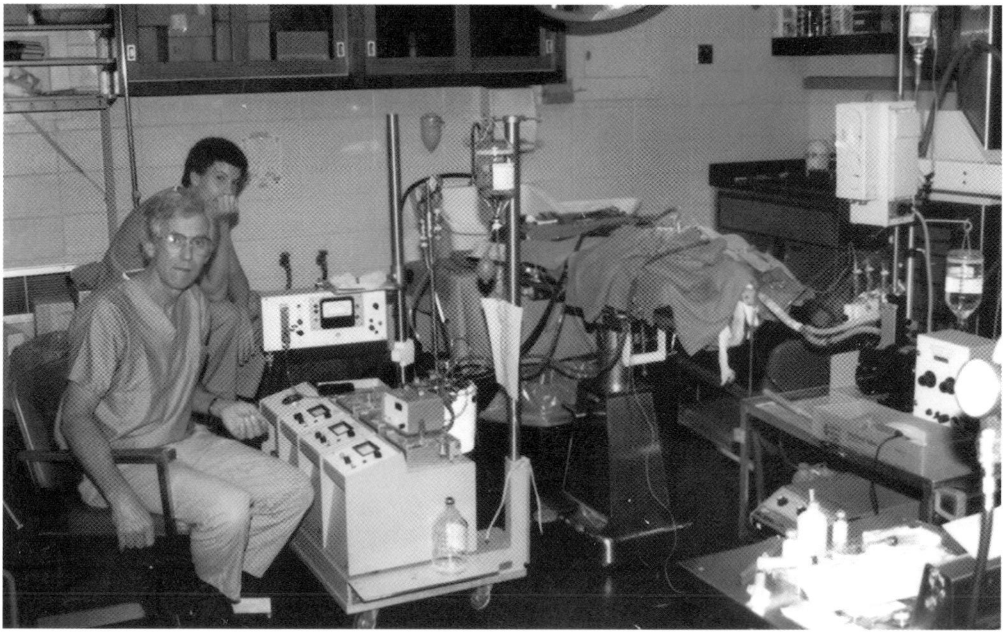

Above: The animal laboratory at the University of Alabama Medical School. The wonderful senior laboratory assistant Mr Bill Tracey in the foreground. Behind is the son of one of the thoracic surgical consultants, deriving lab experience before deciding to train as a medical student. (*Author's collection*)

Below: The author, the new recruit with consultant colleagues John Wallwork, Terence English and retiree Ben Milstein. (*Author's collection*)

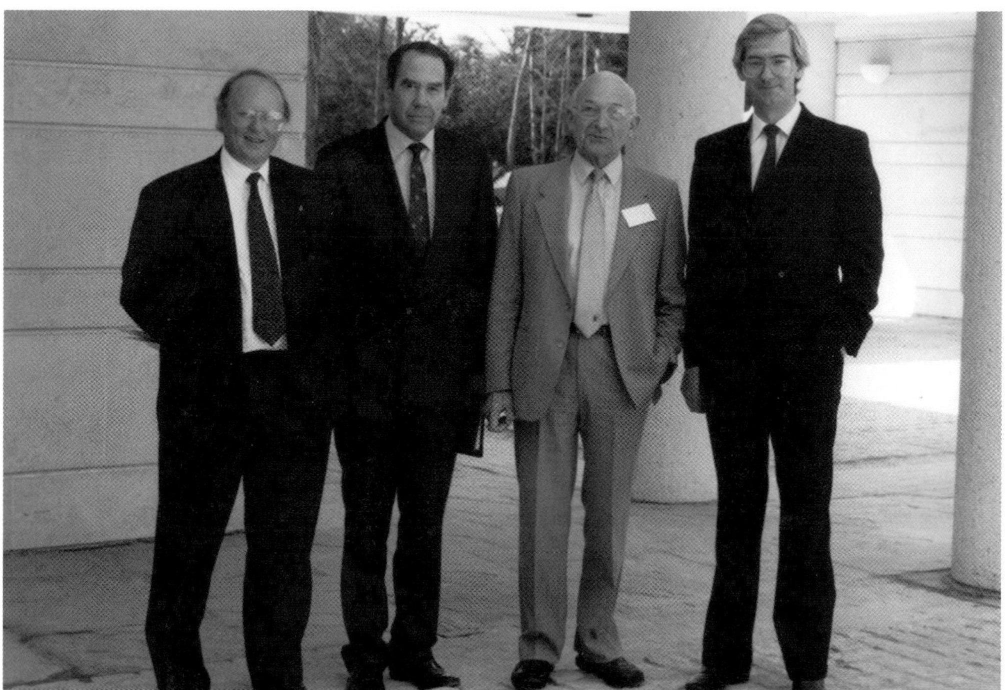

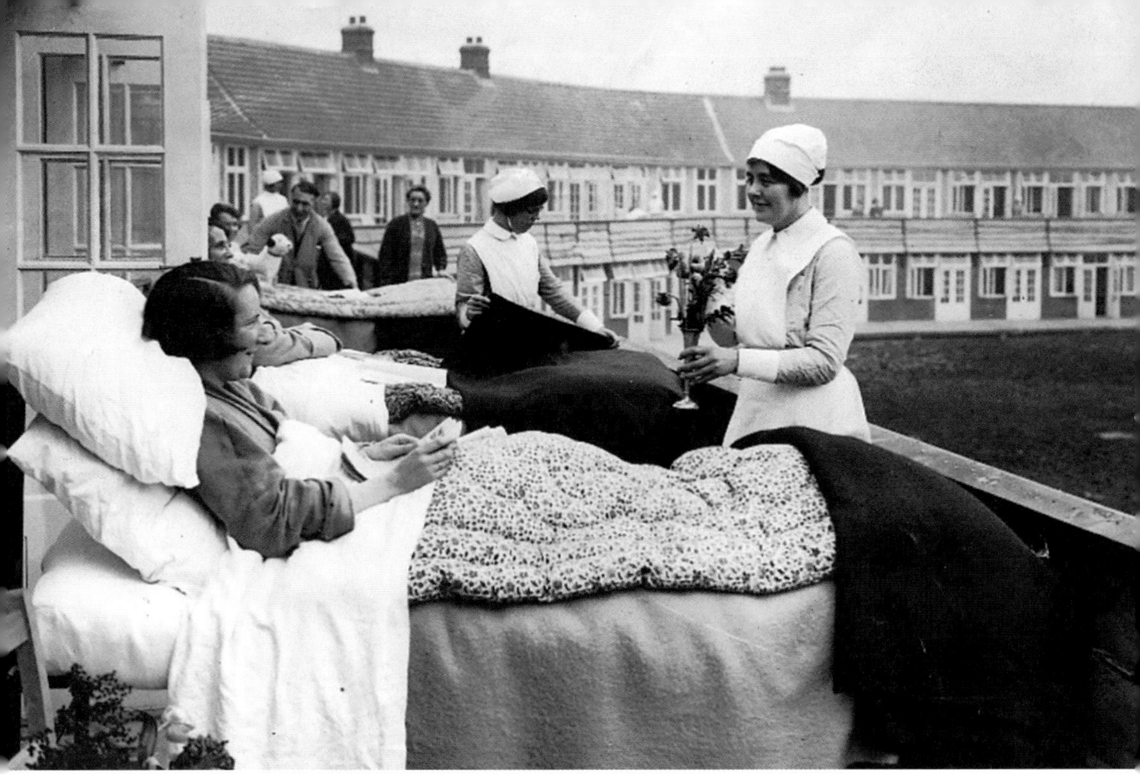

Above: Recovering tuberculosis patients receiving the fresh air treatment on the balcony outside what became my office seventy years later. (*Photograph Copyright Royal Papworth Archives*)

Below: Her Royal Highness Queen Elizabeth II meeting Matron on her visit to Papworth Hospital in 1962. (*Copyright Royal Papworth Hospital*)

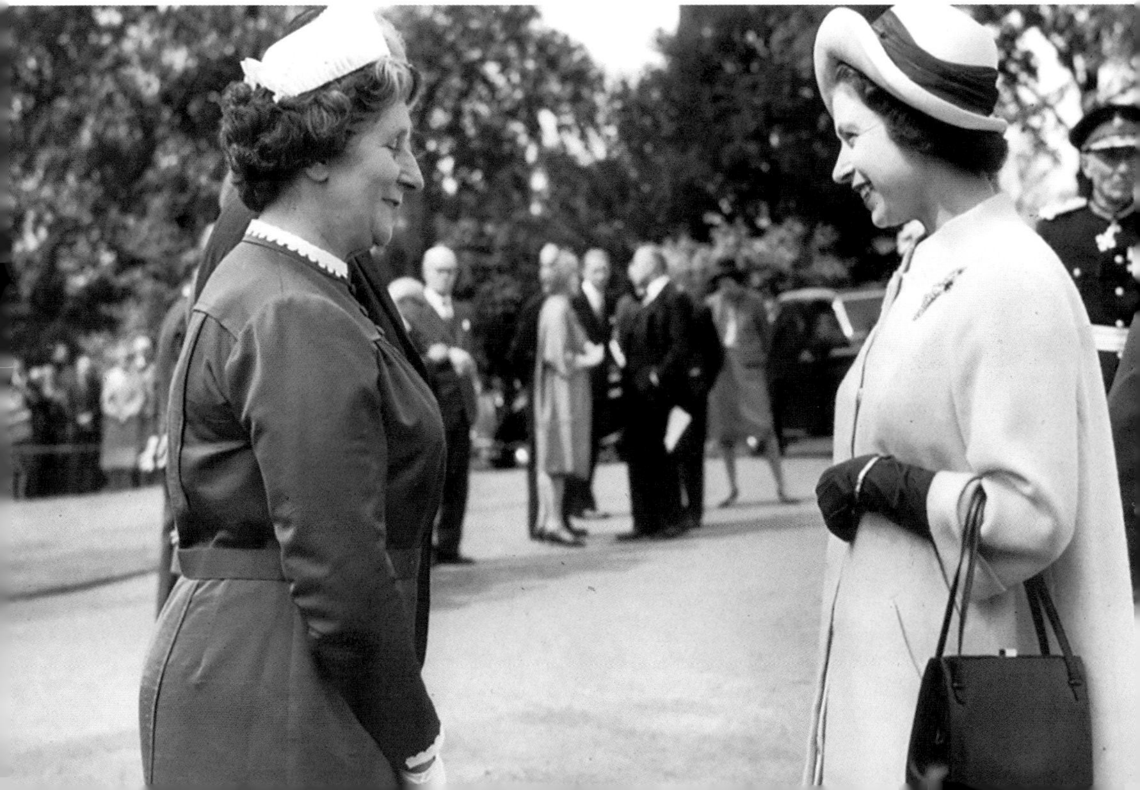

6

Demonstrating Anatomy and Physiology

The first academic step to a surgical career was to pass a tough examination: the Primary Fellowship of the Royal College of Surgeons. It was basically anatomy and physiology to a more intense level. There was a fixed pass rate of around twelve percent, acting as an initial filter to select those who were perceived to be trainable and with some degree of acuity. A common route to achieve this was to act as a demonstrator for the undergraduates in the department of anatomy.

With my house jobs coming to an end I made an appointment with Professor Glenister, who was still the head of the anatomy department. He seemed pleased with my request and granted me the post, he also spoke to Professor Julius Lee, the head of Physiology, suggesting that I cover both departments. Both men were very supportive and suggested to me that I demonstrate for six months rather than the usual full year, as they thought that I could pass the test in that time. This would also enable me to catch up some of the lost time that Harding Rains considered an obstruction to a surgical career. I eagerly accepted, although with some trepidation as it was a significant task to master both subjects to the required level in only six months.

Now that I was on the medical register, I was able to practice on patients. Occasionally in the interim between graduation and beginning work 'on the house' and to supplement my meagre salary I did several brief locum general practice jobs in high street lock-up surgeries. One I remember with affection was on the North End Road in west London. A single relatively anonymous door with a small brass plaque next to it signifying its designation opened directly onto the street. There was a tiny patient waiting room just inside the door on the left, and straight ahead was the small consulting room. It smelt heavily of cigarette smoke, old journals and sweat. Inside the consulting room was a very old partner's desk, with a chair in front and a swivel chair for the doctor behind. Behind that was a rather mangy examination couch, almost certainly from the Victorian period, but more recently untouched as it was covered, several feet high, with old *British Medical Journals* and copies of *The Lancet*, mostly unopened. There was a further door to the right-hand side of the consulting room which I didn't open. I was to find out later where it went. I had several air stewardesses booked in for vaccinations for foreign travel. One morning a young woman entered the consulting room for her 'jabs'. I asked her if she wanted them in her arm or her bottom. She elected for her Gluteus Maximus to prevent any visible lesion on her arm as her uniform had very short sleeves.

Once I had taken the vaccines from the fridge and checked them in the usual way, the young lady adopted the position over the partner's desk and lowered her underwear to allow appropriate access. At that point the phone rang and caught me by surprise. I picked up the receiver to find an extremely excited Indian-sounding gentleman on the line desperately telling me that his son had his head stuck through some railings close to the surgery and would I please come quickly to help. I tried to explain that this would not be appropriate and that he should dial 999 for the emergency services. However, he would not be put off and kept getting more and more excited, insisting that I attend. At that point I recognised an intonation in the voice that gave away the stunt that was being pulled by the also newly graduated Dr Davidson. Realising what was happening, I knew that I was going to burst with laughter and that I had to do something to disguise it, as my patient was patiently waiting with her bottom in the air. An outburst of laughter from me could have been seriously misconstrued. I made a dash for the mystery door to regain control. As I yanked the door open, I was met with a veritable avalanche of mops, brooms and buckets full of cleaning materials and yet more magazines. The game was up, and I had to explode with laughter and then apologise most sincerely to the young patient and confide in her the joke that had been pulled on me. Thankfully the patient was very broad minded and joined in with the fun of it all.

Living in the hospital for house jobs meant that we were a very close fraternity. Impromptu parties were common at weekends. Occasionally things got pretty wild and on one occasion I remember a fire-extinguisher fight on the top floor of the hospital which caused a bit of a mess and got us into huge trouble with the matron, but it was all soon forgotten.

At the end of the year I needed to find somewhere else to live than the hospital accommodation at Charing Cross. Sally Furbanks was a fellow student in our clinical years. She had bought a beautiful bijou apartment on the bank of the River Thames in Chiswick. Sally and her partner and fellow student John Williams had decided to go to work in Canada for a year and she was looking for someone to rent and look after her new home. I was delighted to seize the opportunity and the day after ending the medical houseman's job I moved in with my few possessions and little red Austin Healey Sprite. It was an enjoyable drive to the hospital each day, across Chiswick Bridge with its lovely view of the River Thames.

Demonstrating to the undergraduate students in both anatomy and physiology was an intense experience However, apart from my relationship with Helen, it was a somewhat lonesome life as there was so much work to cover in such a short period of time but one that I thoroughly enjoyed. Being back in the anatomy department with Reg and his brother Fred was fun. Since the formaldehyde-fume-filled days of second MB 'health and safety' had stepped in and insisted that changes be made in the dissection room, now on the top floor of the new hospital in the medical school wing. The prosected body parts were kept in large metal tanks and Reg and Fred had to wear huge full-face masks with breathing tubes and air filters. They often had heated verbal exchanges, but with those masks on, they couldn't really hear what each was saying so these rapidly escalated to shouting matches. The sight of them both going hard at each other with their visors steaming up and their faces becoming redder and redder was hilarious.

This time around I was teaching anatomy and had to conduct the bi-weekly viva tests for the students prior to them moving on to the next anatomical region. My work rate to keep up was intense but having had such a good grounding the first time around, the detail seemed to return fairly easily. I had to conduct supervisions in physiology as well so there was very little time for play. However, as the old saying goes 'If you can teach it, you know it.' This certainly rang true for me in that situation. Life consisted of games of squash, lots of study and endless supervisions of the first and second year students.

My other preoccupation was my unreliable little red sports car. I seemed to travel more miles on the back of an Automobile Association relay wagon than under my own steam. Late one Friday evening in the wintertime I set off on the 167-mile journey to Clun for a weekend at home. I got as far as the White City stadium in west London when the car broke down yet again. I called the now familiar number for roadside assistance and waited. Eventually a lovely AA man arrived and after much grunting and heavy breathing by torchlight under the bonnet declared that it was unfixable. He asked where I was going and didn't seem at all phased when I told him,

Clun in South Shropshire. After making a call on his radio he informed me that he could take me as far as the Newport Pagnell service station where another driver would meet me and take me the rest of the way. As we drove north the fog came down and visibility steadily diminished. By the time we had reached the designated service station the fog was quite dense. My poor little Austin Healey 'Sprout' was off-loaded in the middle of a very large car park, and I was directed to the cafeteria to keep warm and have some nourishment for the journey ahead. Some hours passed and the cafeteria (thankfully an all-nighter) emptied out until there were just the cleaners, the bar staff and me remaining. Eventually I was roused from a half sleep by a gruff voice calling out my name. My relay man had arrived. The only problem was that when we went outside to find the car, the fog was so dense that you could hardly see your hand in front of your face. Where was my car? After wandering about for what seemed ages with a torch beam reflected at us by the fog, we walked straight into it. Having found it, my helpful relay man loaded it onto the back of his truck and off we went into the murky night at a very slow speed. The journey took us over the Clee Hill. There were steep drops on our left-hand side, which caused me some concern. By now it was after 3.00 a.m. In the journey over the hill, the driver kept nodding off and I had to keep digging him in the ribs to keep us on the road. Finally, we arrived in silent and sleepy Clun.

My knight errant set about off-loading my troubled motor car. The first thing that he had to do was drag two metal ramps to the ground. The metallic screeching noise was horrendous, and as I looked around the square, I could see lights coming on in the bedrooms and the curtains twitching as the locals peered out to see what on earth was happening. The car was successfully unloaded in front of the shop and the lonely AA driver set off to his own bed. I was quite worried about him with his somnambulant state. I retired to bed and slept soundly until the mid-afternoon on Saturday. When I woke the car was in the same place that we had left it the night before and I went into the shop to ask Dad when it might go the garage to be fixed. To my amazement Mr Edwardes the Garage (as in Dylan Thomas's *Under Milk Wood*, each of the tradesman in the village was identified by their occupation, viz, Wells the Butcher, Evans the Milk and Edwardes the Garage) had already taken it and replaced the water pump and returned it. This was just one of several adventures that the Sprite and I experienced together.

My studies for the Primary were intense and I also had to take steps to organise my next job, presuming success in the Primary examination. I now just had to do the work. I don't think that I have ever worked so hard before or since. The exam came around quickly. Fortunately, it went well, and

I passed with proxime accessit to the Hallet prize for the pooled national results. The Hallet prize for the highest mark in the examination, which has to be above 90% at the first sitting, was introduced in 1927 by Mr Hallet, who had been the secretary to the examination board of the Royal College of Surgeons since the inception of the examination in 1884. It is funded by the money that was to be awarded to him for his long and distinguished service to the college. His generosity of spirit led him to donate the money as the prize for the student. The entry in my diary reads,

> Tuesday June 14th, Vivas all day. 1.50 pm Pathology, 2.30, Physiology, 3.30, Anatomy, 4.40, RESULTS! PASSED!! Waited until 5.30 for them to be announced. Only 8/76 passed, ~6%.

It was a deliberately tough test to negotiate as it was the first filter on the way towards surgical practice. As I was to discover, and as recounted in Richard Gordon's novel *Doctor in Love*, multiple attempts were common. One of the senior house officers in my next job in A&E had sat and failed it eight times.

The casualty department in King's College Hospital, Denmark Hill was part of my fast-track master plan. It was (and still is I believe) recognised as the busiest and most intense in London. I made my application to start that July, on completion of the Primary, and was fortunate to be accepted.

Once again, on completion of the demonstrator's job, I had to change roles and accommodation overnight. I had begun my next job at King's College Hospital on 1 July. I moved into hospital accommodation just off Denmark Hill. The address was Binfield Court, and it lived up to its name. It was a small, second floor, one-bedroomed apartment. The previous occupants had left it in a terrible state with excrement on the walls. It stank of old food, long ingrained into the fabric of the walls. This was to be the first home following my marriage to Helen, not exactly the way that I had wanted to start married life together, but Helen, stoical as ever, knuckled down to make it as habitable as possible.

7

Marriage and Surgical Training

I had met Helen, who was to become my wife, in my last year as a student. Her parents were dairy farmers in Cheshire. My parents were very accepting of her because of our common backgrounds in the countryside and with finals now passed and the house jobs out of the way, we planned to get married after my hopeful passing the Primary Fellowship in the summer of 1977. Her parents were very welcoming and I found a warmth and comfort in their home that I had not experienced in my own. Being dairy farmers, they lived in a classic Georgian-styled farmhouse in the lush countryside of Cheshire. Helen's local friends were a nice and fun group of people with whom we developed strong friendships. Their lives were varied and included a judge, a plasterer, several farmers, and diverse other occupations. A favourite meeting place was the pub in Crowton, or The Pheasant close by. Mr Stubbs senior was a large and jovial man who loved smoking his pipe, shooting and horse racing; he was frequently to be found watching the latter on the television. He introduced me to my first TV remote control, a long bamboo stick with which he could press the buttons to change channels without leaving his armchair. When not required for that he would use it to poke the embers of a dying fire in the grate. A simple multipurpose remote control. I don't remember him doing a lot of farming. My brother-in-law Philip, a bit of an Elvis Presley lookalike, was married to a lovely girl Liz, who was extremely tolerant of his obduracy and a wonderful mother to her children. Liz's mother ran a pub and was a glamorous and chatty lady, always interested in everything that I got up to in my career. Christmases in Crowton were always enjoyable. It seemed frequently to snow or be very icy. Visits to the local pubs to meet friends, all of whom were very gracious to me, or hearty meals in the farmhouse kitchen by the Aga cooker with a real fire in the grate, gave to me the homely feelings that I had infrequently experienced before. I will always be grateful to Helen's family for that.

In keeping with the mores of the times, Helen and I did not live together prior to our marriage but kept our separate accommodation. Helen had an apartment in the Bohemian area of Queensway, west London, right next to the tube station of that name. A highlight for me was going to Queensway, where Helen was sharing a flat with another British Airways stewardess and hearing of their adventures. We planned for a classical but simple wedding on the farm, which was a short walk from Crowton church. The date set was for the beginning of August.

I asked Andy, my impressionist friend, to be my best man, a risky decision in light of his previous pranks; however, he could scrub up quite nicely when the need arose, and we had been through a lot together. Helen and I were married on 16 July 1977. Many of my medical school friends made the journey up to Cheshire for the occasion. I was particularly touched by the fact that Dr Scott, for whom I had been houseman on my medical firm, had accepted my invitation to the wedding and duly arrived with his wife and a generous wedding present, a silver Victorian engraved salmon knife and fork. The inscription accompanying it read, 'A bit of Victoriana from your late and ageing boss.'

Afterwards we honeymooned in Corfu and enjoyed the rest that I desperately needed. On the way, we stopped for a couple of days in Athens to visit the Parthenon. It was a sunny and restful break. The return from that beautiful island to Binfield Court in the depths of south London was hardly salutary. From a brief sojourn in paradise we were back in reality with a bang.

Following the wedding Helen continued working at Heathrow but had switched to South African Airways. Her father had bought her a blue Renault 5, considerably more reliable than my little Sprite. It was needed for her journey from Denmark Hill to Heathrow.

Accident and Emergency

There were six of us casualty officers covering all shifts in the department. We regularly saw in excess of 400 patients in a 24-hour period. There was an emergency receiving room for major trauma, heart attack victims and other serious life-threatening conditions. The walking wounded were booked in and given a ticket with a summary card placed in a wooden card holder in the consulting rooms reception area. There were two of us on at any one time. Strictly in turn we took the top card out of the box and saw that patient. This prevented anyone sifting through, to find the easiest or most appealing case. As a result, frequent surprises lay in wait for us.

One day, intruding into the early afternoon routine of sprained ankles, chest infections and other serendipitous injuries we began to receive some people with serious lacerations, who had been attacked by a wild man wielding a machete. With the help of the plastic and general surgeons the injured were moved to appropriate wards for surgical repair. About an hour later, I pulled out a card with no information on it other than a name and number. I called for the patient to come in and a man in a brown overcoat entered with his right hand hidden in the fold of the coat. He sat opposite me and I began to ask him what his problem was. At first, he would not answer, but then I noticed what looked like blood stains on the front of his coat. He followed my eyes and suddenly brought out the blood-stained machete, shouting that he had come to finish the job that he had begun in Peckham. Under the desk was a panic button which connected to the local police. With my left hand I pushed the button frantically, and at the same time yelled for help and lunged forwards to grab the wrist of the hand holding the weapon. I managed to get both my hands onto his wrist and my lunge across the desk threw him onto the ground. We had a little Chinese sister in charge that afternoon and she came running to help. Her bravery was amazing, and she threw herself onto him to help hold him down. Others piled in to help. Together we overpowered him and shortly afterwards three burly police arrived and took him away handcuffed. After a quick restorative cup of tea together we all carried on.

On another occasion a schizophrenic woman had wandered away from the nearby psychiatric hospital, dressed only in her nightgown. She entered casualty clearly wanting help. I went up to her and began to talk to her. She was very agitated and suddenly ran out of the department onto Denmark Hill, shedding her nighty as she went. I set out after her. Heads turned as I gave chase in my white coat with stethoscope swinging wildly from my neck. I managed to catch up to her by the traffic lights at the bottom of the hill and tried to grab her and to wrap her in my white coat to protect her modesty. She resisted violently and the expression on the face of a policeman who appeared around the corner was worth a picture. A young male wrestling a naked woman to the ground in broad daylight was not a common sight. Once we had covered her and calmed her down an ambulance arrived and we were able to move her back to the psychiatric department.

On another occasion I found myself being chased around an examination room by a burly psychotic patient trying to kill me with a full oxygen cylinder. There was a trolley in the middle of the room, and he was running around it trying to catch me, swinging the cylinder wildly. Once again I was rescued by the nursing staff and the department porters. Jamming the trolley against him and pinning him to the wall we were able to disarm him and to calm him down. This was not before I had sustained some fractured ribs, but the situation was brought under control.

There were frightening, traumatic events. The weekend nights were often the scariest, with loud and aggressive drunks and drug addicts. One young man was brought in fighting drunk with blood pouring from a large and deep laceration in his scalp. He had attacked his father with a knife. His father, being sober, avoided the knife and hit his son over the head with a full bottle of beer, leaving a deep and long laceration with the skull bone showing beneath. Luckily there was no skull fracture. The wound needed stitching, but he would not let us anywhere near him. He was threshing around and spraying blood everywhere. We happened to have two police officers who had called in to see that everything was under control. Their timing was perfect. They could see the problem that I was having and came over to help. 'Don't worry sir' one said, 'we can sort this out'. There was a metal bar running across the room about one foot below the ceiling. Swiftly they pinned the man between them and lifted him up simultaneously placing a handcuff on one wrist. This was passed over the bar and the other wrist fixed in the other end of the handcuffs. He was now slung from the ceiling with one officer supporting his chest and the other holding his legs still. 'There you are Doc', they said, 'now you can sew up his head.' I stood on a chair and proceeded to do just that. Once done he was unpinned and placed on a gurney where he quickly fell asleep and was wheeled off for a head scan. Thankfully there was no surprising damage to the brain and no sign of internal bleeding. He was allowed to sleep off the alcohol before returning home, probably to repeat the process.

One week in six we had to work night shifts. If memory serves me well, we began at 8.00 p.m. and worked through until 8.00 a.m. the next morning. The workload was variable but never dull. The worst part about it, from my point of view, was that there was serious building work going on right next to Binfield Court and the noise level was high. Added to the building site cacophony was a very noisy Alsatian dog that seemed to bark at anyone and everything. It seemed to spend most of its life attached to a lamppost in the yard on a heavy chain. Its owner was a burly, aggressive, and uncouth man. Sleep was elusive, to say the least, under those conditions.

At that time, we had a 'very' senior house officer who had sat and failed the primary fellowship many times. On the last occasion of failure, out of spite, and under the influence of a considerable amount of alcohol, he had brought in a wheelbarrow full of bricks and bricked up the entrance to the dean's office. Needless to say, that was his last act of defiance, being ejected from the training programme.

It was later in that year that my interest in the anatomical works of Leonardo da Vinci were rekindled. My interest had begun whilst studying art at school, albeit before I realised that I would be studying medicine, but more of this later.

Brompton Hospital: Real Cardiac Surgery

My first real venture into the world of heart and chest surgery began at Brompton Hospital, recognised as one of the trail blazing hospitals in the world in that specialty. I had been encouraged to apply for a post there by Dr. Maini who knew Christopher Lincoln, Brompton's paediatric cardiac surgeon. I applied for the resident surgical officer's (R.S.O.) post and with Dr. Maini's help had been offered the job, following an informal interview by Christopher. Now with my next job secured and another of my planned posts ticked off the list, the remaining time at King's passed quickly in a blur of trauma and mayhem. I had learnt a great deal but was pleased to leave that post behind. Christmas passed happily, again being only allowed a two-day break, as we were on the move to new accommodation in Neville Street for the post at Brompton.

10 B Neville Street is a regency-style townhouse owned by the hospital, just off the Fulham Road, very much up-market from Binfield Court. It was a one-minute walk from the hospital, also making Helen's journey to Heathrow much easier than from Denmark Hill. However, I wasn't to spend much time enjoying the surroundings. On arrival I was informed that the other resident surgical officer that was supposed to be working with me Dr Sam Basu had failed to arrive. I was asked whether I would mind covering until such time as he did? Clearly there was no option, and I willingly agreed. One-in-one on call, that is every day and every night, for paediatric and adult cardiac surgery for a novice such as me, was daunting, but what could a budding young hopeful say to such a request? The next six months were fascinating and hellish at the same time. The workload was enormous, but the clinical cardiology that I witnessed was exhilarating. The hospital was wonderful to work in. It had a tight family feeling and the nurses were generous with their help and teaching. One of the perks we were allowed was cans of beer bought by the consultant staff for us juniors and placed on the table in the dining room for dinner every evening. Difficult to imagine now in this wokist world that we inhabit.

I was working with two charismatic surgeons, as different from each other as could be imagined. One, Christopher Lincoln, brilliant and an outstanding, was some way off-field on the spectrum of personality extremes. He was a tall and elegant man with large hands that made you wonder how he could possibly work on such tiny hearts. He often spoke gazing upwards as though to the heavens with his eyes half closed. His words carefully judged, relatively sparse and enunciated with the effort and clarity of a classical Shakespearean actor. His bedside manner was somewhat lacking to the extent that the registrar and I would return to the parents of the children at the end of a consultant ward round to translate and to reassure them that their child was in very capable and experienced hands. Chris worked hand in glove with Professor Robert Anderson and Dr Elliot Shinebourne. Dr. Anderson, or Bob, as he was affectionately called was another Shropshire lad like me and a world expert in cardiac morphology and development. He would often come to theatre to guide Chris through the complex anatomy of congenital cardiac anomalies. Elliot was the first in-house paediatric cardiologist at Brompton, at a time when the subject was in its infancy. A short man with tousled hair and a somewhat stammering speech, he was always kind and informative to patients and us junior staff. The knowledge and experience of that triumvirate seemed extraordinary to me in this other world of paediatric cardiac anomalies. Complex, awe-inspiring and exceedingly challenging, it was really still in its infancy of development.

Chris could be quite fierce in surgery. I remember in one complex and difficult case he had draped several sutures over my hands separately when a problem arose and he had expected me to make some manoeuvre or other without explaining what it was that he wanted me to do. Before I could move out of the way I felt a sharp wrap on the knuckles of my immobilised hand. He had hit me with forceps for not having yet another spare hand. I suggested politely to him that there was little I could do other than to put down all of the sutures that he had draped over my hand, and perhaps we would get on a lot better without the physical assault. He took it in good part and we carried on. He was always polite to me after that. We were not vexed by things such as this as we all knew that he was trying his best for these, oh so young, frail children, when a single slip could cost the life of the child.

One night, after a long and difficult operation together Chris, who was always available for his patients, had spent a long time on the intensive care unit getting a baby stable; finally, being quite exhausted he had retired to his apartment, which was not far away. I was left to supervise the care overnight. The child had complex transposition of the great vessels and other intracardiac anomalies with poor ventricular function. In this condition the aorta, the main artery supplying the body under high pressure, remains connected to the right ventricle and vice versa. This puts enormous strain on a chamber not genetically designed to be able to withstand it and creates a pressure in the lungs that is also much higher than normal. It is a life limiting condition and one that cannot support typical development. The operation had been to correct the malalignment of the great vessels and the ventricular pumping chambers. As the night progressed the baby was not doing well and was deteriorating. It was the practice then that we RSO's would stay by the bedside all night if necessary. As the night wore on and we entered the small hours, the baby's condition began to deteriorate further and I had to make several calls to Christopher to ensure that we were doing the correct things. Finally, when I had the child on maximum support and had had to re-open the chest to relieve compression on the heart, I called Christopher back for help. The phone was answered after a few more rings than before, which ought to have alerted me, but didn't. I launched straight into a cascade of information,

> ...the left atrial pressure is this, the filling pressure on the right side is very high, the chest is open and there is no bleeding, etcetera, etcetera. What do I do next please?

There was a long pause and a deep drawing of breath before speaking. The response went like this,

> Goodness me what a very exciting life you lead. I'm sorry but I cannot help you, you have the wrong number, I'm an accountant.

One can only imagine the stories that the unfortunate recipient of the call told at future dinner parties. After the right call had been made, Christopher came back into the hospital. We took the child back to theatre and were able to reverse the decline and I am happy to be able to say that a full recovery was made – by all of us – although I cannot vouch for the anonymous recipient of my somewhat hysterical call.

During my time with Chris, I was given a project to study the mental development of children who had been subjected to profound hypothermic circulatory arrest to allow complex cardiac surgery to be performed on the still and bloodless heart. The child would be placed on cardio-pulmonary bypass and the whole body cooled down to around sixteen degrees centigrade. The circulation would then be stopped, as at that temperature the metabolic rate is slowed to almost imperceptible levels and the complex surgery undertaken. At the end, the circulation would be restarted and the child re-warmed. It remains a very well-established method of organ protection and adjunct to safe surgery in very complex situations. However, the effect on brain development and function was little known. We designed a study where the children's cerebral function would be tested by trained professional child psychologists when they reached the age of five years. We compared the findings with those for a control group of children operated on without the circulatory arrest. What we found was that there was no discernible difference up to a circulatory arrest time of forty-five minutes. After that point, steadily worsening effects could be identified in the circulatory arrest group. It was slow and painstaking work, done in conjunction with the psychology department of University College London. I was able to complete most of the work during my time with Chris whilst at Brompton. There was a considerable amount of processing of the data that had to be done following this and the work was not ready for presentation until 1982. We submitted the paper to the American Association of Thoracic Surgery, where it was accepted for presentation at the 1983 annual meeting in Atlanta, and afterwards for publication in the prestigious *Journal of Thoracic and Cardiovascular Surgery*, more of which later.

The other consultant on that firm was Matthias Paneth. A tall, slim, elegantly dressed man, always in a well-fitting pin-stripe suit. He always drove a Porsche. Each morning we looked for it in the car park to register his arrival. He was always in the hospital by 7.30 a.m. Doing ward rounds with Matt was always an amusing affair. His wry sense of humour was in evidence with all of his interactions with patients and staff alike. He was very knowledgeable and highly experienced and was an excellent cardiologist as well as surgeon. His favourite sport was baiting the cardiologists on the ward. The only two adult cardiologists who could compete were Derek and Ronnie Gibson. Derek had many of the traits of autism and was brilliant. He did much of the original work in developing the technique of echocardiography. He would visit theatre with Matt and they would competitively recite the poems of Hilaire Belloc across the drapes. One of his favourites was 'The Water Beetle', taken from Belloc's *Moral Alphabet*. It goes like this:

> The water beetle here shall teach, a sermon far beyond your reach. He flabbergasts the Human race by gliding on the water's face. With ease celerity and grace, But if he ever stopped to think of how he did it, he would sink. Moral: Don't ask questions.

Matt would frequently quote it at me if I was perceived to be asking too many questions, to which he may not have always known the answer. Ronnie Gibson was the complete opposite of Derek, suave and always well dressed in broad pinstripes and with a red handkerchief flamboyantly dangling from his top pocket. He had a large private practice and would deign to visit from time to time for ward rounds and outpatient clinic. Needless to say the two hardly saw eye to eye.

Matt was nothing if not a pragmatist. One day, we entered the room of a patient who had undergone surgery for an extensive abscess in his chest, otherwise known as an empyema. The infection had eroded through into his lung and his progress was steadily downhill. As we entered the room with the ward sister, he began to cough violently. Suddenly the wall opposite him was spattered with bright, fresh, red blood. Clearly it was a terminal event. As cool as a cucumber, Matt clasped my forearm and said 'Wells this is no place for a boy. Sister the morphine if you please'. The poor man was eased of his misery and we moved on.

Matt was an inveterate chess player, and he would always have a game in progress during the operating lists. His opponent was invariably a wonderful quiet anaesthetist Dr. Ian English, who had previously worked at Papworth in its early days. When interrupted by a case ready to be operated upon they would pause the game, only to resume as the registrar closed the chest.

Matt knew that my father had a butcher's business and asked one day if I would bring him some of our meat the next time that I went home. Of course, I agreed and asked Dad to prepare his best cuts of beef for me to take to the Paneth family. The next time I went to Shropshire, I brought back most of a side of beef for the Paneth's deep freeze. They were very appreciative and frequently commented to me that they had enjoyed some Wells' sirloin, or stewing steak the night before and that it was some of the best beef they had ever had.

In return, Matt asked if my father might like to come and to watch some heart surgery. When I asked him, he jumped at the chance and the date was arranged. The day dawned and Dad was escorted up into the viewing gallery, and with the patient's full consent (as I recall he, the patient that is, found it rather amusing) we set about the procedure. Afterwards we repaired to the excellent Italian restaurant, sadly no more, San Frediano's just up the street from the hospital. As lunch progressed Matt turned to my father and asked him, 'Well Mr Wells, what do you think of our surgery?' Dad thought for a moment before saying, 'Well, Mr Paneth, the surgery was all very well, but your operating theatre would not pass our slaughter house regulations. The dust on the theatre light was at least an inch thick.' They laughed and

Dad went on to extol the difficulties of his business over that of Matt's by saying 'and of course Mr Paneth, we have to sell our product at the end of the day'. Needless to say, they got on extremely well. On the strength of that relationship, the Paneth's frequently invited me to their home for dinner.

My birthday that year ended on a sour note. It was a snowy late Monday afternoon, and feeling quite exhausted after a long weekend on call with multiple surgical procedures and endless intensive care unit work, I returned to 10B to find the front door of the house wide open with snow drifting into the hallway. Helen had gone to visit her parents in Cheshire and wasn't expected back for several days. I made my way upstairs to our first-floor apartment to find the door open and swinging in the wind. As I entered, I saw that the flat had been badly damaged with drawers lying emptied onto the floor, clothes strewn all over the place and all my expensive medical books scattered about. To my absolute horror I then saw that ink had been thrown over them and clearly someone had urinated on the pile of books and clothes. We had few luxury items, but our small colour Grundig television that I had bought in the pre-Christmas sales had gone, as had my camera and some of our wedding gifts. A miserable end to an exhausting long weekend. I called the police who came along and took details. Whilst they were there, we noticed that a window on the first floor had been prised open; the method of entry was clear. Neighbours across the street had seen two young, scruffy individuals climbing a ladder to that window but had thought little of it at that time. The police were not hopeful of solving the crime but said they would do what they could. Surprisingly, some weeks later I had a call from the Kensington police telling me that they had retrieved our stolen items and apprehended the individuals. Apparently, they were drug addicts looking for money or items that they could sell to sustain their habit.

The police invited me to their station, where they said that they had items for me to identify. I was taken to a back room which, on opening the door, appeared to be a poor Aladdin's cave with many items stacked haphazardly around the room. The jolly policeman directed my attention to what looked like our television but its plastic surround was melted into stalactites drooping down one side. They clearly had some hot item standing on it for some time. I said that it was ours and began to thank him for the retrieval, but was not sure whether it would work. Those concerns were alleviated when, after asking me if we had home insurance, which we did, he put his size eleven policeman's boot through the screen. Turning to me with a big grin he said, 'I will write a report to state that it was smashed by the thieves. You can get a nice new one from the insurance.' The theft and its resolution appeared on the front page of the *South Kensington Gazette* later that week.

Those days at Brompton set the seal on my desire to practice cardiothoracic surgery. The dynamism of the heart and the circulation fired my imagination. The fact of operating on the human heart and all that it entails was magical to my mind.

During that time several well-known world authorities visited and lectured to us. Professor Binet was a distinguished paediatric surgeon from Paris. I was despatched to Heathrow airport to meet him and to take him to his hotel. To have personal time with such distinguished people was priceless. Similarly, I met Professor Hermes Grillo. He was an anglophile and the father of tracheal surgery, based at Harvard Medical School. His societal orientation was European and he exuded a profound classical knowledge, delivered in a soft Bostonian accent that was very engaging. That meeting led to being invited to spend a week with him at Harvard, time that I will never forget. Being taught tracheal surgery by the master and being able to bring the skills back to the UK was wonderful. Sadly, Professor Grillo died in a road traffic accident in Italy whilst being transported in a taxi from an international meeting.

Another great name that I was able to meet was Professor Dwight McGoon. He was the head of surgery at the Mayo Clinic. He spent the day in the hospital and gave an outstanding lecture on aspects of paediatric cardiac surgery following which he gave me a considerable amount of his time considering my lowly position at that point. He was an important pioneer in mitral valve reconstruction before replacement valves were available, and before valve preservation was popularised by Professor Alain Carpentier. In later years I gave lectures entitled Mitral Valve Repair: the American Correction, as opposed to the French correction proselytised by Carpentier and was able to celebrate McGoon's early important contributions to mitral valve surgery. Carpentier had largely ignored McGoon's work in his presentations. Carpentier had so dominated the area in the early 1980s, that even the American surgeons had lost sight of McGoon's important contributions. I was delighted to be able to say a personal posthumous thank you to him by presenting his work back to the American surgeons. Their gratitude to me for doing so enhanced my credibility in North America immeasurably

Despite the reputation of cardiac surgeons as being highly arrogant there were, and still are, a few of great humility. I can remember sitting in the surgeon's room in Brompton, just outside the theatre area one late afternoon, going through a presentation for the department academic meeting that same evening, when a white haired and softly spoken gentleman sat beside me. He reminded me very much of my grandfather. He knew my name, which surprised me and said:

> Please forgive me for interrupting you in your work but I understand that you are giving a lecture this evening on empyema. I am so sorry, but I cannot be there. Would you be kind enough to tell me what you are going to say?

Naturally I went through my talk for him not realising to whom I was speaking. When I had finished, he thanked me very much, said that he thought that I had prepared well and that his name was Ralph Tubbs. I was stunned and delighted at the same time. Mr Tubbs was one of the seminal pioneers in our specialty at the time of its earliest development. He had pioneered the work on mitral valvotomy, an operation to open up the narrowed rheumatic mitral valve before the era of valve replacement and his name was known all around the world. There is a surgical instrument named for him: the Tubbs dilator, used to open the stenosed mitral valve. Later, when I was in Alabama talking to the celebrated Dr. Jim Kirklin, I discovered that he was a great admirer of both Tubbs and Lord Brock, another great pioneer of those times. Like so much in science and technology in those early days, British cardiac surgery was at least the equal, and perhaps superior to much of North American surgery.

Lord Russell Brock was the son of Herbert Brock, a professional photographer and his wife Elvina Carmen. He attended Christ's Hospital School, leaving in 1921 at the age of seventeen with an arts scholarship for entry to Guy's Hospital Medical School. He won many prizes and qualified in 1927. He was married a year before graduation, which was quite unusual for the time. Brock was a fearless surgeon who had the aura of highborn stock, and who latterly admitted to having never travelled on the London underground until the day his chauffeur driven Rolls Royce broke down. He had to be guided through the maze of passages and shown how to purchase a ticket by the 'proletariat' as he would regard the populus of London. Although he was reported to have a good bedside manner with patients and was said to be very caring, equally he was a difficult man to work for and the stories told by his trainees and contemporaries, such as Matthias Paneth and Terence English, recall a strict man who did not suffer fools lightly. The stories about him are laced with memorable one line pearls of wisdom. 'Wounds heal from side to side man, not end to end', explaining the importance of adequate exposure in an operation for safety and control.

Quite what he would have made of today's minimal access surgery can only be imagined. Another such saying was 'Things are awfully simple or simply awful, always choose the former'. He was made a life peer for his contribution to British surgery.

Yet another great name that I had the privilege of meeting at that very early stage of my career was Donald Ross, a South African surgeon and contemporary of Christian Barnard. Donald was a superb technician and made many original contributions to the specialty. The Ross procedure, an ingenious idea of transferring the pulmonary artery valve into the aortic position in children is still used today. Done well it is superior to the replacement of the valve with an artificial or xenograft valve.

During my time at Brompton, I had made clear to my superiors that cardiac surgery was my goal, and I was humbly gratified that they all encouraged me in that endeavour.

Throughout that six months the work had been intense, with an average of more than 100 hours a week spent in the hospital. This was very hard on Helen my new young wife, but she bore the isolation with great fortitude.

As the weeks passed by, I was very aware that my next move was going to be extremely important. I needed a job wherein I could gain the necessary experience in the generality of surgery to pass the second part of the Fellowship of the College of Surgeons, and more importantly to gain the skills needed to be a good and competent surgeon. I had heard that the registrar rotation in Cambridge was probably the best in the country at that time, combining a lot of exposure to surgery as well as academic principals. I applied and duly went for the interview. During this the lovely Bill Everett, an abdominal and general surgeon of considerable skill and humble personality pointed out to me that I really needed more exposure to surgery to cut the mustard in a full-blown registrar job. He suggested I found a busy job at senior house office level and then to reapply. Helen and I drove back to London somewhat downhearted as we had both liked the idea of spending time in Cambridge.

However, fate took a strong hand. On arrival back in Neville Street the latest edition of the *British Medical Journal* was lying on the mat in the entrance hall. This is the journal where all of the vacant posts, or those soon to be vacant, were to be found. In the job advertisement section I found a senior house officer's post in Winchester, another lovely town with a very busy general surgical department. I applied that same evening, rushing to catch the first post in the morning.

Another post that had interested me was in Swindon, known for its very busy accident and emergency department, taking lots of road traffic accident victim from the nearby M4 motorway. I noted that if I failed to get into Winchester that would be my next goal.

Within a week, I was informed that I had been shortlisted and was invited down to Winchester General Hospital for interview.

I had not visited Winchester since briefly passing through with my parents many years before. We were very pleasantly surprised as we drove around before going to the county hospital for the interview. The hospital is on a hill near to the prison, somewhere I was to grow to know quite well, for all the right reasons I am happy to state. My visits there were to conduct the occasional outpatient clinic for the prisoners.

My interview in Winchester went well. It was chaired by Mr Mosley, the senior surgeon, who was to examine me in the final fellowship some years ahead. We had a brief tour of the hospital and after a hearty meal, as the saying goes, we drove back to London. In less than a week I received the letter offering me the job as senior house officer for six months. Just what I wanted. As the month of June 1978 dawned it was time yet again to think of packing up our meagre belongings ready for the move from London. It was going to be another midnight change over between jobs as I had to work up until the end of the last day in June. Sam Basu had never appeared and other than a few temporary locum SHOs to help me, it had largely been a job where I was on every day and weekend. I had learned a huge amount and thoroughly enjoyed the environment of that world renowned hospital. I would return.

8

Winchester, Cambridge and London Again

As previously noted, in my master plan to reach consultant stage within ten years, I had listed the surgical registrar rotation in Cambridge as a desirable destination. I was also interested in the general surgical job at St James' Hospital in Balham, where a renowned surgical educator Mr Kirk worked. Both seemed to fit the bill but a life in the university town of Cambridge held a somewhat higher appeal than the suburban reaches of London south of the River Thames. My idea was that by doing a full rotation through several specialties I could shorten the length of my training. I applied to both. However, it was Cambridge that offered me the post first, starting in January of 1979. I eagerly accepted their offer.

The remainder of my time at Brompton was hard work but it cemented my desire to train in cardiothoracic surgery.

We left our lovely house in Fulham and overnight moved into a condemned house in Winchester. It was in the middle of a row of terraced houses, built many years previously by prisoners from Winchester jail, which was just at the top of the road. Once again, we were moving at the end of the six months, and I started in Winchester on 1 July . There seemed to be very little concern for the well-being of us young trainees. The attitude was that we should count ourselves lucky to have found another job on the steep pyramid of surgical training. The higher one progressed in training, the more trainees fell off the pyramid and, with no help, had to find other routes to a life in practice. Many opted for general practice, others, in extremis, a life at sea. The idea of a run-through training programme had yet to be thought of, rather like restricting the hours worked by doctors in training.

The next six months were excellent with a real immersion in general surgery. Winchester is a beautiful old town with a huge history. The Royal

Hampshire County Hospital was at the lower half of a steep hill. The wards radiated at right angles from a long downhill corridor. Amusingly the surgical wards were at the highest point and the operating theatres were at the bottom of the hill. Wheeling the patients down to theatre could be a fraught business with the ever-present threat of a runaway trolley and the image of the porter giving chase never far from my mind. Some of the patients were clearly concerned about that possibility.

It was there that I worked with one of the most impressive surgeons of my entire career. Miss Marie South was our senior registrar, on rotation from St George's Hospital. With the glass ceiling for women fully operational she was on her second or third time around the four-year rotational period. She was vastly experienced and a wonderful pair of hands. Marie was also infinitely patient with us trainees. With her across the table from me I was taken through a huge amount of surgery in an ever-increasing complexity.

During the six months at Winchester General, I completed over 120 cases. They included: gall bladder removal, thyroidectomies, colonic resections, splenectomies, countless numbers of hernia repairs in all their guises and appendicectomies of increasing difficulty such as high retro caecal presentations. Marie finally went on to be a wonderful general surgeon in Hastings. I felt that she should have graced the hallowed halls of a top London teaching hospital. I shall never be able to thank her adequately for all that she did to train and to encourage me.

The consultant that I was working for was Mr Jim Mousely, another excellent general surgeon and real gentleman. Mr Mousely was very generous with his time and seemed to really enjoy supervising us juniors. The manners of both Jim Mousely and Marie South on ward rounds and in the clinics was exemplary. We were so fortunate to have them as our teachers. Later Jim Mousely would examine me in the final F.R.C.S. examination. Amongst his many distinctions, Jim was the ship's doctor on the second transatlantic crossing of the QE2. In his national service in the RAF he rose to the rank of squadron leader, unusual in that setting. Winchester is a relatively small city (it has a cathedral) and I remember saying to him that it must be rather nice strolling around the town on a Saturday afternoon and seeing many of his surgical successes back in normal life. His amusing answer was rather more sombre. With a wry smile he said, 'Actually you can spend quite a bit of time hiding in shop doorways avoiding your disasters.' I doubt that was true, as he was such a good surgeon, but it was a different perspective on the life of a district general surgeon. I learnt so much from him.

One of my duties was to visit a small cottage hospital in Andover to carry out a varicose vein clinic. On the first Monday of each month I would set off to spend a happy morning there. The primary management for most of them was with injection of sclerosant agents to encourage the veins to scar down. On arrival all the ladies (for the vast majority were women) would be standing on a bench with their bandages removed from their legs, ready for me to inspect the results and to plan the next stage. When this was complete, I was served with tea and toasted teacakes on a silver salver by the senior nurse and made to take a thirty minute break before seeing the second group, who were there to have their veins injected and their legs bound. Then it was back in the car and a return to the county hospital through lovely countryside for an enjoyable surgical list in the afternoon. Life was good.

As I have already mentioned, Winchester jail was close by and we were called in occasionally to help the inmates. I remember being sent to reduce an inguinal hernia that was threatening to strangulate one poor reprobate. His relief led to the promise that if ever I needed a bit of muscle, he was my man. A few days later we admitted him under prison guard for the operation. I was assured of personal protection for life. Thankfully thus far it has not been needed. The genial personalities of many of the inmates struck me time and again. For so many, the bad starts and false turns in life had led them behind bars, when what they really needed was help, education and people to take an interest in them as functional human beings, and a leg up to restart their lives in a more meaningful way. I enjoyed meeting many of them and never felt threatened.

Winchester is steeped in English history. One of the star attractions is advertised as King Arthur's round table with the names of the knights bold inscribed around the circumference. Whilst myth and legend demands that it is the original, carbon dating places it in the thirteenth or fourteenth century. It is still a magical sight. The gardens in the hospital of St Cross were peaceful and quite beautiful. Founded in 1132 by Henry of Blois, grandson of William the Conqueror, it is one of England's oldest alms-houses with continuous use for that purpose. It is described by Simon Jenkins in his book *England's Thousand Best Churches* as England's most perfect alms-house.

At Christmas we put together a show where all the hospital characters were taken off by the junior staff. Of course I took the part of Mr Mousely. I kept watch on his reactions to my shenanigans through the corner of my eye, but he took it all in very good part. In my experience there was something different about district general surgeons as opposed to those in teaching hospital academia. They felt more akin to good family GPs to me, immersed in the community that they served, rather than point scoring over other academics as was so much on show in the London teaching hospitals in particular.

During the latter part of my tenure in Winchester, the Cambridge surgical rotation was advertised and once again I applied. Again, I was short-listed for the job and invited for interview. I remember driving up to Cambridge in the late autumn for the interview, this time feeling more confident about the likely outcome. I badly needed a haircut and found a barber's shop inside the now defunct old store Joshua Taylor's, a mini-Harrods in the centre of town. The barbers were in the basement and run by a very charismatic Italian man named Domenic. He had Italian co-workers who spoke no English. Domenic would only cut your hair if you were one of the elites of Cambridge. As a newcomer I was decanted to one of his new recruits. Forty-six years later, I had my final haircut with Remi, who is retiring to return to Italy. Later he had set up his own chairs with a colleague Toni, and they rotated every six months between Cambridge and Italy where Remi had his own vines and olive trees. He will be sorely missed. One of his compatriots Franco was an extremely colourful character and almost certainly a Mafia functionary and many of the tales that he would tell have to remain sub judice. He would disappear for months on end before returning once again to Cambridge. He seemed to have connections everywhere from New York to Milan. Very sadly, whilst he survived his likely dodgy connections, he died a premature death with prostate cancer.

Resplendent with a fresh haircut, the interview went well, and we returned to Winchester fairly confident of the outcome after the encouraging words I had received from some of the consultants on the panel, particularly Professor Sir Roy Calne. I was offered the job. Now I really was making progress. On receiving the offer I could not resist allowing a self-satisfied smile as the unsupportive words of Professor Harding Rains from two years earlier went through my mind: 'You are too old to do surgery.' More than ever I thought, 'I will show you.' It became a great motivating force.

Cambridge

Once again, we found ourselves packing up to move on New Year's Eve. For the first part of the rotation we had been offered a small terraced house in the grounds of Papworth Hospital. The hospital is quite isolated in the countryside, 12 miles from Cambridge, which made it quite a change from the hustle and bustle of London and Winchester.

There were six posts, each five months long. They included cardiothoracic surgery at Papworth, orthopaedics, urology, general, vascular, and endocrine surgery, and general and transplant surgery all at Addenbrooke's. Cambridge was to be our home for the next few years. Little did I know then that this strangely and unromantically named hospital, Papworth, in the village of Papworth Everard, was going to become such a major part of my life. In truth I hated the name Papworth Everard. It conjured up tasteless images in my mind: the word Everard being the catch phrase of the 1970s comedian Larry Grayson, who often began with the phrase, 'What a gay day', and followed it with, 'Everard, shut that door.' Pap is an archaic word for a female breast, or soft unpalatable food. The derivation of the name is the farmland of Papworth which was granted by William the Conqueror to a Norman Knight, Everard de Beche. Papworth means the enclosure of Papa's people. Those same Anglo-Saxons were probably instrumental in founding the hamlets of Papworth St Agnes and Papley Grove. Running directly through the village is the old Roman road of Ermine Street, which ran from London to Lincoln and York. It became known later as the Old North Road. As with Watling Street from Dover through London to St Albans and Wroxeter, they were the main arterial routes for trade and military dominance. To this day there is an ancient feel to the area.

The turning from the main Cambridge to Bedford Road to the village is marked by the Caxton Gibbet. This was an old hangman's gibbet from which were strung highway robbers and sheep thieves in the Middle Ages. A thought that has latterly crossed my mind is that perhaps it is a solution for failing and wasteful modern-day managers of the NHS. The thought quickly evaporates out of concern for those promoted way beyond their true capacity.

There remains an incongruity to the place that was Papworth Hospital; finding an important sub-specialty hospital in such a relatively poor village may be considered strange until its history is appreciated. Why was the hospital placed there? Well, the answer lies in the fact that its health care role began as a sanatorium in the era of tuberculosis (TB). It was sited far away from conurbations to minimise the chance of disease dissemination and to give the patients the benefit of good fresh country air as there were no other meaningful treatments apart than good nourishment at that time. Others sprang up elsewhere in the country, such as Harefield in North London and Wythenshawe in Manchester.

At first the Cambridge tuberculosis colony, as they were referred to then, was started in the nearby village of Bourn by Sir Pendrill Varrier Jones in 1916. Following on from its early success in Bourn, and with a donation of

£5,000 from a wealthy philanthropist, Varrier Jones was able to purchase the pre-existing estate in Papworth Everard and to move his enterprise to that site in 1918.

The early interventions to deal with tuberculosis and its complications were limited. They were dealt with, as far as was possible, within the wards of the converted Georgian house. It had become appreciated that the bacterium was what is called a microaerophilic organism. In other words, it doesn't like too much or too little oxygen. Hence fresh air was seen as good therapy. To that end, as soon as it was thought reasonable, the patients were moved out into little huts in the grounds of the hospital. Prior to this they spent much of the day in the 'fresh air' on the balconies of the wards to saturate their infected lungs with oxygen. By the time of my arrival things had moved on somewhat, and there was just one hut preserved in the grounds for posterity.

Thoracic medicine, and later thoracic surgery, grew out of this primitive start. Collapsing the affected lung within the chest was done to compress the lung and to starve the bacillus of adequate oxygen causing its death. This was done in three ways. The first was by introducing air into the chest outside the lung, causing a pneumothorax. There is a special instrument to achieve this called a Maxwell Box. A needle is introduced into the pleural cavity and through valved tubing air is pumped into the pleural space, compressing the lung. An alternative approach was to surgically place table tennis-like Lucite balls into the chest (known as plombage). Over many years these balls could migrate up into the neck through longstanding pressure, risking injury to the blood vessels there and occasionally breaking through the skin allowing the introduction of infection into that important junctional part of the body. I had to surgically remove these Lucite (polymethyl methacrylate) balls in some patients many decades after their placement for those reasons, the patients being cured of their tuberculosis by this simple remedy. The third method was to compress the chest from below by pumping air into the abdominal cavity, driving up the diaphragm. This technique still has its use in speeding up the resolution of an air leak following lung resection although known by very few thoracic surgeons in the modern era and prevented in most places by the loss of the Maxwell Boxes. Remarkably these seemingly primitive procedures worked for many people.

The next stage was to help the afflicted patients back into a normal life. This was another remarkable project of Varrier Jones. He begun to develop a small industrial base in the village, which became known as the Papworth industries. They varied from high quality leather goods that were sold in the best shops in London's fashionable West End, to mail bags for the Royal

Mail. In addition, housing accommodation was developed for the families of the patients who mainly came from the deprived areas of east London. A movie was made describing the whole patient journey with several distinguished actors and was shown at a major film premiere in London in 1926 in front of the King.

As a result of his good works Varrier Jones was knighted, and the hospital has been visited by every reigning monarch since Queen Victoria, most recently receiving Royal ascent to the privileged title of Royal Papworth Hospital. The latest visit was from Queen Elizabeth II who graced the institution by opening the new hospital in 2019 as one of her final acts. It was her second visit, her first when still a very young Queen in 1962.

Gradually those simple forms of thoracic surgery expanded into surgery for lung cancer and benign conditions. Before this could happen, however, reliable general anaesthesia with safe lung positive pressure ventilation needed to be developed. Surgical treatments could then extend into removal of part of, or the whole lung.

The logical next step was to develop surgery on the heart. Norwich Hospital had beaten Papworth in this and were already carrying out closed heart procedures with some good success in the early 1950s. This was countered in Papworth by the appointment of Christopher Parish, a surgeon from Liverpool. He began the closed heart programme, but progress was slow. At that time Lord Brock, based at Brompton hospital was visiting Papworth in a supporting role in the development of the sub-specialty. As a result, Papworth became known as 'Brompton in the country.' Lord Brock had a feisty senior registrar Ben Milstein. Ben would travel to Papworth with his lordship and as I understand it, would sort out the problems after the great man had left. It became a natural progression then, for him to be appointed alongside Christopher Parish to a consultant post at this somewhat anomalous hospital deep in the countryside.

Ben was clever and very hard working and soon had the unit buzzing with activity. He, with Parish, introduced profound hypothermic arrest cardiac surgery. This entailed cooling the patient in a bath of ice before transferring them to the operating table for the open-heart procedure. The results were surprisingly good. It was most effective in heart surgery in children. At Brompton, Ralph Tubbs would cool the babies down and then transfer them to his knee where he would open the chest and do the surgery. Again, some excellent results were obtained.

At about that time the early heart-lung machines became available. The machines were crude and the damaging effects on the blood caused significant problems for the patients, with haemolysis (breaking up of red blood cells) and severe perturbation of the clotting cascade. Mortality was high, approaching fifty percent, not helped by the fact that patients being offered surgery were extremely late in referral.

Things took a big turn for the better when Ben and Christopher were joined by a fairly mature South African surgeon Terence English. Terence, now Sir Terence KCB, had begun life as a mining engineer and had decided to pursue a career in surgery quite late. Studying at Guy's Hospital, he had become friendly with another great pioneer in cardiac surgery, also of South African origin, Donald Ross. Being of non-English origin and having a later start, subjected him to something of a glass ceiling, in that he was the last of his generation to get a consultant job. He was offered to Ben who took him under his wing, first as a locum and then with a permanent appointment in the early 1970s.

At that time, Ben had been working on heart transplantation in pigs with Sir Roy Calne, the eminent transplant surgeon in the University of Cambridge, based at Addenbrooke's Hospital. Following the early sorties into heart transplantation pioneered by Christian Barnard, another South African, but with poor results, Roy was trying to bring his knowledge and experience in kidney and liver transplantation to bear on the heart. Roy had been engaged in animal work but with little success as he really didn't understand the more subtle aspects of open-heart surgery. Roy invited Ben to help him and between them they began to make the project work. When Sir Terence arrived, Ben suggested that he become involved, as it would be a good project for him to be part of. During this period arrangements were made for Terence to spend time with Norman Shumway in Stanford, a part of the University of California. Dr Shumway had been the real pioneer in this work, and many felt that Barnard had jumped the gun in carrying out the first human to human heart transplant as the immunosuppression was inadequate at that time. Indeed, Barnard's intervention was criticised in the wider circle of academic transplant cardiac surgeons as it was thought by many that he had simply been opportunistic. The truth lies somewhere in the middle, as Barnard himself had carried out extensive animal work at the Groote Schuur Hospital in Cape Town.

The triumvirate of Roy, Ben and Terence worked well and with the very determined organisational attributes of Terence the programme began to take shape. Roy had pioneered the immunosuppressive regime of azathioprine and steroids in his kidney transplant patients and thus it was cleared for human use. Patients were screened as recipients and a protocol was prepared for execution of the plan.

It was at this point that I joined the party. It was January 1979 and I was the most junior member of the team. Although the rotation was at registrar level, for this job we were regarded as senior house officers at Papworth, cannon-fodder in working terms. It was back to the 110 hours per week, with lots of form filling, blood taking and patient clerking. However, I now had an ace up my sleeve. I had done a huge amount of operating for my age and stage, and dear Ben recognised my experience very quickly. I was soon opening and closing chests, taking saphenous vein for coronary artery surgery and learning other surgical skills. I rapidly became familiar with a very wide range of thoracic surgical techniques.

Andrew Thorpe was the surgical registrar and with Ben had developed the first oesophageal physiology laboratory for assessing malfunctioning oesophagi. Giving it the grand name of a laboratory was something of a euphemism as there was no designated room and the equipment was wheeled from place to place on a purloined trolley from the canteen. One of the tests was to persuade an unsuspecting patient to swallow a pH probe to assess whether there was acid reflux from the stomach into the oesophagus. As Andrew was learning how to use this and needed to standardise it, he persuaded me to be a guinea pig. Of course, being the new boy on the block I agreed. Swallowing the fine probe wasn't pleasant but bearable.

I thought no more of it until that night I woke with saliva pouring from my mouth and rapidly worsening pain in my upper abdomen. I managed to get through the night, albeit with no sleep and to struggle into work. The first person I met was our lovely radiologist Dr. Bob Verney. He instantly saw that there was something very wrong with me and asked what was going on. I told him my symptoms and he instantly said 'We must do a chest radiograph and a barium swallow to check you out.' These were duly done but then came the shock. Bob had not liked what he saw on the barium swallow and without speaking to me had called Dr. John Hunter, a first-rate gastroenterologist in Addenbrooke's, and booked a gastro-duodenoscopy with him. I was dispatched in a taxi and before I knew it, I was lying sedated on the endoscopy table swallowing the probe. Once again there was shock on his face, and he told me that he wasn't sure what was going on but within my stomach my gastric ruggae (tissue folds) looked highly suspicious and he had taken multiple biopsies. The list of possibilities included gastric lymphoma. I was sent back to Papworth and to bed. Over the next few days of frantic worry things seemed gradually to improve spontaneously. I returned to work. Bob continued to look worried which didn't help me at all. Finally, the result came through. It wasn't malign, but a viral gastritis. My new buddy Andrew admitted that he had not cleaned the pH probe since the last patient and had infected me with their virus! I was relieved but angry at the same time. Certainly, it caused Andrew to be more careful over cleaning his apparatus in the future.

On 13 January, my first full weekend on call, I received a telephone call from Terence English informing me that we were going to do a transplant the following day. In my naiveté I enquired, 'What organ?' Was it to be a kidney? There had been no heart transplants in the UK since early in 1971. Because of the bad results a moratorium had been placed on the practice within the NHS. The reply came, 'No, it's a heart transplant. Go to my office and in the top right-hand drawer you will find the protocol. Take it out and read it.' I was extremely surprised as no one had mentioned the programme to me in my first few days in the hospital. I did as was asked. Things began to move quickly after that. The patient, strangely, was another South African gentleman who had worked extensively with horses, a fact that was to become vitally important very quickly. He had severe coronary artery disease and had had two previous operations, but now he was rapidly deteriorating with unremitting heart failure. A new heart was his only option.

I admitted, clerked him and gained consent. Interestingly I cannot remember any family present. The immunosuppressive agents that were in use then, were equine (horse) anti-thymocyte globulin (ATG), azathioprine and steroids. I administered the latter two drugs and began the infusion of the ATG, when suddenly he gasped and lost consciousness. I could find no pulse and on looking up at the monitor saw that his heart had stopped beating and it was fluttering in ventricular fibrillation. I immediately began cardio-pulmonary resuscitation (CPR) and gave adrenalin whilst calling very loudly for help. The crash team arrived and together we were able to get his heart back to a regular rhythm. It transpired that he was hyperallergic to horse protein, from which equine ATG was generated! We had no idea that was the case. It had not been declared nor tested in the past.

We moved him swiftly around to the anaesthetic room and called Mr English who was at Addenbrooke's Hospital where the donor was being prepared. He had already begun to remove the heart from the donor patient. Horrendous dilemma. What to do? Terence being made of stern stuff quickly made the decision to proceed as we were able to tell him that the recipient patient had regained consciousness in the anaesthetic room.

We quickly prepared the patient for surgery and began to open the chest. As he already had two previous operations through the same incision, access was difficult and the usual dense adhesions between heart and surrounding structures were encountered. Going was slow, even though our senior registrar at the time, David Cooper, was an excellent and very experienced surgeon. He had worked with Barnard in Groote Schur Hospital. As we were progressing, I noticed from a reflection in the glass portal of the operating theatre door that once again the pressure was falling, and the heart was fibrillating. Our anaesthetist at that time liked to conceal the information from the surgeons. He had missed the fact that this was happening. I immediately alerted David who was able to quickly place the necessary tubes into the heart and great vessels to allow the use of cardio-pulmonary bypass (the support from the heart and lung machine). We could not know what effect that the cardiac arrest had on the recipient's brain because of low perfusion for a period of time. Shortly after that Terence arrived with the explanted heart, scrubbed into the case, and quickly removed the old, now huge and useless, heart. His movements were well practiced from the animal laboratory and quite soon we were beginning the four long suture lines securing the new heart. On completion it was re-perfused and then we witnessed the beautiful sight of a stranger's heart beginning to beat inside the chest of another human being.

It is still one of the most humbling sights in modern medicine. It requires the immense generosity of the family of the deceased, who at a time of such immense grief have the kindness in their own hearts to agree to the donation. Even though the donor will have given their permission in advance of their death, it still requires a hugely emotional and generous act for those left behind. Then there is the sheer beauty of the sight of this life-sustaining organ beating under its own strength and resilience after being removed from one body and placed in another. At a basic physiological level there is wonder that this can be made to work so successfully and repeatedly.

We were all ecstatic at the sight of this profound medical innovation. There was a palpable sense of an immense release of tension and satisfaction palpable in the room amongst us all. Little did we know, however, what was to come.

Aside from this medical drama, another was unfolding of a professional and political nature. I had noted that in the middle of the implantation, our other consultant Ben Milstein had appeared at the theatre door in his outside clothes. He asked Terence if everything was alright and if he needed any help. Without looking up from the table, Terence stated quite abruptly, that he didn't. I was facing Ben across the table and saw him thinking deeply for a moment before turning and leaving the theatre. This was the beginning of an unspoken state of dissonance between the two of them which was to last throughout their time together at Papworth. Also, unknown to me, there was an agreement between Professor Calne, Ben and Terence that when the programme was to start that all three would be involved in the first operations. Moreover, because of the expertise in immunosuppression that already existed in Addenbrooke's surgical department, arising from the kidney and liver programme, Sir Roy had tried to insist that the heart programme should be carried out at Addenbrooke's. To the contrary, there was no expertise in the management of open-heart surgery at Addenbrooke's as a result of the geographic separation of the two hospitals. An uncomfortable compromise had been reached that the surgery would be done at Papworth, but that all three would be involved. At the time of this procedure, Sir Roy was returning from a skiing holiday and at that time of limited communication possibilities, had not been contacted. Perhaps less forgivable was the fact that Ben who lived near to Terence, only twenty minutes away, had not been contacted either. This led to a furious row behind the scenes between Terence and Roy which, sadly, was never resolved. Also Ben, who had introduced Terence to the heart transplant programme, withdrew from it and played no further part in it. A sad consequence of surgical ego.

The transplanted heart worked beautifully and the patient was transferred to the intensive care unit where he remained physiologically very stable. Later that day, the drugs keeping him asleep were withdrawn and expectations rose as we looked forward to giving him the good news. Only he didn't wake up on that day or the next, nor in the next ten days.

The depressing realisation set in that he had suffered irreversible brain damage through the low perfusion caused by the fibrillating heart at the commencement of the procedure. With massive pain and regret, the life support was withdrawn and the patient declared dead. Such a massive irony was being played out. After all the years of the moratorium, the actual transplant had been accomplished with great success, only to be dashed by a quirk of fate, placing a patient's life in the hands of a complication derived from his passion for horses. This could have ended the new attempt to resuscitate the heart transplant programme, but the tenacity of Terence eventually won the day, and the programme continued but there were no more transplants in my remaining five months on the house, but more of that later.

Both Ben and Terence did cardiac and thoracic surgery. Ben's practice was enormous, encompassing oesophageal, vascular, pulmonary and all other surgery in and around the thoracic cavity. In addition, he was an excellent, if somewhat easily angered, cardiac surgeon. Terence majored more in cardiac surgery but helped with the thoracic cases as well. At that time, Terence also did some paediatric cardiac surgery. In the absence of any in-house paediatric support this was limited. There was a third consultant Christopher Parish, whose presence was sparse. He had a pig farm nearby in Elsworth, and this seemed to keep him pre-occupied. However, when he did operate, he had beautiful surgical technique and I regretted not being able to learn more from him. After his retirement he became the librarian for Gonville and Caius College (the alma mater of William Harvey, the author of *De Motu Cordis*, the first concise description of the human circulation of the blood). Many years later, after I had become a consultant on the staff at Papworth I received a request from Christopher asking if he could come in to observe some surgery. Of course I was delighted to see him. He watched a couple of procedures and then quietly commented that not much had changed and left. I never saw him again.

Very quickly I was allowed to do quite large procedures with the help of the consultants, Ben in particular. David Cooper, our senior registrar, was also a great teacher and supported me a lot. We were joined by another senior registrar, a James Robertson Justice look alike named Richard Cory Pearce. Richard had a very rich, gravelly voice, and oozed wit and charm from the entirety of his considerable frame. He rather liked alcohol and had a very relaxed attitude towards life. The first contact I had with him was a very late Saturday night phone call. I had no idea who was calling, but a deep, drawling voice enquired to whom was he speaking. I introduced myself and asked the same of him. He gave me his name and said, 'I'm your senior registrar.' I asked him where he was and he replied, 'I don't really know, but I will call you in the morning.' This is going to be interesting I thought. He was a highly intelligent man and an extremely good raconteur. His stories were legion. He would come to work in a large pick-up truck with a chainsaw in the back and wearing cowboy boots, often accompanied by a Stetson hat. In later years he could be found in the woods at the back of the hospital with one of the transplant patients and their ferrets, pursuing rabbits and other vermin.

Infuriatingly he would rarely approach the same procedure in the same way twice. In closing the chest or cannulating the heart for cardio-pulmonary bypass he would change his technique, making it difficult to predict his next move. At the end of the case he would stand resting against the anaesthetic pole, regaling the theatre staff with stories. He was an excellent surgeon but loved the camaraderie of the job. I once asked him why he didn't do things the same way allowing the rest of us to know what was coming next. He fixed me with his beady eyes and enquired as to whether I drove the same way to work every day. I said that I did. He responded by saying that I must lead a very boring life. Two years later, when I returned as the registrar on the firm, he was still there but had been joined by a new consultant John Wallwork. Both were extremely strong characters, but Richard was rather sharper of mind, wit, and intellect. In the clinical meetings, debate would break out between them, but Richard would always win out with great humour and a greater depth of understanding of basic science which continuously amused and amazed us juniors. He was a huge talent which, channelled well, should have ensured a golden career. Sadly, that didn't materialise.

As the months passed by my experience grew rapidly. Ben was an excellent surgical mentor but also had a big interest in the arts. We spent a lot of time discussing music and literature. He was also a passionate gardener, and if he came across a knowledgeable patient his eyes would light up and he would enjoy indulging his knowledge in Latin terms for the plants and flowers of the season.

Perhaps the most outstanding thing about him was his interest in making violins and other string instruments. As previously mentioned, when he retired a concert was organised for him and the students from the Cambridge University music department played a string quartet on the cello, viola and violin that he had made.

Operating just about every day gave me huge experience both in the operative procedures but also in the post-operative care. Being in theatre all day meant long nights catching up with the ward work. There were no ward clerks to help with form filling and no haematology technicians to take the bloods from the patients. It all fell to us junior doctors. Thursday afternoon was clinic at Addenbrooke's with Ben. We saw a huge range of cases and when the clinic was finished, we started roaming the wards seeing cases referred by cardiologists, oncologists and gastroenterologists. Ben loved to tease the junior staff on the different wards to the extent that several of them used to dread his arrival. It did mean, however, that they were well prepared in presenting the cases for discussion. It was a splendid education in physical signs and how not to interact with colleagues. A style that simply would not be tolerated today.

At that time we bought our first house. It was a terraced house in Comberton, quite well placed between Papworth and Cambridge. The price was £12,000, which approximates to £50,000 in today's money.

It had been a terrific five months but now it was time to move on to orthopaedics, or as the uninterested would call it 'awfulpaedics'. A completely different challenge awaited. Murray Mathewson was a larger than life, hugely popular New Zealander who specialised in hand and back surgery. He introduced to Addenbrooke's a relatively new procedure for the correction of kyphoscoliosis (twisted spine). It involved using metal rods, called Harrington Rods, to progressively straighten the spine. It was a long, painstaking procedure and often would take most of the day. The results were progressive as the rods could be lengthened and straightened slowly over several months. His approach to hand surgery was also cutting edge work and he became highly sought after. Whilst a very genial man he had an irascible side to his character which was accommodated because of his recognised skill. His overtly logical mind did not suffer fools easily.

Our senior registrar at the time was a delightful Welsh surgeon named Tudor Thomas. Every Monday morning the three of us would go in two separate cars to Huntingdon Hospital. Tudor and I together in his or my car, and Murray in his Volvo estate car. We would do the fracture clinic whilst Murray operated. If we got on with the clinic we could finish in time to call at an excellent hostelry for some lunch on the outskirts of the town before heading back to Cambridge for an afternoon clinic. We had a regular window seat to watch out for Murray. As soon as we saw his car pass by, we would make a run for it to be back in time. The day continued into the late afternoon with another fracture clinic followed by a lengthy ward round to review the patients for the next day's operating list. This in turn was followed by operating all night on trauma patients. The morning led straight into theatre for the long Harrington Rod list. This surgery was complex and fraught with the potential risk of paraplegia if not done correctly. It meant that my role in retracting tissues and holding instruments was long and drawn out. This was tedious and following a night with little or no sleep meant that staying awake was a challenge.

On other days I was quite quickly taken through basic hip surgery and the use of the 'Watson Moore' prosthesis to replace a fractured neck of femur. One day I admitted a lovely elderly Scottish lady who had fallen, breaking her hip, on a visit to Cambridge. She had fallen whilst walking in the town. I prepared her for surgery and called Murray to inform him. He was already involved in a case at another hospital and so he said, 'You know what to do, just get on with it', and so I did. Thankfully it went well. Soon it was time for her to go home. I was going on holiday the following day, and on the ward round I asked her if she had family to take her home and she said that she hadn't. I offered to order a taxi to take her home at which she looked delighted, on reflection, almost too pleased. I thought no more of it and left for my short break. When I returned, I was summoned to the office of the hospital chief executive. I was presented with a bill for a taxi ride to Edinburgh and an overnight stop for the driver. I had forgotten to ask where she lived. The pain of paying the bill, a significant financial hit for a junior registrar's salary, was mitigated somewhat by the effusive thank you letter from the lady and her family. She expressed the wish that the Scottish NHS was as kind and supportive as the English one, a rare compliment.

From orthopaedics I moved to general surgery with an absolute gentleman Bill Everett. Bill's temperament was expressed in his surgery. He had a lightness of touch that I had not seen before. His fingers danced over the tissues and the dissection planes were clean and almost bloodless. Bill had been developing the somewhat difficult operation of forming what was known as a Koch pouch using a loop of small bowel shaped into a 'J' to reduce the number of bowel movements following an ileostomy, where the bowel is brought out onto the abdominal wall. It was ground-breaking at the time. His practice ranged over the full gamut of general surgery with a wide referral base. He was also a very good watercolourist, an interest that we shared. His daughter became a professional artist, and they hold regular exhibitions to this day.

Several surgeons are good artists and Bob Whittaker, the senior urologist, was also excellent. Bob would take his sketch pad and watercolour palette to theatres and illustrate his operations. Sir Roy Calne took his art to another level and practiced oil and watercolour painting as well as sculpting. Coached by an important contemporary artist John Bellany he developed a reputation of his own in the art world. Bellany had been a patient of Roy, undergoing a liver transplant by him. They struck up a close relationship as a result. Surgery requires excellent hand to eye co-ordination and the ability to see in three dimensions. Also, good imaginative thinking for reconstructive work is essential in all aspects of surgery, an important attribute also found in the arts. Several surgical meetings have exhibitions of work by surgeons as a part of the proceedings.

There is a significant role for the humanities in medicine. It was ever thus, but as science had taken a rightful stronger hold on the profession, the role of the humanities was being forgotten. This is slowly being rectified in the modern world and an appreciation of the arts is growing again. The College of Surgeons has run courses in sculpture, and art courses are common. Several medical schools are now incorporating a course unit on the humanities. There are many aspects to this, from the intellectual exercise of appropriate ethics to the relevance of an appreciation of the arts in general, and the execution of artistic modalities in the influence on looking and seeing deeply and cogently.[1]

The arts also have a considerable role in patient well-being. This appreciation was expressed as far back as the very early Renaissance. Frescoes on the wall of the hospitals during that period were heavily religious, but they also illustrated life in the hospitals at that time. There are particularly beautiful examples in the hospital of Santa Maria della Scala in Sienna. Giovanni d'Andrea della Robbia produced beautiful ceramic wall mountings for the Ospedale del Ceppo in Florence.[2] This has been appreciated once again in modern times. The Chelsea and Westminster Hospital took this on as a serious project. As a result, they have turned their hospital into a gallery of beautiful art.[3] We will return to this subject later.

Although life was busy, we managed to find time to enjoy music concerts, the opera and ballet. Nureyev was still dancing, and I saw him perform several times.

During this time, we also bought our first house. 52 Harbour Avenue was a middle terrace house in the nearby village of Comberton. The drive to Addenbrooke's through Grantchester was relaxing and an easy commute. Having our own home for the first time was a huge relief after the poor-quality hospital accommodation that we had to endure previously.

The remainder of the attachments on the rotation flashed by. Urology with Patrick Doyle and Bob Whittaker was an enjoyable diversion, but definitely not what I wanted to do. An abiding memory is of Bob ducking and weaving, resectoscope in hand with his eye fixed onto the eyepiece as he cut out strips of brownish prostate gland to remove prostatic obstruction. This took a huge toll on his cervical spine, resulting in the serious consequence of a prolapsed cervical disc whilst lecturing in New York, precipitating an emergency flight home for surgery. I was taught how to do an open prostatectomy, which involved taking up some very rakish poses, with your back to the patient, between his legs and your arm internally rotated and hand flexed behind you to scoop out the prostate within its capsule. Bleeding was profuse and repeated bladder washouts necessary after the procedure.

Patrick Doyle, the other urologist on the firm, was a completely different character. Softly spoken and immensely kind, his pastoral care of us trainees was the most genuine. His gentle manner and soft gaze resembled that of a very benign priest. He was hugely missed when he died prematurely whilst out walking alone in sand dunes during a urology meeting.

A highlight of the firm was a punting trip on the River Cam arranged to entertain a visiting professor from Stanford University. We had two punts for the surgical teams and inevitably a race between us ensued. Bob was piloting one punt and I the other. All was going well until, distracted by the perpetual Japanese tourists, I rammed the punt head-on into a projecting wall at Queen's College and propelled the visiting professor into the cool and muddy waters of the Cam. We fished him out and took him back to his hotel for a change of clothes. Luckily, he seemed to see the funny side of it, but I suspect that I wouldn't have been offered a job in Stanford had I applied.

The next two firms, first with Mr David Dunn, Alastair Smellie, and ultimately Professor Calne were packed with operating every day of the week. My experience grew rapidly and was perfect preparation for the final fellowship examination of the English Royal College of Surgeons. I sat this exam in May 1980. I felt a huge relief when my name was read out on the pass list in front of John Hunter's statue in the entrance lobby of the College. The numbers of those who had passed were called out and we walked forwards to confirm our identity with the College official, a portly and friendly Cockney gentleman, who carried out his responsibilities with dignity and a quiet humour. Those who passed were ushered around a corner, out of sight of the others waiting, whilst the many who failed were able to leave quietly having not heard their number. My number was 62. The numbers called out went something like 8, 15, 22, 34 and then I heard sixty... the candidate next to me with that number took a step forwards only to be halted as the official continued, 2! Sixty-two, my number. I strode forwards without looking back. A somewhat inhumane process, carried over from more ancient times, when the attitude was that we were lucky even to be there. When all the names of those who had passed had been read out, we were then ushered into the main hall of the college, formed into a line and presented to the college president and the council. The president read out a short piece of congratulations for having achieved the seemingly impossible, bowed to us along with all of the council members and then walked in procession along our line to shake our hands, followed by the council. When this was all over, I remember walking out through the hallowed hall of the college and into the early summer sunshine to stand on the steps and to reflect for a moment on my achievement. The words of Harding Rains came back to me telling me that I was too old to do surgery. Well, here I was at just thirty years of age and now, in the centuries old tradition of referring to surgeons as Mister, Mr Wells.

The surgical training on the Cambridge rotation was superb. We were exposed to so much pathology, with a great deal of time in the operating theatre, that can only be imagined today. I remember Mr Smellie asking me what procedures I was light on. I said that I would like to become more rehearsed in thyroid surgery. He sent me to the waiting list office to pick several thyroid cases and to book them on each of the lists for the coming few weeks. By the end of that time, I was proficient in thyroidectomy. This was something that came to stand me in good stead when I began thoracic surgery. It meant that I didn't need to call upon a thyroid surgeon when removing enlarged intrathoracic thyroid glands (goitres). Indeed it enabled me to teach E.N.T. surgeons that procedure when I became a consultant thoracic surgeon.

Every Sunday morning in the summer months, Alistair (affectionately known as WABS by us registrars in the light of his initials), would come onto the surgical ward in his tennis clothes to do a ward round with us before going off for a game. His other eccentricity was to wear a monocle. The only other mentor that I had met who wore one was Professor Glenister. Both men wore a wry smile with the eyepiece as if to say, 'I know I am eccentric and I enjoy it.'

The other consultant that I worked for on the rotation was David Dunn, also an excellent surgeon. He was one of the first surgeons in the country to develop minimally invasive laparoscopic vagotomy and gall bladder removal. On the final Friday evening of each month, all of us surgical registrars were invited to David's house to present our latest research. Sustenance was provided for us by his lovely wife Anna, in the form of beer and sandwiches. We were a very competitive bunch and continually trying to outdo each other. Through David's encouragement we all succeeded in building a solid CV with multiple publications and presentations. Probably the smartest of us was John Shaw, who went on to a very successful general surgical career. Following the meeting we would adjourn to the Little Rose pub on Trumpington street for more beer and a game of Space Invaders. It was with David that I presented my first surgical paper at a European gastroenterology meeting in Garmisch-Partenkirchen. It was April 1981 during the firm with Alastair Smellie and David. Despite my anxiety, my presentation on the esoterically named subject of highly, highly selective vagotomy for gastric ulceration went well. The procedure was named highly, highly selective as there had been a progression from vagotomy, the division of the Vagus nerve before its branches separated to innervate the stomach, to selected branches and then highly selected branches and finally highly, highly selected, dividing only the nerve of Latargé branch, found to be the main culprit in neurogenic acid secretion. Since the discovery of the fact that most of gastric ulceration is caused by colonisation of the stomach by the bacterium Helicobacter Pylorii, which can be treated with antibiotics, this surgery has disappeared along with gastrectomy for advanced gastric ulceration. Following our presentation in the session I was able to relax and enjoy the rest of the meeting.

For the final five months of the programme I was attached to the Professorial transplant and general surgical firm with Roy Calne. Professor Calne was a wonderful mentor. He was very trusting of his registrars, who in turn worked extremely hard for him and our patients. One evening on call a young man came in with severe abdominal pain, the early signs of which suggested appendicitis. However, the pain had settled in the right upper side of the abdomen under the liver, quite atypical for this condition. An x-ray of the patient's abdomen revealed a stripe of gas along the edge of the colon. I predicted that this would be a burst appendix high in the abdomen, a high retrocaecal appendix, which is quite rare. Surgery confirmed the finding. Roy insisted that I write it up for a surgical journal and that the stripe of gas at the side of the abdomen be called 'Wells' Sign'.[4] It was accepted for publication and my first eponymous attachment was established. Without his encouragement it would not have happened.

At about that time, fortuitously as it turned out for me, we had operated to good effect on the local chief of traffic police. I had been on call all weekend and was on my way home at four in the morning after a night of emergency surgery. Just as I entered the house, the phone rang (no mobile phones then). A young woman had been admitted with a ruptured ectopic pregnancy and was bleeding into her abdomen profusely. I was asked to return as quickly as I could. I jumped into my car and set off at high speed. I was drifting nicely around a roundabout on the Barton Road when I noticed a police car whose blue lights came on and gave chase. I was faced with a dilemma. Do I stop and try to explain or keep going? I kept going. I reached the front of the hospital with the police car not far behind. I leapt out of the car and rushed to the operating theatre where the woman was being prepared for surgery. Quickly opening her abdomen, I was able to bring the bleeding under control and to stabilise the situation. As I walked out of the theatre, by now quite tired, I was met by the two police men who marched up to me and seized both of my arms, one on each side saying, 'You're coming with us.' My mind flashed forwards to the likely court scene and the loss of my driving license and what that would do to the family and my work. As we got down to the entrance lobby, instead of walking to the outside and their car, they turned towards the restaurant which was just opening. I asked where we were going, and they said, 'to buy you breakfast. We understand that you helped our chief recently, and he has told us to look after you.' We had a full English breakfast together and then I was escorted home to ensure my safety, and nothing more came of it. It is difficult to imagine that happening today.

As mentioned, Roy was a talented artist in the style of John Bellamy, who had been a patient of his and latterly became a close friend and artistic mentor. In the late spring of 1983 Roy recruited me to join him and other surgical colleagues on a weekend of big brush water colour held by Ron Ranson at his home. The other friends on the trip were Bob Whittaker,

David Dunn, Roy and Esther Rantzen. Esther was great fun to be around but enjoyed the sunshine on the riverbank more than the painting. I remember her asking me to complete one of her paintings for her. She had developed a friendship with Roy over some children that he had helped with liver transplantation. They had worked together on Esther's Childline project and her association with Children in Need. Roy was deeply serious about his art and set the pace for the rest of us.

In contrast with the restricted hours that today's trainees are subject to, all surgical trainees were expected to attend a Saturday morning teaching session presented by one of us, followed by a teaching ward round that Roy led. Not only was this educationally excellent, but it led to close cohesion in the surgical units. Something that is often sadly lacking today. During the thirty months on the Cambridge rotation, I had learned a huge amount and gained massive surgical experience.

I kept a detailed record of all cases done on the various stages of my rotation. On referring back to this the first thing that struck me is the fact that we were operating almost every day and every other night and weekend being the era of over 100 hours a week. In my first four months as a junior registrar I carried out 220 cases, which is 55 cases per month. This included eighteen gall bladder removals, thirty-seven appendicectomies, forty-two hernias of one kind or another, four peripheral vascular reconstructions and twenty-two breast procedures, including mastectomies. The second firm was in urology, during which another large number of cases were completed. Back in general surgery another 240 cases were done in the next five months. These included a further thirty-eight cholecystectomies, thirty-four appendicectomies, twenty-eight breast lumps, fifty-four hernia repairs and eighteen pairs of varicose veins. The following five months saw another 303 cases, including many cholecystectomies, hernia repairs, mastectomies and anal procedures. My final stint with Professor Roy Calne yielded over 400 cases, including stomach, pancreas and hepatic procedures. By the time that I had finished the Cambridge rotation my general surgical, orthopaedic and urology experience was huge by modern standards. It amounted to over 1,000 cases. Prior to this rotation in Cambridge, I had also done over 250 cases at Winchester as a senior house officer. It meant that on moving on to more specialist training, we were very familiar with the handling of human tissue and surgical instruments. All of this was done before we embarked on our specialist surgical training in cardiothoracic surgery.

Current surgical training programmes demand and allow for far less. It is so sad that in the modern period the trainees receive much less experience meaning that the modern NHS is training surgeons who are more like proceduralists and not properly experienced surgeons, able to turn their hands to many different scenarios. This has resulted in multiple 'specialists' dealing with different aspects of a single procedure, delaying management, slowing the process of surgery and raising costs significantly. It also exposes the security of surgery as a career for properly trained people to the invasion of surgeon assistants, able to do small parts of the specialty without the depth of knowledge that a classical education gives to practitioners.

During the last months I received a phone call from Terence English asking me if I would like to return to Papworth as his surgical registrar. At the time, I had begun to think of pursuing training in general surgery as I had enjoyed it so much and Roy had invited me to continue in that role with his team. This offer made me reconsider and I decided to continue along my initial ambition in cardiothoracic surgery. And so I accepted his offer and prepared to move back to Papworth on completion of the rotation in Cambridge.

Return to Papworth and Cardiothoracic Surgery

My return began in July 1982. Despite the lauded reputations of two of the consultants, Ben Milstein was, in my opinion and experience, the best and most widely experienced surgeon at Papworth at that time and it is an ongoing sadness to me that his huge contribution to the generality of cardiothoracic surgery remains unrecognised within the hospital. Ben, as described earlier, had been brought up to the hospital from Brompton to accelerate the implementation of cardiac surgery. He was a vastly experienced thoracic surgeon and combined both aspects of the specialty in great style. Something of an irascible character, and somewhat in the mould of his mentor, Lord Brock, he didn't suffer fools gladly. However, hard work and diligence won him over, when he could be utterly charming.

By that time my surgical experience was large. This meant that Ben quickly took me into his trust and helped me to develop my thoracic surgical experience. He had set up the first peripheral vascular surgery practice and the first significant oesophageal service in the region. Quickly, I was doing two and three stage oesophagectomies, a whole range of benign oesophageal surgery, peripheral vascular procedures from abdominal aortic aneurysms to peripheral vascular reconstructions, and the full range of lung resections for cancer and other conditions. It was an experience that is currently unavailable for trainees or consultants. I loved it and it prepared me extremely well for the career that lay ahead of me.

Ben had relinquished his role in transplantation as a result of the somewhat predatory nature of his younger colleague. As a result, he really led the teaching of heart valve surgery as well as all things thoracic. Coronary surgery stretched the limits of his patience and was the one area in which he didn't excel, happily leaving it to his trained junior staff and later to John Wallwork, a very fine coronary surgeon. His teaching of endoscopic techniques was excellent, and I rapidly built up a big experience in both rigid and flexible endoscopic techniques. The rigid endoscopes demanded particular surgical techniques, especially the oesophagoscope. The position of the head of the anaesthetised patient should be positioned as for 'sniffing the morning air'. In other words, neck flexed on the torso and the head extended on the neck to open up the pharynx and allow easy passage of the scope into the upper oesophagus, just like a sword swallower as Ben would tell us. The difficulty of wielding the rigid endoscopes was well illustrated by the famed American heart surgeon Dr Denton Cooley who had been a surgical fellow at Brompton Hospital with Ben under the tutelage of the Lord Brock in the early 1960s. On his arrival at Brompton, Cooley had done little or no thoracic surgery but was expected to be involved in the practice during his year there. Early after his arrival he was asked to carry out a rigid bronchoscopy on a patient and was having severe difficulty in passing the endoscope. At which point the theatre porter said to him, 'You hold the bronchoscope still Dr Cooley and I will thread the patient over it' and proceeded to do so.[5] During my time with Ben, Cooley came to visit him and I had the opportunity to ask if the story of the bronchoscope was true, and indeed it was.

I didn't know that Dr Cooley was visiting Papworth and only discovered one day when I was operating on a patient doing coronary artery bypass surgery. There is a point in that procedure where a clamp needs to be placed on the aorta to sew on the vein graft. The clamp was designed by Dr Cooley and named after him. At the relevant point in the procedure I asked for the Cooley and a voice came quietly over the top of the table 'present'. My astonishment and anxiety at having such a huge name in cardiac surgery observing me can easily be imagined. Afterwards we struck up a conversation in the changing room and I noticed a large, branded scar on his chest in the form of the University of Texas in Galveston. I couldn't resist asking the origin of such a thing, He told me that he and some fellow graduates went out into the desert, got really drunk on tequila and decided to brand each other. It was then that I was able to ask him about the bronchoscope story.

Having got to know each other a little, Denton invited me to visit his centre in Texas at the Heart Institute. On arrival in the hospital, I was greeted by his assistant and taken up to his grand office where we chatted and drank American coffee. He spoke very affectionately of his year in London and his respect for Lord Brock and Oswald (Os) Tubbs. During his time there, Tubbs needed a lung resection for tuberculosis and Denton had been the assistant on that procedure. Tubbs had asked him to ensure that Brock crushed his phrenic nerve (the nerve that stimulates the diaphragm to contract), to temporary paralyse the diaphragm to rest the operated lung whilst it recovered. Brock said that it was unnecessary, but whilst he wasn't looking, Denton quickly pinched the nerve with a forceps, satisfying Os' request.[6] He also spent time with Norman 'Pasty' Barrett, another thoracic surgeon and Sir Clement Price-Thomas, who was knighted for operating on King George VI. He had removed his lung for cancer. At the end of that operation, performed in Buckingham Palace, he stepped away from the operating table after removing the King's lung, but before the chest had been closed. The anaesthetist asked him why he was leaving the table and Price-Thomas replied, 'Good God man I haven't closed a chest for thirty years, why practice on the King?' During the conversation Cooley reminded me of some of Lord Brock's famous sayings when referring to a surgical procedure that things can be 'Awfully simple or simply awful', and that 'Wounds healed from side to side and not end to end', when extolling the virtues of adequate surgical exposure. Brock's words had spread far and wide.

When I arrived at the Texas Heart Institute, Dr Cooley had a meeting of the hospital board to attend and asked his secretary to take me down to the operating theatre to meet his friend and associate Dr 'Bud' Frazier. Standing at the top of the operating table, I introduced myself to Bud, who in his wonderful Texas drawl enquired where I was from. I replied that I was born and had lived my early life in Shropshire. With no prompting he immediately began to recite long screeds of poetry from Houseman's *A Shropshire Lad*. I felt immediately at home. We began a long friendship in that instant.

Bud is a surgeon with a heritage like no other I have met. One of his nineteenth century cowboy relatives had been a gunslinger in West Texas. He had a sepia photograph of him strung up on a makeshift gallows with other gang members following the infamous shoot-out at the OK Corral. Bud had seen combat as an assault helicopter flight surgeon in Vietnam and had survived being shot down. For his valiant efforts he received several distinguished service medals. He and Denton Cooley had an extremely cool manner about them and reminded me very much of the characters described in Tom Wolfe's book about Chuck Yeager and the astronaut programme, *The Right Stuff*. They were an unusual and impressive team.

After he had completed the operation, Bud took me to his office and asked if I was interested in rare books. I replied in the affirmative, and he began to show me some of his collection. These included stunning first editions of Vesalius's *De Humani Corporis Fabrica Libri Septem* (*de Fabrica* for short). At that stage in my life, and with all the preconceptions of the American mindset, I was truly surprised to find such learning of medieval literature in a surgeon's office in downtown Houston Texas.

Later that evening, we went to a Texan steak house. I was wearing a shirt and tie but noticed that the others were not wearing a necktie. I soon discovered why. On entering the restaurant there was a man at the door with a huge pair of scissors. Apparently if seen sporting a tie the scissors were wielded, and the body of the tie was cut off and pinned to the wall with many others of all shapes, sizes and colours from other patrons who had made the same mistake. That fact had been withheld to amuse the rest of the party. Mine followed suit. I was told that I should order the house steak. The shock on my face when I saw the size of it brought the others to tears of mirth. It was on the biggest plate I had ever been given and even then, this massive piece of meat was overlapping the edges considerably. As they say everything in Texas is bigger than anything anywhere else in the world. It was also the most delicious steak I have ever eaten, and coming from a butcher's son that is quite an admission. The meal over, the true amusements began. I was told that I had to try my hand, or perhaps I should say my backside, at the bucking bronco, a life-size mechanical beast in the centre of the restaurant. It lived up to its name as few stayed on it for more than a few rounds. However, to my pleasure and self-pride I manged to ride it to the end with huge cheers from the whole restaurant, and the gift of a new tie from the proprietors.

The following day, I attended Dr. Cooley's operating room to see him carry out a complex aortic root replacement. His manual dexterity and fluidity of movement was utterly mesmerising. Without appearing to rush, and with no wasted movements the operation was completed in lightning quick time and with minimal blood loss. The reason for his reputation as among the best, if not the best surgeon in the world at that time, was clear to see. As assistant to Michael DeBakey, Denton had been involved in the very first replacement of the aorta with a Dacron Graft, cobbled together by DeBakey's wife, a dress maker. This then, my earliest exposure to American cardiac surgery had been all that I could have imagined and more. The can-do attitude of everyone around the department in the hospital was truly infectious, but also a source of depression on re-entering the restrictive world of the British NHS. We British love to run down the American system of medicine and there are problems of access for the poor and uninsured, but for those adequately covered, it is a fast, efficient and expert service that is to this day world beating.

During my time spent with Professor Calne, I had been intrigued by the developments in the understanding of the control of blood flow within the vessels by the presence of the prostaglandin compounds prostacyclin and thromboxane A2. Thromboxane is a vasoconstrictor and platelet aggregator, that has evolved to allow healing of an injured blood vessel. Prostacyclin is a vasodilator and an inhibitor of platelet aggregation. These two substances work in beautiful harmony to maintain the integrity of the circulation in the normal and abnormal states. Sir John Vane had shared the Nobel Prize for Medicine for his work on the prostaglandins and their effects on vascular physiology. Reading about this I was struck with the possibilities that it threw up in patients with vascular disease. I was seeing several people who had extreme versions of Raynaud's phenomenon, when the peripheral blood vessels undergo exaggerated spasm in response to the cold. This can endanger the tips of the digits and seriously limit the capacity for the individual to work with their hands. Reading about the effects of prostacyclin as a dilator of blood vessels, I suggested to Roy that we get hold of some and give it to such patients and to observe the effects. Roy's adventurous spirit gave me permission to do this and moreover, he contacted Professor Vane to access off-licence use of the drug. We admitted several patients and set up an infusion of the drug and observed the results. In every patient their vasospasm dissipated and along with it their pain. The only catch was the very short life of action of the drug. We therefore gave it over a few days. The effects were sustained and for the rest of the winter these patients were greatly relieved. We noted side-effects of abdominal pain and diarrhoea in some patients, headache and facial flushing in others.

Not long after beginning my registrar job at Papworth, Ben had operated on a middle-aged lady, who after the operation had repeated emboli of clots to her lungs and we could not wean her from the ventilator. I suggested to Ben that we try an infusion of prostacyclin. After I had explained to him the experience that we had had with Raynaud's patients at Addenbrooke's, he agreed. As if by magic the lady's problems abated and we were able to wean her from the ventilator.

At the same time, in the bed next to her was a patient with severe thrombotic obstruction of her pulmonary blood vessels. This is a chronic problem and causes an early death through advancing failure of the right ventricle of the heart to pump blood against the resistance in the lung arteries. Following the success with the previous lady I suggested that we try it in this patient also. It worked beautifully. Steadily her colour improved, with her hands and face turning from a purple-bluish colour with hypoxia to a rosy pink. The problem once again was that when we stopped the drug the blood vessels became obstructed again and the hypoxia returned. It was not clear what to do. It was difficult to ignore the effect of the drug, but could we use it continuously? Again, fresh from my general surgical experience, wherein we treated general surgical patients with problems of absorption of food from the bowel with continuous infusion whilst up and about, I suggested that we tried the same in this situation. Once again it worked. We were able to stabilise the patient for thirteen months with a continuous infusion, eventually enabling her to live independently at home. This treatment has gone on to be a mainstay in the therapy of that condition.

There was, however, a distasteful episode that arose from this. Despite having the idea in the first place and administering the prostacyclin and monitoring it, as a lowly registrar I found myself excluded initially from the paper reporting the treatment. Shortly after I had treated that patient with prostacyclin, I had gone to Alabama on my senior research fellowship. Whilst I was there, John Wallwork and Tim Higginbotham came to visit me in Birmingham, Alabama. They let it slip that the prostacyclin work had been written up and accepted for publication in the prestigious journal, *The Lancet*. I discovered that I was not on the paper, despite being the person who had suggested the idea and produced the wherewithal for it to happen. I was quite distressed and complained strongly that this was not acceptable. By then I had been offered and accepted a consultant job back in Papworth and felt able to argue my case with more strength than if I had been a surgical trainee with them. I had to threaten to inform the editor of the journal of the omission if not included and ultimately they gave way and I was included on the paper.[6] But it was a lesson in how academia can work to the detriment of junior training medical staff. Sadly, it is something that continues to this day in too many institutions, including academic units of repute, even in the 'great' universities at large.

My research fellowship in Alabama came about when early after my return to Papworth, Terence English suggested that I should apply for the post of Senior Research Fellow with Dr John Kirklin at the University of Alabama in Birmingham. Several British consultants, including himself, had passed through this important department of cardiac surgery with one of the most impressive research and development portfolios in the world. John Kirklin, who had been brought down from the Mayo clinic where he was the head of the department of surgery, was one of the most respected pioneers in the specialty. Famously John Fitzgerald Kennedy, the thirty-fifth president of the United States of America, had called him up and asked him to move to the south to set up a major centre for cardiac surgery in that relatively deprived area. Whilst at the Mayo clinic 'Big John' as we referred to him had pioneered the use of the heart and lung machine, first devised by John Gibbon. After an initial successful case closing an atrial septal defect (a hole in the heart between the two upper chambers), Gibbon lost the next two children that he operated on. The distress of this caused him to stop and he placed a moratorium on the use of his device. He also removed himself from the field of cardiac surgery, never to do another heart operation.

Although this appeared to be the end of the road for this technical development, the cool headed and brave John Kirklin, when still at the Mayo clinic, began to research and to develop it to a state of clinical readiness. Known by close colleagues at the time as 'The Ice-man', Kirklin applied hard-headed scientific thought and hard work with remorseless documentation and determination, transforming what had been vital initial work into a viable solution to the problem of operating within the heart and yet to keep the patient alive. Out of respect to Dr Gibbon, the group at Mayo named it the Mayo-Gibbon pump. Those early days were fraught for Kirklin also. Following successful experiments in dogs he and his team set out to repair ventricular-septal defects in neonates and young children within a rigidly defined protocol. Eight children were selected. The first child survived but the next four died. He was instructed by the hospital management that he should cease the experiment. He forcefully responded that the protocol had stated eight children and that was what would be done.[7] To his credit and as a tribute to his courage the remainder survived to produce one of the most important series in the history of cardiac surgery.

The hallmark of John Kirklin's work was rigorous scientific planning, adherence to protocol (something that I was to discover later when carrying out my own research in his department) and detailed measurement and documentation of everything, producing vital databases. He brought this rigour to the post-operative care of the surgical patient by setting up the earliest intensive care units, where all vital signs were monitored and recorded along with all therapeutic interventions. Whilst seeming such an obvious thing to do these days it was novel in his times. His department at UAB (University of Alabama) was the first to implement this. Terence, quite correctly, identified this unit as the ideal one for a young cardiac surgeon to develop discipline in his/her practice and so it proved to be. Whilst other units in the developed world, such as that of Walt Lillehei in Minnesota and Viking Björk in the Karolinska for instance, were exciting places to work, they all looked to Kirklin's unit for rigour and excellence in scientific development. I have a quote from a letter from Oswald Tubbs, who was working at St Bartholomew's hospital in London, to Bill Oliver, a pioneering thoracic surgeon at the Norfolk and Norwich Hospital in England, dated 28 December 1959, wherein he writes:

> The proper treatment of Fallot's Tetralogy is still worrying everyone. Obviously total correction using a pump is ideal, but even Kirklin (Mayo) still has a mortality of 25%.

Whilst Kirklin was recognised for his scientific approach and tenacity he wasn't necessarily recognised as the most dextrous pair of hands. That accolade rested with another North American hero of cardiac surgery C. Walton Lillehei. Tubbs, in recognition of this, goes on to state in his letter that:

> I am going to America to work with Lillehei next year and then we will do a few more dogs and then we will be ready to start these cases here [Bart's].

As the technicalities of a working heart and lung machine were being overcome, another problem raised its head. That was of the damaging effects of passing blood through the plastic piping of the machine and the exposure to large synthetic surface areas in the various forms of oxygenation that were necessary for gas transfer during the procedure. It wasn't until the seminal work of Kirklin in the early 1980s that the molecular biology of this problem was unravelled. At that time, all the surgeons knew was that even on completion of a successful surgical correction of the heart defect, patients died with lung, kidney and bowel failure. Chest radiographs revealed lungs that had turned completely white with massive fluid infiltration into the air spaces, a condition that became known as respiratory distress syndrome or post-pump lung. Kidneys stopped working with internal micro-haemorrhage. Trauma to the patient's blood was causing the release of aggressive substances which attacked the lining of blood vessels causing them to leak blood and molecules of super-oxide radicals into the tissues, leading to extensive tissue disruption. This happened to a greater or lesser extent in all patients but was exacerbated by extended periods of support on the machine.

To resolve this problem, Lillehei developed and performed perhaps the most remarkable solution. The child was sustained by a parent's circulation, the cross-circulation method. His revolutionary idea was to use a parent (usually but not exclusively the mother's circulation) to support the child.

To achieve this he simply connected a major artery of the parent to that of the child, for arterial flow. Similarly, using another plastic tube, a major vein was connected from parent to child to allow venous drainage. The lungs and kidneys of the parent then did the job of vascular homeostasis for the child whilst the surgery was being carried out. This procedure held the possibility of causing the death of both parent and child. However, this technique of cross-circulation was extraordinarily successful.

Lillehei was the grandson of a Norwegian fisherman, a good looking and fast-living risk taker. He was also a problem solver. Being refused a motorcycle by his parents, he simply bought all the parts and assembled one for himself. He was in charge of a mobile surgical unit (a MASH unit, fabled in the 1970 movie by the same name) in North Africa in the desert war against Rommel, from whence he won a bronze star. At the age of only thirty-one, he was cruelly struck down with a malignant disease of the parotid gland, a lymphosarcoma. Recognised as being highly malignant, with only a five to ten percent chance of surviving five years, his boss at that time Owen Wangensteen carried out an extremely radical resection of all lymph nodes and surrounding muscular structures in his neck and upper chest. Whilst very deforming, the procedure, which was followed by radical radiotherapy, was successful in clearing that dreadful disease. Lillehei went on to live until the age of eighty. During his long life, Walt Lillehei became one of the world's foremost cardiac surgeons, an original thinker and teacher. Out of respect for his enormous contributions to our specialty, he became known as the father of cardiac surgery, hence the desire of Oswald Tubbs to experience working with him in trying to resolve the problem of complex cardiac surgical corrective procedures.

Sadly, later in life Lillehei encountered legal difficulties over tax avoidance and had to endure an extended and embarrassing trial, at the end of which he was convicted. As a result he was shunned by many in the medical profession. Those two great men of Cardiac surgery Kirklin and Lillehei came together, however, when at a large gathering of international cardiac surgeons, Lillehei's seminal contributions were recognised. Dr Kirklin, who was on stage at the time spotted Walt in the vast audience and called him to his feet and began to applaud him, following which the whole audience rose to its feet and joined in with what became rapturous applause for a great scientist, innovator and surgeon. The great man had been rehabilitated at a stroke by another hero of the specialty. I was fortunate to spend quite some considerable time with Dr Lillehei later in my consultant's role.

He was the inventor of the replacement heart valve, the St Jude Bi-leaflet Mechanical Valve, which revolutionised valve design. A tongue-in-cheek name for such an important device, as St Jude is the patron saint of hopeless cases and lost causes; one wonders if this was the work of the tearaway Lillehei. The valve was manufactured and marketed by the company of the same name. The company sponsored a series of courses for cardiac surgical trainees which I was fortunate enough to be asked to organise and run. They were held in a splendid country park hotel in the middle of England. The idea was to bring together all or most of the trainees in the UK for a series of short presentations, to be followed by extensive discussions of the subject mimicking what we consultants discussed in the coffee room after an interesting or challenging procedure. In the midst of it all was Dr Lillehei, who patiently listened and encouraged the discussions. At the end of the day and after dinner he would sit in the bar surrounded by eager trainees and he would hold court into the early hours of the morning. The following day a series of events were organised to enhance a sense of companionship. Events such as archery, clay-pigeon shooting and off the road driving were enjoyed by everyone. During those times I found Dr Lillehei to be an immensely warm and giving man who enjoyed the company of the coming generation of cardiac surgeons.

After just over a year at Papworth as surgical registrar, the senior registrar job was advertised back in London on what was considered to be the senior training programme in cardiothoracic surgery. The post rotated through Brompton, the London Chest Hospital and the National Heart Hospital, working for such luminaries as Donald Ross, Sir Magdi Yacoub, John Wright, Jack Belcher, Christopher Lincon and Matthias Paneth, for whom I had worked before. Whilst I was enjoying my time at Papworth and getting lots of experience, my goal was to return to Brompton for the final part of my training. I was not expecting to get the job but decided to apply. Discussion with Ben and Terence met with their support. The interview went well, and to my amazement I was offered the job. In competition with me was a superb registrar, already at Brompton, Alan Wood. I knew him to be a very competent surgeon and expected him to get the post. When the role was given to me, I felt somewhat embarrassed, but Alan was extremely generous towards me and became an excellent colleague.

Brompton: Here We Come Again

Once again, we were on the move. The house in Comberton needed to be sold and another found in London. Shortly after I had begun the job, I was operating with Mr Paneth when a theatre porter came to the head of the table and asked to speak to me. He was carrying a message from my wife Helen. She had found a terrace house in East Sheen, near the river, at the point of the end of the Oxford/Cambridge boat race. We had sold the house in Comberton for approximately £15,000 and the house that Helen was found was on offer for £52,000. This seemed a huge amount to me. I swallowed hard and sent a message to place an offer. Out of the corner of my eye I could see Mr Paneth smiling behind his mask. We succeeded in purchasing the property and were able to move in quickly. Driving in to work from Sheen was relatively easy in those days. Mr Paneth lived close by and occasionally I would see him in his Porsche headed in the same direction.

I began the rotation at Brompton with Peter Goldstraw, an excellent thoracic surgeon whose star was very definitely in the ascendancy. I had hoped to have been able to return to Mr Paneth's practice, but his post was already taken. I soon realised what a golden egg Peter's practice was for learning. He had strong links with the Royal Marsden Hospital, next door to Brompton. Every Monday we went to a multi-disciplinary meeting with the oncologists. This produced many challenging cases with a multitude of malignant conditions. My experience continued to grow rapidly. Peter was an excellent teacher whose practice was at the cutting edge of the specialty. He granted a lot of freedom with many difficult cases, and I was honoured that he would give me such responsibility.

After six months, I rotated to work with Stuart Lennox. As mentioned earlier, despite Stuart having a somewhat prickly character I enjoyed working with him. He had novel ideas for the management of the cardiac patient but had difficulty implementing them through the obduracy of others around him. He had been the surgeon who had introduced coronary artery surgery to Brompton amongst other things.

I loved working at Brompton. It sits in a wonderful part of London and was steeped in the history of cardiac and thoracic surgery. The nurses were of a very high calibre and many of them had worked there for a long time and knew the foibles of each of the consultants well. It always paid to listen to them. The hours were long, but the rate of learning through the sheer volume of work and the expertise around us meant that the learning curve was very steep.

Some events stand out in my mind. I had helped Matt with a particularly nasty coronary bypass operation late on a Friday evening. The vessels were narrow and heavily calcified. We managed to complete the operation and get the patient to the intensive care for recovery. All seemed to be going well, and he was transferred to the ward on the Saturday afternoon. However, around 7.00 p.m. the following day, a cardiac arrest call went out. It was our patient. I was on call and in the hospital, as was my long-term friend and colleague Len Shapiro. We both arrived at the bedside simultaneously and began cardiac massage. The beds were old and springy, therefore, to get effective heart compressions, we moved him to the hard floor. The heart was not responding despite all of the usual measures of drugs and repeated cardioversion shocks. We decided that the only other resort was to open the chest for internal cardiac massage. By then the theatre nurses had arrived with a surgical set and I removed the sutures holding the wound together and exposed the heart. I could then take the heart in my hand and apply direct pressure on the ventricles to get good emptying and vascular perfusion. We had tried direct intracardiac injection of adrenaline as well as all other manoeuvres. There was some return of activity, but repeated episodes of massage were necessary.

I had felt the vein graft to the right coronary artery, and it seemed to be the cause of the problem, being blocked with clot. I was able to detach it, empty the clot and to sew it back onto the aorta. That seemed to improve the situation and so we decided that the time had come to move the patient to the intensive care unit. Len went ahead to call the lift as the ICU was two floors above us.

With the anaesthetist ventilating the patient, a porter at the head of the bed and a nurse at the foot we were ready to move. I was kneeling across the open chest of the patient ready to resume cardiac massage as it became necessary. The lift was the old, gated type with two sliding metal gates. The patient was wheeled in with me still astride him. Len closed the gates form the outside and pressed the button for the lift to ascend. As we rose to about 4 feet off the ground the lift shuddered to an abrupt halt. We called for Len to come back and to get the thing going again. Despite all his efforts the lift was stuck fast. At that point Len disappeared for about fifteen minutes. Our calls for help seemed to fall on deaf ears. I had had to resume open chest massage and thigs were looking very bad. Finally, Len appeared with another couple of porters and with a lot of grunting and rattling suddenly the lift began to ascend once again. We eventually reached the ICU and moved the patient to a bed space and connected him to all the necessary monitoring and intravenous infusions. I was then able to close the chest and in the early hours of the morning we were able to retire to bed, leaving the patient in the capable hands of the night staff.

The next morning, I was up at 5.30 and set off to the hospital across the Fulham Road to the south side building where the surgical and intensive care units were. Len appeared, and we began to walk over together. As we came out onto the road, we noticed a long line of vans parked all the way along the front of the hospital. They were lift engineers. At that point Len shouted, 'quick, make a run for it'. He sprinted across the road with me in hot pursuit. Once we had gained the safety of the hospital, I asked him what all that was about. Apparently when he had disappeared during the lift episode, he had got the yellow pages and phoned every lift company that he could find to get help. Naturally all were off duty and so he had left messages in desperation. First thing in the morning the desperate calls for help from Brompton Hospital were heard and they all set off to bring help. We slunk off to do the ward round on ICU, following which I went to theatre for the day's surgery and by the time we emerged late into the afternoon all sign of them had gone. The patient rallied for several days but sadly subsequently passed away. Matt Paneth found the whole event macabrely amusing. We escaped without a reprimand.

During my latter time at Brompton, I had begun to feel that it was the place that I would like to settle as a consultant but was too unsure of myself to think that I could achieve this, as my colleagues were very bright and I was still very junior. The next part of my senior registrar rotation was going to take me to the London Chest Hospital to work with an exceptional coronary surgeon John Wright. The issue for me there was that he was quite an aggressive man and spent much of his time in the private sector. When I had gone to meet him before the interview for the job, he was in the scrub room, preparing for an operation. I introduced myself, and he asked what I was doing there. I said that I had come to discuss the senior registrar post with him as I was applying. Barely looking up at me he barked, 'Can you run an adult cardiac surgical practice?' I replied, 'No, that was what I thought I was coming here to be taught.' He snapped back, 'Well, you are no damn use to me then,' and strode off, arms raised to gown up for the procedure.

Clearly I was not going to learn much working for him and it felt to me that my future career would be in jeopardy if I couldn't perform adequately, and more than that I would potentially be putting the lives of patients at risk. I left feeling quite downhearted. The third part of the rotation was at the National Heart Hospital with Donald Ross and Magdi Yacoub. That was very appealing to me and so I continued, successfully, with my application. The concern about working with John Wright played a very significant part in my applying for the consultant job at Papworth, where I had mixed feelings about working. Central London was my first choice, but the words of Harding Rains kept ringing in my ears. My concerns about Papworth were partly because there was so much emphasis on transplantation, in which I had only a moderate interest, and partly because the research possibilities in London seemed much greater. However, fate was to play a strong hand in what happened next.

I had been accepted onto the programme with Dr. Kirklin, to start in January of 1984. However, before that there was to be another momentous event. Ben Milstein was about to retire, and the hunt was on for a replacement. I had returned to Brompton as senior registrar and was contacted by John Wallwork, suggesting that I should apply for the post. Still quite green in experience in cardiac surgery I was somewhat taken aback, but close friends advised that even if failed to be appointed, at least it would be good interview experience and encouraged me to go for it. Somewhat in trepidation I put in my application. To my great surprise I was short-listed and called for interview. At that time, I was senior registrar to Stuart Lennox at Brompton. Stuart was a moderately controversial character, somewhat irascible and on occasions argumentative. However, he was always very supportive of me, and I found him to be very caring of his patients. The day before the interview, we were walking through the tunnel beneath the Fulham Road following a ward round. He turned to me and asked where I was going to be the following day. I told him of the upcoming interview. His response was prompt and quite disarming. He asked me what on earth I was doing going for a job outside of London. It seemed to him that the only natural place to be was in central London. I explained that I was fairly certain that I would not be appointed but was going for the interview experience. What I didn't know until several years later was that he and others had thought of me as a good candidate for a job at Brompton. I suspect that had I known this was the case I probably would have withdrawn and waited for a year or two to see when a post would become available. Several years later, I met by chance the then chairman of the board at Brompton, John Plant. He came to see an exhibition that I had mounted with Caitlin Edwardes (then Ben). It was titled 'A Week in the Life of a Cardiac Surgeon' and consisted of very large format photographs of me in all aspects of my work. After the usual pleasantries, he asked me why I hadn't waited to apply for Matt Paneth's job at Brompton, as they had me lined up to take over from him. I suspect that my surprise was clear for him to see. I told him that no indication of that possibility had been passed to me, for if it had I would not have applied for Papworth as Brompton was my first choice. It remains a regret for me as it would have fitted my personality much better, and I could have avoided a major part of my life being tied up in transplantation which held only marginal interest for me.

At Papworth I have met with much resistance to my development of mitral valve reconstruction and the development of thoracic surgery. To this day, there is no recognition of our contribution internationally to the surgical management of the regurgitant mitral valve, although it is widely recognised around the world. Unlike many London hospitals and other major institutions, Papworth's institutional memory is poor and selective at best. It does not reflect the numerous developments from its surgical consultants outside of transplantation and latterly pulmonary thromboendarterectomy, both quite marginal activities in the greater scheme of things, but profitable in management's eyes.

The day after my brief conversation with Mr Lennox, I drove up to Cambridge with Helen for the interview. My fellow short-listed candidates included Chris McGregor, the senior registrar at Papworth at the time, Stephen Westaby, who was at the Hammersmith, and Phil Spratt, who was a senior fellow from Australia, an excellent and very experienced surgeon. Both Phil and Chris had significant transplant experience and would have been first rate appointees to work with Terence and John. I really saw myself as interview cannon fodder. What happened next was quite extraordinary. The interview committee consisted of thirteen people. Prior to my turn, I had heard laughter and energised conversation coming from behind the closed doors. This simply reinforced my thought that I was just there to make up the numbers. Prior to my turn, one of my competitors walked me outside with his arm around my shoulders, informing me that the job was his, but he was sure that I would get something very soon. For my part the interview seemed to pass quite uneventfully. I had quite a strong CV with perhaps more published papers that many others. However, I left the room with little hope of a positive outcome. Indeed, I had begun to think that not getting the job would be positive for me as more experience would be nothing but a good thing.

Finally, the deliberations were over, and the hospital secretary came out to announce the result. As she began to speak and call out the name of the successful candidate, 'Mr…', two of the candidates leapt to their feet expecting it to be them. The secretary finished her sentence, with '…Wells.' I did not look sideways, nor behind me but followed her into the room where all thirteen interviewers stood and congratulated me, offering me a proleptic appointment, so that I could take up the post after my forthcoming year in Alabama. After conversing with them all and expressing my thanks I left the room to find that all of the others, with the exception of Phil Spratt, had left. Phil had stayed behind to congratulate me, a measure of him as a gentleman of character. I was disappointed for him, as I truly felt that he was the best man for the job and would have fulfilled the post, in a way, much better than I would have been able to at that juncture in my career.

Ben Milstein had invited me to his house in central Cambridge following the interview. Helen was waiting there with him to hear the result. On the way, I parked my car on the road at the back of the colleges. What I had just done was beginning to sink in and I was in a state of mild shock. I really hadn't expected this outcome, and the enormity of what was ahead of me with my inexperience felt quite overwhelming. After several minutes to reflect I drove on to Ben's house where the Champagne was already flowing. John Wallwork had phoned ahead to let Ben know the result. It was then that Ben confirmed that he had agreed to work the extra year to keep the post open for me. The final chapter in that particular story was that a few months into my year abroad, Ben fell into a large pothole outside the transplant portacabin in the grounds of Papworth and fractured his patella. As a result, he couldn't work for the remainder of the year. But at least his generosity had earned him a gold merit award, making a substantial contribution to his pension.

My remaining time as senior registrar at Brompton hospital was entertaining and productive. The work that I had done with Christopher Lincoln on the effects of profound hypothermic circulatory arrest on cerebral function in children had been accepted for presentation at that year's American Association of Thoracic Surgeons meeting in Atlanta. Georgia. This was a huge event for me in two ways. The first was having a major presentation at such a prestigious meeting, and the second was that the paper that followed mine was the honoured guest lecture, given that year by Professor Alain Carpentier and titled 'The French Correction.'[8] This was to become one of the most important presentations ever given at that meeting as it set the scene for the international expansion of programmes of mitral valve reconstruction around the world, which up until that time had been a niche sub-specialty often accompanied by poor results.

The discussant on my paper was Sir Brian Barratt-Boyes, a world expert in the subject, but also known for his aggressive responses. In his obituary in *The Independent*, Barratt-Boyes was described as aggressive, autocratic, patriarchal and tough. His peers felt that he was opinionated and intolerant, while his juniors found him aloof, demanding and intimidating. He had trained with, and was very close to John Kirklin, my future research boss, so my performance was under great and meaningful scrutiny. The presentation went well and despite his formidable reputation, he was surprisingly charming to me and supportive in his comments.

Professor Carpentier's presentation followed. As a result, the hall had been packed for my presentation, which added to the stress. Terence English, who had come to support me, had offered me a dose of a beta blocker to calm my nerves, but I refused, being concerned that I might suffer a hypotensive collapse during the presentation.

Carpentier's honoured guest lecture was seminal in my career as, having only done one mitral valve procedure on my own in my training, I found the presentation on mitral valve reconstruction fascinating, and was determined to develop this skill myself. It became the bedrock of my practice to the present day.

The end of the year was approaching rapidly with a lot of planning for my trip to Alabama yet to be completed.

I flew to Birmingham in late November to discuss my project with Dr. Kirklin and to find somewhere to live. My first sight of the university campus was impressive. The buildings were of a higher quality than anything that I had experienced at home and the campus covered a large area in the south of the city. My first meeting with Dr. Kirklin was warm and invigorating. He wanted me to become involved in the work that they were developing trying to understand the role of inflammation in the damaging effects of cardio-pulmonary bypass. Work that had begun with Stephen Westaby, a senior trainee who had also been a student at Charing Cross Hospital, two or three years ahead of me. They had demonstrated that the passage of the patient's blood through the plastic tubing of the bypass machine, and the traumatic effect of the roller pump in mashing up the cells triggered a huge initiation of the complement system causing cell damage in the lungs, brain and gut. My project was to delineate the damaging effects on the lungs in particular. I was shown around the considerable laboratory space and introduced to the lab. technicians Stanley Digerness and Bil Tracey, as well as the various components of the pathology department that I would be working with. Everyone was welcoming and charming. A key person that I met was Eugene Blackstone, the department statistician who enjoyed an international reputation.

The following day I drove my hired Cadillac out into the suburbs to find living accommodation. I had focussed on a few condominiums and finally settled on one called Arboretum. There was an outdoor pool, and the ground floor apartment seemed comfortable. I quickly signed the rental agreement with the manager and, very pleased with myself, set off back to the centre of the city and my hotel, prior to my departure the following day. I made one very basic error. I failed to notice that the apartment was largely unfurnished as it was already being lived in. This resulted in something of a surprise when we arrived 'en famille' in January but more of that later.

On the way back to the hotel, cruising along the six-lane highway at a comfortable 70 mph, I was suddenly alerted to a black and white highway patrol car with siren blaring and lights flashing rapidly approaching me from behind. A large STOP sign was flashing on his roof. I rapidly slowed down and pulled over to the hard shoulder and waited with hands clearly visible on the steering wheel, as I had been instructed to do if stopped.

At first, I lost sight of the police officer, but then I could see him approaching very close to the side of the car with a shotgun in hand. I carefully wound down the window and in my best and most polite English, asked him what the matter was. He growled, 'You were speeding. It's only fifty miles per hour on this stretch of road. Show me your driver's licence and papers.' I duly produced them, and he asked me where I was from and what I was doing there. I answered dutifully and stated that I was visiting Dr Kirklin at UAB. Instantly his attitude changed, and he lowered his shotgun. In as stern a voice as he could muster, he said:

> We all admire Dr. Kirklin in this town but Dr. Wells, you drive too fast. You can go this time, but I will be looking for you when you return in January.

I thanked him profusely and, greatly relieved, drove off to the hotel within the newly recognised speed limit.

The rest of my trip was uneventful.

9

Fun with the Arts

> To develop a complete mind, study the science of art. Study the art of science. Learn how to see. Realise that everything connects to everything else.
>
> Leonardo da Vinci

> There is an art to science and a science to art; the two are not enemies, but different aspects of the whole.
>
> Isaac Asimov

As far back as I can remember I have been drawn to art, but my excitement over graphic art in particular was primed by a wonderful teacher at school Mr Chambers. A hugely colourful character and trombonist, he was a favourite of everyone. He had encouraged me to take art at O level (this test preceded G.C.E.s) and instilled in some of us a real love of drawing which he held to be the foundation of everything. As mentioned previously, he overcame the natural reluctance to make marks on paper which many have, by strolling around the classroom saying loudly, 'Waste paper boys, waste paper. Don't be afraid to make a mess, just waste paper.' It was through him that I discovered Leonardo da Vinci. I couldn't have imagined then the world that would open up for me in the future.

A note in my diary for 1977, states that, 'On Thursday 29 November I visited an exhibition of anatomical notes and drawings by Leonardo da Vinci, in the Royal Academy on Piccadilly'. It was notable for several reasons. First is the fact that, apart from two showings in the United States of America in 1976, this was the first time that they had been shown as individual sheets to the British public. There had been an exhibition in Burlington House in 1952 celebrating the quincentenary of Leonardo's birth, but at that time they were still bound in the book in which they had been mounted by the Madrid based Italian artist Pompeo Leoni. On his death, Leonardo had bequeathed most of his belongings to his faithful young student and companion Francesco Melzi, the son of a wealthy Milanese nobleman. Leonardo left instructions with Francesco to catalogue his notes and drawings. Francesco's attempts were poor and little of importance arose from his work. Indeed, it is likely that many pages of notes were lost whilst in his possession. On Francesco's death all was left to his brother who had no interest in them and seemed to be happy to be rid of them. Pompeo Leoni bound the pages into at least one large, leather-bound book. Many of the pages were cut into smaller fragments and mounted in that reduced form. It was this bound volume that was on show, with the pages turned on a regular basis and accompanied by photographs of the pages.

The second point of interest was that Sir Anthony Blunt, Curator of the Queen's Pictures, became infamous as the fourth man in the Cambridge Russian spy ring, along with Kim Philby, Guy Burgess, Donald Maclean and latterly, John Cairncross. Blunt had been dramatically exposed by Margaret Thatcher using Parliamentary privilege on the floor of the House of Commons early into her premiership in 1979. Each of these treacherous spies had somewhat colourful code names: Maclean was Homer, Burgess was Hicks, Philby was Sonny and Cairncross was Liszt. Cambridge graduates all. Blunt, as the keeper of the Queen's pictures, was at the heart of the establishment, making the scandal even more salacious. Suspicions had been raised earlier but the idea of a spy being so close to the heart of the establishment was ridiculed for a long time and almost certainly covered up by some of those establishment figures who knew the facts but were keen to avoid embarrassment.

Walking along Piccadilly, I had found myself passing the grand entrance to Burlington House, the home of the Royal Academy since the mid-nineteenth century. I knew the building well, having passed it many times whilst at the old Charing Cross. However, what grabbed my attention was a poster advertising the exhibition of Leonardo's anatomical drawings from the Royal Collection. I knew of his manuscripts and drawings but, until that time, was only familiar with his paintings, few though they were. I had studied Leonardo's life as a painter, along with Vincent van Gogh, for my O level exam. (A more dissonant pair of artists is hard to imagine). Learning anatomy for my medical studies, I had spent many hours studying contemporary anatomical illustrations in the textbooks of Henry Gray, as well as Last and Cunningham's dissection manuals and Frank Netters illustrations. Knowing something of the diversity of Leonardo's interests,

I was intrigued to see how his anatomical work would stand up against modern accepted anatomy. What I found was refreshing and vibrant in a way that, to my eyes, no contemporary illustration could match. Not only are they extraordinary feats of draughtsmanship and quite beautiful as works of art, but it also became instantly clear to me that there was a great deal of accuracy to be found there. This experience began a lifelong and deepening interest that has led me to many interesting places and to meet many people that I would not have otherwise.

To make meaningful sense of it all, the first thing that I knew I had to do, was to educate myself in the history of the Renaissance and Leonardo's place in it. This goal produced a fascinating reading list for the next two decades. I had been impressed by a quotation that I thought originated from Winston Churchill, 'Never read anything to do with work after ten o'clock at night.' I took this to heart, and began to devour books by Kenneth Keele, a physician with a practice in Windsor, for whom Leonardo studies had also become a lifetime interest. Keele was also a cardiac specialist. Others of influence were Carlo Pedretti, the scholar with perhaps the most encyclopaedic knowledge of Leonardo's manuscripts, and latterly Martin Kemp, professor of History of Art at St Andrew's and then Oxford Universities. Little did I know that I would have the great fortune to get to know and become friends with the latter two men.

The life and times of Leonardo are fascinating and involve many of the great characters of the period. From Michelangelo to Machiavelli, Bramante to Botticelli, the Medici to the Sforzas, and Pope Leo X to King Francis I of France, the cast of personalities of that time was large and massively influential. It was a time of war and plague making life difficult for the ordinary man. Leonardo moved around a great deal in his lifetime, from Tuscany to Northern Italy and further south to Rome pursuing work and commissions. Born in Vinci (hence the name, da, *from*, Vinci) in the hills north-west of Florence to the hot beds of academia in Florence, Milan and Rome. In learning about his life and the pressures causing him to move so much, I bought every book that I came across on the subject and began to learn of the structure of the great courts in those cities and the geopolitics generated there in quattro- and cinquecento Italy. A study that I found utterly absorbing.

In the winter of 1992, I decided that I wanted to see first-hand Leonardo's drawings of the heart, being by then a young consultant surgeon with a significant knowledge and experience of the heart and lungs. All of the anatomical drawings amongst others came into the hands of the Royal Household through King Charles I and II through the efforts of Lord Arundel, Duke of Norfolk. Therefore I wrote to the Honourable Jane Roberts, then the Curator of the Queen's Pictures and wife of Sir Hugh Roberts, Director of the Royal Collection, to request a visit to the Royal Library. Some weeks passed without a reply, and I began to assume that my plebeian request had been tossed into the royal bin. Then, to my astonishment, I received a grand looking letter with the royal seal emblazoned upon it. In great excitement, I opened it carefully with a paper knife, so as not to damage what I thought was likely to be my only correspondence from the royal household. My wish had been granted. I was invited to attend the library, having first to pass the necessary security clearance.

Early on the morning of Thursday 20 February, a snowy birthday, I arrived at the entrance to Windsor Castle. After carefully inspecting my security clearance, the police at the gate politely allowed me to pass, and I drove up the hill past St George's Chapel towards the royal library, brimming with excitement. The small reception area was staffed by two jolly policemen who checked my credentials. Janie, as she liked to be called, met me at the entrance and escorted me into the library. It is a very beautiful building that readers may remember from that terrible night in November of the same year when fire almost destroyed that part of the castle. Prince Charles (as he was then) could be seen running out of the library with the large box files containing the Leonardo drawings. Indeed, there were many times in the history of those manuscript sheets when they could have been lost forever. This was certainly one of them. Martin Kemp suggests that, probably three to four fifths of Leonardo's manuscripts have been lost across the centuries. Reading his notes, though already without order and much structure, it quite often feels as though the reader comes to a precipice of words that abruptly stop, supporting the suggesting of the loss of pages.

I had asked to see the manuscript pages that relate to the heart. There they all were, in their ultraviolet light protective mountings spread all around one large room. Janie had also put out several other important drawings of the musculoskeletal system and I was told not to be afraid to ask to see any other ones that were of particular interest to me.

I had a plan in mind; to review all the written notes and drawings of the heart, seen through the eyes of someone (me) who spends their life working with the heart. In light of the fact that Leonardo had wanted to publish a magnum opus of anatomy but didn't succeed in it, I hoped to publish them with a modern commentary. The more that I examined them the more my excitement rose. Not only were they beautiful to look at but the accuracy of some of them was astonishing. Reading Leonardo's notes, it became clear that his interpretation of the structure of the components of the heart had led him to physiological conclusions that are importantly relevant to today's cardiological investigations.

I was completely absorbed throughout the day. The hours flew by. Finally, Janie returned and enquired how I had got on. It was hard to put into words the emotions that I felt having had the privilege to have so many uninterrupted hours with Leonardo's handwriting and drawings in my own hands. We discussed my thoughts for quite some time, and a provisional agreement was reached to proceed with the idea of the book. I think that it had become clear to her that there was much more of importance in these drawings and notes of the heart than had perhaps been realised by the pure art historians.

Before leaving Janie asked me if there was anything else that I might care to see. I naively asked her what she had in the library. Her reply was, 'We have around 40,000 old master drawings', and she invited me to take my pick. This was an impossible task for me, with no detailed knowledge of the library holdings, and so I suggested that perhaps she would show me what she thought would be of interest. With a smile Janie produced the anatomical drawings of Michelangelo. My jaw dropped further, and we spent another hour or more comparing and contrasting styles and objectives of those two Renaissance giants. Leonardo the scientist and Michelangelo, the forever artist, sculptor. The former digging ever deeper into the structure of things and then attempting, usually very successfully, to identify form with function in startling modern ways, and the latter, identifying form more generically for artistic interpretation. This difference led Leonardo to describe Michelangelo as producing the muscles in the human frame like a bag of nuts.

We finally said our goodbyes and I left for Cambridge. I felt so privileged as I drove slowly back down the hill passing the great circular castle keep towards the exit and with a cheery wave to the policemen on the gate I left for home. What a birthday it had been. My journey had begun.

There are sixty-four pages of notes and drawings on the heart in the extant Leonardo manuscripts. Kenneth Keele reviewed and interpreted them in his 1952 privately published book, *Leonardo da Vinci On the Movement of the Heart and Blood.*[1] It is relevant to repeat part of the preface to that book because it was that which led me to go on with the work that I pursued. Keele wrote:

> In this book I have attempted to co-ordinate Leonardo's writings on the heart, blood vessels, and movement of the blood, and to present his views in an easily comprehensible sequence. Only a few fragmentary phrases have, so far as I am aware, been omitted, so that it is hoped that the presentation may be considered complete. The task of presentation is not of course limited to the written word. A great number of drawings

and diagrams, some of great beauty, others of artistic insignificance, often express Leonardo's views more clearly than his text.

Almost all such drawings are represented in his book, and their relation to the text noted.

Some, I am afraid, still baffle interpretation.

That last sentence intrigued me. I wondered what extra light could be thrown on Leonardo's deductions fifty years later through the eyes of a contemporary cardiac surgeon. With my interest in the anatomy and physiology of the heart, elements of his descriptions and deductions spoke to me directly. More modern understanding of the way in which the heart works has revealed a dovetailing of Leonardo's descriptions with cutting edge knowledge. Clearly I had to document this, and so I decided to reproduce Leonardo's dissections. A difference between Renaissance thinkers and us in more modern times, is that man was seen then as God incarnate. Therefore, if you could understand man in the fullest way possible, you could begin to understand God. The first step was to appreciate Leonardo's interest and awareness of comparative anatomy. Leonardo placed the same importance on animal anatomy as he did on that of the human. All the known heart drawings, bar one, are of the Ox, whose basic anatomical constituents are similar to that of man, but in exaggerated form. There is one drawing on cream paper from his time in Rome of an opened right ventricle that is clearly human, but all the rest are from the ox heart. My own observation was that in studying ox anatomy, the exaggerated features found therein over those in the human heart, make some of his deductions easier to understand. The anatomical structures are more striking. None more so than those that are to be found in the arterial outlet of the heart (the left ventricular outflow tract, the aortic valve and the sinuses of the aorta) where his observations, backed up by experimental testing, were so very far ahead of his time.

These dissections and drawings were probably made in his time with the family Melzi in Vaprio d'Ada, just outside Milan, where he went following the French invasion of that city. The animal material would be readily available from local slaughterhouses. The exaggerated size of the structures would have aroused Leonardo's architectural and engineering mind. It is my contention that this led Leonardo, the engineer/architect, towards conclusions drawn from his wider experience in hydrology and engineering. His interpretations of his findings were far ahead of his time and are only now being realisable with advanced research, adding weight to Keele's comment on the difficulty of interpretation in the mid-twentieth century before modern imaging had been devised. The prime example is his precise and correct description of the beautifully observed closure mechanism of the aortic valve (the valve that controls the flow of blood out of the heart). His experimental design to test his hypothesis took a further 500 years and modern technology with some complex mathematics to confirm. In fact, the experiment that he designed and almost certainly carried out was repeated in 1968 by two Oxford engineers the Bellhouse brothers. Their work was published in the important scientific magazine *Nature* and it is the only paper that I have ever seen in that august journal with just one reference attached to it, and that being over 500 years old.[2] Fate seemed to play a hand here as one of the authors, Professor Brian Bellhouse, was killed by an angered cow (ox) whilst walking in the fields near his home in Guesting, near Hastings in 2017. A brilliant engineer, Professor Bellhouse was responsible for the development of the needleless injection system and in doing so was one of the first in Oxford university to develop a spin-out company.

As a Butcher's boy, and being familiar with the hearts of cattle, it was a minor step to want to repeat Leonardo's dissections of the ox heart. Access to undamaged ox hearts is not straight forward these days, as meat inspectors incise the removed hearts looking for heart worm before they can be sold. The only way to easily access the material was to collect a heart and lung block from a freshly killed animal before the meat inspectors had access. This was acceptable as the organ was not going to be sold for consumption and incinerated after the dissection. Large abattoirs wouldn't suffice as the organs that they would allow me to buy had to go through their established protocol. I began to phone around several local butchers who slaughtered their own cattle, but none was forthcoming until I manged to locate a small country butcher who was willing to help me, as long as I went to help him with the process. I arrived at 6.00 a.m., and we completed the task and I was able to return to the laboratory with the fresh heart and lung block to do the dissection.

It was at that point that I realised the full enormity of Leonardo's accomplishments. With no books and no meaningful knowledge to help him he had to make sense of very complex anatomy. Here it is important to reproduce his own note on the process of dissection. He wrote:

> And though you have a love for such things you will perhaps be impeded by your stomach, and if this does not impede you, you will perhaps be impeded by the fear of living through the night hours in the company

> of quartered and flayed corpses fearful to behold. And if this does not impede you, perhaps you the lack of draughtsmanship which appertains to such representation; and even if you have the skill in drawing, it may not be accompanied by a knowledge of perspective; and if it were so accompanied, you may lack the methods of geometrical demonstration and methods of calculating the forces and strength of muscles; or perhaps you will lack patience so that you will not be diligent. Whether all these things were found in me or not, the 120 books composed by me give the verdict, yes or no. In these I have been impeded neither by avarice nor negligence, but only by time. Farewell.[3]

From this quotation it can be seen that he was very well aware of his superior skill in draughtsmanship and not slow to proclaim it. He described the attributes needed to do this kind of important research properly, patience, determination to complete the task, a strong stomach and a broad education and experience in engineering, and some facility in mathematics, although it has to be said that he was not an accomplished mathematician.

There were no preservatives at that time and so dissection had to be completed at the coolest part of the day, hence at night, and human dissection could only be carried out in winter. He goes on to stress the importance of repeating studies more than once to check the findings and to ensure that the deductions and descriptions are true representations of the facts, something that is grossly lacking in much research these days where a single study is reported and proclaimed, often through the popular media, as being the last word on the subject. This, too frequently for comfort, is then disproved at a later date by other workers in the field.

Here is his note on the importance of meticulous work and of repeating it to give the information verisimilitude:

> In order to obtain an exact and complete knowledge, I have dissected more than ten human bodies, destroying all the various members, and removing even the smallest particles of the flesh which surround these veins without causing any effusion of blood other than the imperceptible bleeding of the capillary veins. And, as one single body did not suffice for a long time, it was necessary to proceed by stages with so many bodies as would render my knowledge complete; and this I repeated twice over in order to discover the differences.[4]

This marks a true scientist at work, striving for the truth and leaving no stone unturned in the process. Here is a man whose observations must be taken seriously and so it has proved when his work has been studied by experts in many different disciplines. It is also what makes study of his notes and drawings so rewarding. His respect for the heart is revealed in the following quotation:

> With what words will you describe this heart so as not to fill a book? The longer you write on the details the more you will confuse the mind of the auditor. You will always be in need of commentators or be required to return to experience, which in your case is very brief, and gives knowledge of but a few things concerning the whole subject of which you desire an entire knowledge.[5]

Conversations around Leonardo's work usually focus on his paintings and drawing skills, but I have found that his notes are clear, often concise and beautiful to read. Translations of his reversed left-handed medieval Tuscan Italian are readily available, making the notes accessible for all.

Taking Leonardo's advice, I repeated the dissection on two separate blocks of tissue. I was assisted in this by my consultant pathologist colleague Martin Goddard. He found it equally amazing. For the second set of dissections we invited Professor Robert Anderson, (a fellow Shropshire lad) one of the foremost embryologist and foetal anatomist in the world today. It was wonderful watching Robert's face and hearing the excitement in his voice as we proceeded through the dissections. To share my excitement with such an eminent authority on the anatomy of the heart and to see his own amazement at the quality of Leonardo's work, in the absence of any prior knowledge was energising. If ever reassurance was needed of the veracity of Leonardo's work, this was it. It is intriguing to wonder how Leonardo would approach the modern world of science. I suspect that it would be with considerably more rigour that is to be found in some areas of work.

Eventually I had enough material to write the book. The work already had a large public outing. I had been invited to give the prestigious basic science lecture at the European Society of Thoracic Surgeons' annual meeting in Lisbon in 2019. The lecture was broadcast into all three huge halls of the conference centre which were packed with over 6,000 surgeons and associated specialists from all around the world. The basic science lectures are variably attended but this unusual level of interest revealed the respect and veneration that Leonardo continues to generate amongst scientists and physicians. When I had concluded my talk, there was a forest of hands with interested questions from all ages within the audience. Present amongst this vast sea of faces was Dr Andy Wechsler, the president of the American Association of Thoracic Surgeons and editor of the *Journal of Thoracic and Cardiovascular Surgery*, one of the highest ranked medical journals in the world. Immediately after I had climbed down from the podium, he almost ran up to me and invited me to write up the presentation as the opening paper in an edition of the journal. He wanted to get in his request before any of the other journal editors in the audience. I was delighted to accept. My title for the presentation was, 'Leonardo da Vinci as a Paradigm for Modern Clinical Research'. Leonardo made many comments about the conduct of meaningful research which reverberate ever more clearly today. Leonardo stated the importance of not publishing something until it had been verified repeatedly. This is in contrast to the all too frequent rush to publish today, based on thin evidence that does not stand up to serious scrutiny. He wrote abrasively of those who took short cuts in their work.

> The abbreviators of works do injury to knowledge and to love, for the love of anything is the offspring of knowledge, love being more fervent in proportion as knowledge is more certain, and this certainty springs from a thorough knowledge of all those parts, which united compose the whole. Truly it is impatience, mother of folly who praises brevity.[6]

It appears from Leonardo's notes that he was criticised by recognised academics of the day for daring to expound on academic themes, and to challenge others when he had not had a formal education. His reply was direct and highly critical of those academics who only spoke from knowledge derived from the books of others, while his reporting was derived from direct experimentation:

> Many will think that they can with reason blame me, alleging that my proofs are contrary to the authority of certain men held in great reverence by their inexperienced judgement, not considering that my works are the issue of simple and plain experience [experiment] which is the true mistress. These rules enable you to know truth from the false.
>
> I am fully aware that the fact of my not being a man of letters may cause certain presumptuous persons to think that they may with reason blame me, alleging that I am a man without learning. Foolish Folk.[7]

My paper in the journal is followed by a tribute to Dr Francis Robicsek, (1925–2020) a brilliant Hungarian American surgeon, Europhile and medical historian based in Charlotte North Carolina. Francis had written about Leonardo's work on the aortic valve long before me.[8] I was fortunate to become a friend and every time we met, we had hugely entertaining conversations on medical history and the progress of surgery.

Windsor had suggested Prestel as the publisher for my forthcoming book on the cardiac anatomy of Leonardo. However, after quite detailed and indeed intense discussions with them it became clear to me that they didn't really understand what my aims were. They tried to force me into writing something that I did not want to, and after trying to cooperate and re-writing the book several times it became clear that it simply wasn't working so I withdrew from the process. Eventually, my efforts were rewarded with the help of Grant Weston, commissioning editor of perhaps the most important scientific publishing house today Springer-Verlag. He was working with me on another surgical text and, having the manuscript in the top draw of my desk, I produced it and asked if he might be interested. He immediately saw the merits of the book as a cross-over between the arts and science, something that they had been trying to bridge for a while. Talking to someone who could see the point of what I was trying to do was refreshing. It also seemed to me to be another affirmation of the importance of Leonardo's work. Happily, Martin Clayton and Janie Roberts approved of the move to Springer. Windsor were so very kind in allowing me to reproduce all of the relevant manuscript pages, freshly digitised in high definition, and to use the most recent translation of Leonardo's notes by the scholar Carlo Pedretti. Quite quickly the book was put into production.

Royal support did not end there. His Royal Highness, King Charles (then the Prince of Wales) wrote the first of two forewords, the second was by Professor Martin Kemp. I was invited to hold the book launch in the Queen's Gallery, within the walls of Buckingham Palace. The gallery staff moved the standing exhibits from the ground floor room and the Royal Library provided several of the drawings to be hung there for the event. Since that time the lovely staff in the Royal Library have continued to be very supportive, for which I am extremely grateful.

My deeper involvement in all things Leonardo had derived from the generosity of Professor Martin Kemp, then Professor of History of Art in Oxford. In 2003, hearing of my interest in the anatomy of Leonardo, Professor Kemp had invited me to give a lecture at Central St Martin's School of Art and Design. My secretary at that time, Julie Mazzone, received a phone call from Martin, who made the invitation to speak. She immediately gave her default response, which was to say yes and then to tell me what she had accepted for me. At that time, I had not met Professor Kemp but knew who he was through my reading. It seemed an enormous privilege. The day arrived and I delivered the lecture to a room with around fifty people present, mostly elderly or middle-aged men.

The lecture seemed to proceed well enough other than in my general anxiety, my managing to confuse William Hunter, the eighteenth century anatomist and obstetrician, with William Harvey, the sixteenth century physician to King Charles II who had first described the circulation of the blood in his seminal book *de Motu Cordis*. A fairly large mistake which Martin pressed home at the end with the double entendre, 'Aren't we lucky that Francis did not choose to be an art historian?'. Suitably humbled we retired for dinner at an Italian restaurant across the road. There I was informed as to whom I had been presenting. They seemed to consist of most of the important gallery directors in the western world. My embarrassment was amplified considerably, but they were all very nice to me and seemingly truthfully thought that the work that I was doing was worthwhile.

It was at that dinner that I met Thereza, who was to become my wife. Thereza was part of a research group called the Universal Leonardo Project (U.L.P.), an international digital humanities initiative founded by Professor Marina Wallace and Professor Kemp and funded by Stavros Niarchos. It was dedicated to making the work of Leonardo globally accessible. They orchestrated meetings, papers and exhibitions on Leonardo. For the years of our marriage Martin referred to the U.L.P. as an art history research group and marriage bureau. Thereza had spent her PhD years under the tutelage of Martin, studying a famous Leonardo, the Lansdowne Madonna of the Yarnwinder. She researched its history and provenance. She was privileged to have it on her desk for a significant period of time whilst carrying out the research. There are several versions of this painting in existence but two stand out as autograph Leonardos, one in the possession of a wealthy New York family, the Lansdowne Madonna, and the other owned by the Duke of Buccleuch. The aforementioned Lansdowne Madonna was thoroughly researched at the Opificio in Florence under the direction of Cristina Acidini, with Thereza heavily involved in the process.

Leonardos are the highest prized paintings in the art world. As a result they are high on the list of desirable objects by the extremely wealthy. The Mona Lisa was famously stolen from the Louvre in Paris in 1911. It was stolen by a petty criminal Vincenzo Perugia and was missing for two years before being restored to its home in Paris. The story of that theft is well told in books and on film. In 2003 the Scottish Leonardo was stolen in broad daylight from Drumlanrig castle in Scotland. The thieves tore it from the wall and ran outside to a waiting getaway car. It disappeared for four years but was eventually recovered in a solicitor's office in Edinburgh in 2007. Elements of that story remain a mystery to this day. On its recovery the experts on the painting, Martin and Thereza, were invited to the National Gallery of Scotland in Edinburgh to review the painting and to examine it for verification and any damage. This was in the presence of the young Duke of Buccleuch, his father having died before the painting had been recovered. His heart had been broken by its theft. I had the great privilege of being invited along with Marina Wallace, and together we were among the first to see the painting out of its frame, before its return to its rightful owner. It now hangs in the National Gallery of Scotland, courtesy of the duke and his family.

A rather more dubious event was to be invited by the BBC to take part in a giant painting of the Mona Lisa, again in Edinburgh at the foot of the castle and orchestrated by the now disgraced Rolf Harris. Olivia, then a baby, featured in the opening credits in Thereza's arms.

Thereza is an intelligent academic art historian and I had thought that, with my interest in the Renaissance, in particular Leonardo, it would be a perfect match. Sadly, that wasn't to be. However, Thereza has proved to be an excellent mother to our beautiful daughter Olivia.

Professor Kemp is an extremely generous man and following that event he invited me to be involved in several projects with him. We made programmes for Discovery channel, wherein the glider that Leonardo had designed[7] was built and flown by the British hang-glider champion, a very brave woman. With some help and a bit of practice and a slight downhill slope on the Luton Downs it flew further than the Wright Brothers' first flight. Martin had perceived that Leonardo had stumbled upon the need for a cross-sectional shape similar to the aerofoil, which is what gives wings their lift, and that had been built into the leading edge of the wing. The massive catapult (a latter-day weapon of mass destruction) was built and would have worked other than the fact that properly seasoned wood was not available, and the crossbow arm fractured with the force needed to draw it to a firing position[9]

I also had the privilege of helping Martin and his team with a prestigious exhibition at the Victoria and Albert Museum in 2006 titled 'Leonardo da Vinci: Experience, Experiment and Design'. It was an eye-opening experience to witness the care and collegiate academic input that goes into such important shows. Here computer graphics were used to animate some of Leonardo's key drawings. This was done using the expertise of Steven Maher, working for Cosgrove Hall Productions. A star of the show was a beautiful rendering of Leonardo's depiction of a tiny figure wielding a hammer or an axe. I truly felt that I was living in a dream world and thoroughly enjoyed meeting such interesting people in a completely different sphere of life, one that in truth I found more interesting than the repetitious nature of cardiac surgery

Other delights and excitement were to follow. Early in February 2004, again close to my birthday, on a Saturday morning, the phone rang, and a familiar sounding voice with a Yorkshire accent asked, 'Is that Frank Wells?' 'Yes', I answered, 'And who is calling?' 'David Hockney', came the reply. Clearly, from the unmistakable voice, it was David Hockney himself, among the most renowned active artists in the modern world. I stood to attention and asked how I could help him. I fully expected him to want to talk about a cardiac surgical problem, relating to my day job. However, to my surprise he said, 'I hear that you use drawing in your work.' He had been informed of this by Martin Kemp. I answered tentatively in the affirmative. He went on to explain that he was curating the Royal Academy Summer Exhibition with Allen Jones that year and wanted to have a section wherein they planned to include drawings by non-professional artists who used drawing in their work. He asked to see some of my drawings and whether I could bring them down to the Royal Academy the following week for him to take a look. Calmly, trying to conceal my real excitement, of course my answer was yes. I had admired his work since visiting a large exhibition at the Royal Academy two decades before. He had narrated the show on tape of which I still have a copy. On that tape his description of an early portrait of his mother was particularly moving.

The following Wednesday I journeyed down to London and we met in the Royal Academy where David reviewed the drawings that I had brought with me. To my surprise he chose six of them that he wanted to exhibit. They were kept by the staff of the academy to be framed in their house style ready for the exhibition.

At that time, I had some American surgeons visiting me at Papworth to see the way that I repaired the mitral valve. There is a point in the operation when the reparative surgery is complete and the patient is being rewarmed whilst the heart rests on cardiopulmonary bypass. The visitors were asking questions about a particular style of repair that I had performed. I reached for some sterile paper, and using a pair of surgical forceps, dipped them in some blood in the open chest, and began to draw to illustrate the procedure, as I often did. I find thinking and expressing myself through drawing particularly effective.

Dilute blood is readily available in the pericardial space around the heart and the amount used is miniscule (think of the amount of ink flowing from a pen when writing). Also, at that time I had one of a series of artists in residence with me. Professor Jane Profit was producing hearts sculpted in silver and gold from magnetic resonance scans. Jane saw what I was doing and rushed to get her movie camera to film the drawing. After the surgery we were chatting about the forthcoming RA exhibition, and we wondered if David Hockney might like to consider using the footage. I phoned to ask him, He was excited by the idea and asked me to go down again to show him. When he saw the short film, he said that they must show it in the exhibition. So we did. It became the first installation video ever in the Summer Exhibition and the story travelled around the world in the press and on television.

This 'blood film', as it became known, reverberated in many ways. It provoked several articles in the major newspapers. In *The Independent* on 4 June under the heading 'Doctor's Bloody Work on Show', Maeve Kennedy wrote

> For sheer shock value, no shark, tent or kebab is in the same league as the moment Francis Wells dips his drawing implement and begins sketching away on paper. His instrument is a pair of surgical forceps, his medium blood on sterilised white paper, and his inkwell is the opened chest on which he is operating. Yesterday, Mr Wells, consultant cardiac surgeon at the world-famous Papworth Hospital in Cambridge, was surprised to have his work hanging in the Royal Academy summer exhibition, at the invitation of the guest curators, David Hockney and Allen Jones, both champions of the Art of drawing. He was equally surprised at the hardened hacks tottering away from the video showing him at work. 'I must say it's a wonderful drawing medium,' he said thoughtfully of blood. 'It flows beautifully.'

Reflecting the decrease in the teaching of anatomy at art school in the modern era, she went on to quote me saying that there were better artists, but no better anatomists on the walls:

> There's some terrible anatomy in this exhibition, he said scowling at a ballet dancer, her back bent like a bowstring. Analysing the positioning of the vertebrae, he barked: 'It should be at L3/4, not T 12 you know.'

The Times ran a story written by Dalya Alberge, their arts correspondent at the time, headed, 'Academy Show Gets to the Heart of Life Drawing'. She quoted David Hockney defending his decision to allow the showing of the blood drawing video. 'It's not gruesome,' he said, insisting that the subject matter was secondary. 'I just see images.' Allen Jones is quoted as saying, 'Francis Wells draws with absolute clarity. It's like watching Matisse. It's quite compulsive.' Quite the best compliment I have ever been paid, and I must admit that at that moment I wish that my mother could have read those words when she told me to forget being an artist and to get a proper job, although on reflection she was probably right. Dalya quotes me saying

> ...drawing is also an intellectual process: Some people use drawing in their thinking process, communication and teaching. In an operation, it's the drawing activity that helps you communicate and think.'

This reflects my view very accurately. In another piece for *The Guardian*, Allen Jones is quoted in conversation with David Hockney, saying

> ...that in the show there will be three videos and one of them will be of this heart transplant surgeon, Francis Wells, who is drawing in blood during an operation. The camera is in quite close to, and you see the hand there with the forceps. He dips the forceps in the inkwell, which is someone's open chest, and he draws on a kind of white swab. I've seen pictures of Matisse drawing and Picasso, and this man draws absolutely incisively. It's beautiful to behold, to see the economy.

All remarks were not so kind. The work also provoked outrage in some traditionalists. They railed against what was referred to as an 'avant-gardist' take-over from what some saw as the central role of the RA in being a centre of excellence for craftsmanship. The reaction against the introduction of conceptual art by the Brit Art's brash young conceptualists in 2001 was raised by Edna Weiss, a painter and former student of the Royal Academy Schools. Referring to my offering, she was quoted as saying that 'This belongs in the Royal College of Surgeons, rather than the Royal Academy of Arts. Anything goes today, it seems.' Allen Jones defended the decision to show the piece when asked if it was art. He said, 'It isn't. It's drawing as communication', which of course was precisely the point of inclusion of work by non-professional artists. However, I would argue that it is art. After all, isn't all art a form of communication? It also raises the philosophical discussion whether only professionally trained artists can produce art, or if art is the domain of everyone, the arbiter of quality being the acceptance by the observer. The quality of drawing on show by the non-professionals drew higher praise than several of the conceptual pieces on show at that gallery over previous years. Indeed, David Hockney was heavily critical of the fact that art schools no longer teach the basic skill of drawing. He argued that the craft of drawing teases the eye into really looking at the world around us. He drew comparison with the cave drawings of ancient times as some of the earliest forms of communication. His further comment on my contribution in rebuttal of the criticisms was, 'Far from returning to the life room for drawing sessions, this is about going forwards to the life room.'

The surety of the art form demonstrated by us non-artists was celebrated by Laura Gascoigne, who in her article for *The Spectator* in the same month stated that the inclusion of the drawings by the non-artists showed that Hockney and Jones had 'Taken another leaf from the Campaign for Drawing's book'. She wrote

> Lying as they do, outside the self-referential definition of art as done by artists, these working sketches can be judged purely on their own terms. On those terms, they stand up remarkably well. Though few of us could name the subject of a Francis wells ink drawing as 'the repair of the perimembranous ventricular septal defect', it's 'of' something, leaving Antony Gormley's inky abstractions looking aimless by comparison. The non-artists drawings are also refreshingly free of 'style', that sclerosis which can creep up on artists when inspiration wanes.

In our defence at being hung on the hallowed walls of the Royal Academy, I quote E. H. Gombrich, who states as the opening sentence in his book on the history of art *The Story of Art*: 'There really is no such things as art, there are only artists', raising the question once again of how to define what makes someone an artist. It can be argued that anyone who expresses themselves creatively is an artist.

For balance, however, I have to include the rather scathing, but possibly appropriate review by the late, and some would say great art critic Brian Sewell. He wrote in the *Evening Standard* of 4 June:

> The academy's craving for publicity subverts the exhibition's declared theme – a return to drawing. Both Jones and Hockney know perfectly well what drawing is – that it marks the beginning of an idea, that it records the intellectual exploration of that idea, that it is invention, correction and adjustment and development, that it is the foundation of everything in art that is representational (no matter how loosely we use the word) that it is the hidden skeleton of every brushstroke and the preliminary armature of every sculpture and that implying form and volume as weightily as any sculpture.
>
> But for Jones and Hockney all this is not enough- drawings must be exhibited as the medium by which merely technical information is communicated, and into the exhibition must come diagrams drawn by the cardiac surgeon, the mathematician, the poet and old Uncle Tom Cobleigh and all, and all. Of course, we all draw to demonstrate a point- on envelopes, napkins and with a finger in the dust – but this does not make us artists any more than a shopping list makes authors of us. It is absurd to have these two old buffers to have invited non-artists to exhibit in the Summer exhibition (every amateur scribble eliminates a painting by a

> professional) but I have no doubt that it has ensured publicity in vocational journals that would never in the normal course of work and subject, have printed one word about the Academy and will whip in unwonted visitors.

Of course, Sewell has a point, but perhaps he missed the underpinning of the point of the Summer Exhibition which, in my opinion, every year indulges the showing of 'art' by many amateur holiday painters as well as the accepted academicians, whose work is often repetitious and boring. Several of the senior academicians cannot break out of their hackneyed styles and every year, there they are in exactly the same guise, so much so that it is almost possible to cut and paste from the previous year. Much of the entertainment and joy comes from submissions by people one has never heard of and will never hear or see again. In addition, the proclivity of art to be relevant to the wider and important aspects of life, is frequently referred to in all sorts of trade publications. Sadly, Mr Sewell is no longer with us to take up and develop the argument, as I have always regarded him as one of the most entertaining of critics on the art scene.

This, with subsequent events, caused an interesting reaction from the Royal College of Surgeons but more of that later. Most amusing was standing close to the video when the show was open to the public. A large group of ladies from a distant Women's Institute gathered around to watch. Few noticed the progress of the drawing, but many expressed their concern at the use of the patient's blood to draw with. Of course, as a quiet bystander, I was in no position to explain to them what it really entailed. However, if part of the reason for art is to instigate challenge and discussion, this video piece certainly did.

Further on in the exhibition, Tracey Emin had some drawings on show. I overheard another group of ladies comment that they liked 'those drawings by the surgeon' better. They couldn't see the broad smile on my face.

The Tuesday of the week before the opening of the exhibition was varnishing day. On 1 June every year since 1769 (except during the recent Covid-19 pandemic) exhibiting artists were invited to the RA to complete their entries. These days it is more of a celebration and an evening when the prizes are distributed. During the previous week I had received a phone call from Edith Devaney asking me to attend. My initial reaction was that it would not be possible because of clinical commitments. Edith tried several different approaches, but all met with the same response. Ultimately, she said 'Well, I'm not supposed to tell you but you have been nominated for a prize. Can you come now?' I admit rather ashamedly that my response quickly changed and I accepted the invitation.

Late in the afternoon of that day, we all assembled in one of the large galleries and were plied with canapes and champagne. As things got under way the various prize categories were read out. The president then reached the Sir Hugh Casson Prize for Drawing. He announced, 'This year the prize is split three ways. The winners are Frank Auerbach, Paula Rego and Francis Wells.' I nearly collapsed in shock. Frank Auerbach wasn't there but Paula and I walked up together to receive our, quite sizeable, cheque within an envelope labelled Casson. As we returned to our places, I commented to Paula that I thought for her it was just another prize along the way of her glittering career but for me it was the height of mine and would never be surpassed. Paula turned to me and took the envelope from my hand and wrote on it, 'From the heights, Forever Good Luck, Congratulations Paula Rego.' She went on to say, 'I expect you would like me to paint your portrait now.' Before I could reply, my partner at that time, Thereza Crowe, grabbed my arm and whisked me away. Sadly, the moment had gone, deflating an otherwise wonderful moment in my life.

The drawing that won a share of the Casson prize for me was made over a cup of coffee in the surgeon's room, made to explain the procedure to trainee surgeons, thus supporting Brian Sewell's contention. The attestation for the prize stated that the

> ...speed and weight of line, and the selective hatching are integral to the act of emphatic communication, picking out exactly what is essential, filtering out all the visual clutter that would be generated in a photograph or video. Even for someone who has not seen the drawing being made, the sense of motion of the draughtsman's hand, in accordance with the flow of ideas, remains apparent, just as it would in a rapid sketch by Hockney or Jones. Indeed, Wells' drawing shares notable affinities with Hockney's drawings, especially those of the 1960s.

My own words that they further quote, sum up my feelings about drawing consummately:

> Wells himself is fully conscious of the special quality of the act of communicative drawing in time and place: having just completed the operation, drawing one's thoughts feels like an extension of the operation with the hand-eye interworking. It graphically demonstrates the superiority of drawing over other means of visual record, as it is a process of communicating thought and idea as composed in the mind

> without constraints of any equipment limitations and I would add to that the restriction of finding the best words.

This affirmation of the importance of drawing in human communication seemed to underscore the whole reason that David Hockney and Allen Jones had included this section in the exhibition.

As an exhibitor, I was invited to the glittering Summer Exhibition dinner. The guest speaker was Robert Hughes, the long-established Australian art critic. I was sitting next to Bob Geldof who was clearly not in the mood for conversation and looked decidedly worse for wear. Very close to Hughes near the top table was Andrew Lloyd Webber, whose collection of Pre-Raphaelite paintings had hung in the Royal Academy not long before, in place of a late cancellation of an exhibition of Russian art. There had been a call for an end to Fast Art, such as that produced by Damien Hurst and Tracey Emin. Hughes developed the line that it was time for a more aesthetic rather than merely sensational form of artwork. He said that a string of brush marks on a lace collar in a Velasqüez can be as radical as a shark caught for an Englishman some years ago, and now murkily disintegrating in its tank on the other side of the Thames. He went on to say that we have had a gutful of fast art and fast food. What we need more of is slow art, in a word, art that is the very opposite of mass media. He ridiculed the fetishes of art encouraged by collectors such as Charles Saatchi. He railed against the distorting effect of big money on the art world, at which I could see Andrew Lloyd Webber colour up and his head go down, clearly not enjoying the speech, which was turning into a bit of a rant. However, it was interesting to be a fly in the soup of this establishment jamboree.

There was a great deal of publicity surrounding my interest in the work of Leonardo, and as is so often the case, several journalists wrote ever more exaggerated stories claiming that I had drawn knowledge from Leonardo on how to repair the mitral valve. This led to headline news in newspapers such as *The London Times* and *The Guardian*. The truth of the matter was that reading the notes of Leonardo in detail and following his line of thought that all things in nature are as they are for a reason, I began to look at the valve through new eyes and to question the way that we had been taught to reconstruct it. It produced a more empathic approach to the anatomy and a desire to reconstruct in a way that was closer to nature rather than forcing a solution upon it. As a result, a process that became known as respect and not resect evolved. Although this became the mantra of Professor Patrick Perrier, I had first presented the idea in a meeting at Harefield Hospital where, he, Professors Gilles Dreyfus and Magdi Yacoub were present. I was nervous

in presenting these thoughts in front of such a distinguished group. In fact there was some laughter at the ideas which were deviating from the classical Carpentier methods. However, this approach has now become dominant.

A hilarious editorial under the title 'The Code of Life, Heart Surgery is Only One of the Fields Mastered by Da Vinci' appeared in *The Times* newspaper at that time

> Look carefully at The Last Supper. Measure the angle between the sloping right hand side of Christ and the figure-John the Baptist or is it Mary Magdalene? – leaning away on his right. It measures 81 degrees. This is the exact angle at which the hypodermic must be inserted into the aorta for a successful angioplasty. Leonardo da Vinci not only knew the geometry of a quadruple bypass: but he left a detailed set of coded instructions on procedure. Count the number of transverse rafters on the ceiling: seven. Now balance these against the five supporting beams: there you have the precise ratio of camphor and opium required for successful anaesthesia. Finally, note the position of the disciples left hand, held up vertically as a clear sign – or is it a warning? – that a reflux of blood back towards the ventricle alone cannot be the force that closes the valve. As Francis Wells, a consultant cardiac surgeon at Papworth hospital notes: "All cardiac surgeons will know this phenomenon when the valve is tripped open during the infusion of antegrade aortic cardioplegia."
>
> 'This is more than coincidence. The Renaissance artist was so far ahead of his time in anatomy, engineering, botany, geology, geography, hydraulics and aerodynamics that he encoded all his formulae, to await their discovery five centuries later. Extend the legs of a table by a factor of three and you see an inverse map of Latin America. Divide the number of rolls by the plates and you have the coefficient of hydraulic thrust. The cloak of the second disciple on the right slopes at precisely the angle required for take-off. Astonishingly, invert the whole picture and you find a giant pasta cutter.

At least one journalist understood the ridiculous nature of the reporting of the subject.

Another spin off for me were the Summer Exhibition Lectures, a series of four on varying subjects in the world of the arts. The lecturers were David Hockney, renowned composer Sir Harrison Birtwistle, choreographer Siobhan Davies and me. David spoke of drawing in the age of the camera, a fascinating review of his photo montages and i-pad drawings. Harrison Birtwistle explored the theoretical relationships between the writing of

Paul Klee and his own music. Siobhan, with artists David Ward and Bill Woodrow compared their different practices in the mark-making process. Siobhan described the influence of calligraphy in her choreography. I discussed the anatomical drawings of Leonardo in a modern context. They were a fascinating series of lectures and each of us attended the others'.

Following this, Siobhan asked me if I would like to be involved in the preparation for the next dance piece that she was choreographing. Being a fan of dance, both modern and classical ballet, I jumped at the chance, without having an idea of what I could contribute. Along with landscape designer Dan Pearson and linguist Susan Hitch we met with the dancers regularly on a Monday afternoon in Siobhan's dance studio near the Elephant and Castle. Siobhan explained to me that my role was to go through the physiology of breathing and how this was manifest in bodily form and movement. During the process several of the dancers visited Papworth and came into the operating theatre to see the vital organs of the body in their natural state. It was quite an emotional experience for all of us. The nurses in theatre particularly enjoyed the association and many of them still talk about it today. I have always found this cross over between the arts, science and medicine fascinating and a form of continuity from the Renaissance where there was such integration.

The dancers were all very experienced, several of them from the Royal Ballet. I particularly remember Matteo Fargion and Pari Naderi. Their movement was exquisite. What amazed me was their ability to memorise complex moves from one week to the next just as if it had been written down, but of course it was all in their muscle memory.

When complete, I was asked to do an opening night pre-performance talk along with Juliet Stevenson. I remember that I was somewhat overcome with emotion by the event, and this is reflected in the review in *The Independent* newspaper written by Jenny Gilbert.[10] She wrote

> I'm not sure surgeon Francis Wells should give up the day job yet, but his little spiel about core consciousness and extended consciousness ('the galaxy of our minds') was stirring as well as apt.

Another little reminder that perhaps straying too far into the world of the arts was beyond me. However, she went on to say that

> Part of Davies' idea is that these talks will focus the audiences' minds in a different way and encourage them to make new connections with what

> they see. But also, it's about Davies and her dancers gaining insights too. And 'In Plain Clothes' suggests she's on to something.

This exposure led to some very interesting developments. I was asked to contribute lectures for the Prince's Teaching Trust to state school headmasters and mistresses. I was invited to take part in one that was in Cambridge. Lecturers included Stephen Hawking and Roger Penrose, far more distinguished guests than me, but it was exciting to be in such company. The idea was to allow these excellent teachers to open their minds amongst each other and to hear from the horse's mouth as it were, about a huge variety of subjects. My contribution was again on Leonardo and his anatomical works.

Eventually, I was asked to lecture at the Royal Institution for the same body. Standing behind the desk of Faraday, the discoverer of electromagnetic induction and the electric motor, was an amazing feeling. Following this I was invited to dine with the now King, then Prince Charles and his wife Camilla at St James's Palace. At the same occasion was the great British playwright Tom Stoppard and his wife, who were generous in their conversation. I was deeply honoured to find myself sitting opposite His Royal Highness at dinner. When he rose to speak, the first person he referenced was Leonardo and my lecture and work on his anatomy. He proclaimed that it had touched him personally.

My enjoyment of the Renaissance has taken me to places and events that would never have otherwise happened. The people that I have met have enriched my life greatly. Perhaps rather than being an artist, my earliest desire, I should have followed the arts into a career in the history of art. I suspect that I would have had a more fulfilling and interesting life. I spoke about this with Martin Kemp over a drink one evening in Italy where we were at a meeting on Leonardo. He was not impressed and reminded me that I had done much more for humanity in surgery than ever he had in academia. Perhaps he is correct although his work has influenced many in his field over several decades.

Artists in Residence

Cailin Edwards

It all began in 1996 when I met a photographer and artist Ben Edwards, recently transitioned to Cailin. She had worked in many environments as both a documentary and artistic photographer from Cambodia to the heart of Texas. We rapidly became friends. Cailin wanted to photograph the intersection between technology and the human being and what better situation was there than the interface of these two specialist areas than in cardiac surgery. On completion of the original project, one day she said to me that she would like to film a week in my working life as a cardiac surgeon. To spice up the request, she told me that she had recently completed a similar project with the singer Sting. I agreed, but my eagerness was tempered by Cailin telling me that it was not going to be that easy as she would insist on being present in every aspect of my environment. Initially I wasn't concerned by this statement. However, Cailin suggested that we have a trial run to see how it would go. She came up to Cambridge and moved in with me for a couple of days. Sure enough, whenever I said that I was going to this meeting, or that clinical session, there she was by my side. It was more uncomfortable than I had first thought that it would be. Of course, we had sought permission from all of the patients and my colleagues in advance, and somewhat surprisingly no-one objected. Once we had arranged a method of working, the start date was fixed. Cailin is a lovely person, with great skills in communication and a kindness that is rare to find. Her empathy with the patients and their condition instantly transmitted itself to them and they took her to their heart. It was astonishing how she was able to blend into the background, even in the most intimate of settings without causing any interference in the consultative process. It was a testament to her natural humanity, that she was so readily accepted.

The result was a stunning series of photographs reflecting the complexities of the job in communication with patients, the stresses of it and also the beauty of living a life wherein every day it is possible to make a huge difference to more than one person's life and their families. One evening on call for transplantation, the phone rang in the middle of the night, and I was amazed to see Cailin appear at the foot of the bed, camera in hand, which resulted in what has been referred to as my Marilyn Monroe styled photograph. At first, I hadn't even noticed her presence. At first sight, embarrassingly, I am lying in bed, chest naked, with phone clamped to my right ear, left hand behind my head, eyes closed in a sincere attempt at concentration having just been woken from deep sleep. Perhaps overly dramatic but factually correct. So much of the role of transplant surgeon on call entailed many often unproductive calls in the dead of night.

The resultant fifteen selected photographs were printed in large scale format, 6 by 4 feet, on gelatine prints and made a very bold statement. A touring exhibition called 'The Surgeon: Behind and Beyond the Hands' was organised by, then retired, Dr Geoffrey Farrar-Brown on behalf of the charity A Picture of Health. This charity aimed to use art as a means of relieving distress and hardship experienced by patients suffering from cancer and other serious diseases. The accompanying text explained that the general public view of the life of a surgeon, as glamorous, powerful and well rewarded was not quite as it seemed. Few people look at the person behind the surgical hands. Our personalities will differ, but all of us are using our skills in a self-chosen career, which is fulfilling. However, the constant demands, the excessively long hours, the increasingly heavy workload, combating tiredness and the rapidly increasing administrative burden are largely unseen. The stress of difficult operations, the loneliness of decision making and at times the feeling of failure is usually hidden. The exhibition also focussed on the importance of teamwork amongst the health professionals and the importance of placing the patient and family four-square in the centre of things.

It was a great success and was well received wherever it was shown, including in the House of Commons. I have huge admiration for Cailin, whose recent life changes have, I think, liberated her spirit in the most remarkable ways. We have remained close friends ever since, a friendship that I cherish.

Jordan Baseman

Not long after this followed an approach from Wysing Arts, an artistic community on the edge of the village of Bourn, near Cambridge, to ask if I would be interested in working with the New York visual artist and film maker Jordan Baseman. Jordan has won several important prizes, such as best film in the experimental film category at the 53rd Venice Biennale, with other prizes in San Francisco, Melbourne and London. He had been awarded an Arts Council grant to work with Wysing Arts. Wysing is quite close to the old Papworth Hospital. When we met, Jordan clearly had an idea of what he wanted to do but really didn't share with me the detail. However, I was intrigued to experience working with him and sought permission from the hospital management. At that time, we had an excellent chief executive Stephen Bridge, who was very supportive of the consultant staff and what we were trying to do for the hospital and our patients. He came on board very quickly, trusting my instincts that it would be a good experience for Papworth. Jordan became a regular fixture in my working week and had the gift of being able to blend into the background as well as to integrate well with all of the staff. In total he filmed seventy-five hours of open-heart surgery and took sound recordings from the operating theatre environment, all with full patient and staff consent of course. Also, he filmed interviews with heart transplant patients before and after their surgery. These he then edited into two films.

The first was called *Under the Blood.* After spending three summer months with me, he left for his studio in London to work on the editing. About three months after that I received a phone call from him inviting me to his studio to have a private and personal first view of the finished piece. Jordan's studio was the vast upper floor of a large warehouse in East London. He had screened off one end where there were no windows and fashioned a room with black drapes all around. He seated me in front of a large screen, started the video and left the room.

I was enveloped by a silent blackness on the screen and all around me. Softly at first, an eerie sound began, building in crescendo to that of a high-pitched stringed instrument-like sound. Into this were threaded sounds like tiny bells and then a very ominous orchestral sound in the minor key. As if that wasn't enough drama, the images of the patient being prepared for surgery appeared, and a sermon called 'The Blood of Jesus' by the American evangelist Billy Graham began to boom ominously around the room. Many years before, whilst in New York, Jordan had recorded it from National Public Radio, thinking that one day it would have a purpose. The film that Jordan had made did not portray an operation in any logical sense but consisted of images extracted from the footage that he had filmed. Throughout the film, Billy Graham's sermon on the necessity of the shedding of blood for life boomed out. Our voices can be heard quietly in the background without being able to really make out what is being said. It was shocking and captivating at the same time. Although filmed from my work in theatre, it was not in any way recognisable, but a vehicle for perhaps a greater statement. He had blended the mixture of sounds from the ambient noises in theatre to produce the continuous unsettling background. I had seen nothing like it before. When it had finished, I sat stunned into silence. Eventually Jordan appeared quietly to hear my thoughts. The way he had used the images was intensely engaging, and the sounds that suddenly interjected on top of the background, horror movie sounding accompaniment, jolted me back to look again at what I was seeing. I was intensely intrigued to discover what the neutral viewer might make of it. That information was to come later at an exhibition that I had co-curated for the Wellcome Trust with Ken Arnold, Melissa Larner and James Peto. Jordan had managed to take what was, for me, an everyday occupation and turn it into an original and gripping out-of-body experience.

The work was shown in many places including at the Cambridge Arts Picture House under the guise of the Cambridge Science Week.

Professor Jane Prophet

The next artist that I worked with was Professor Jane Prophet. Jane's father was already known to me through the world of motor racing. I had watched him hurl a Ford GT 40 around various racing tracks and was a huge admirer of him from my teenage years. Sadly, he was killed in a helicopter accident at the young age of forty-three. In 2004 Jane approached me to do a joint project. We spent many hours together inside and out of the operating theatre. My interest in Leonardo surfaced many times. Our project was called Silver Hearts. Its sense was to investigate some of the social, technological and psychological aspects of transplant surgery. We used Magnetic Resonance derived images of the heart. Here, I quote Jane from her web-site description:

> The raw data was translated into a digital three-dimensional model. From this, real objects were produced using rapid prototyping technology, which is not normally used to reverse engineer existing objects. The transference of data from one field to another and the act of reconstruction echoes the process of organ transplant. Reproduced at two different scales the polymer objects were gold-leafed or silver-plated. The structure and detail of the heart can be seen fully, as it would be in situ in the human body. Silver Heart twists the idea of transplant, turning a vital human organ into a precious art object.

It was during this time that Jane filmed the blood drawing video which I have described earlier in the text. It had been another fascinating collaboration.

Combinations of the work produced in these collaborations were shown in a variety of venues. At the Cornerhouse Gallery in Manchester in a show entitled 'WONDERFUL: Visions of the Near Future' curated by Clare Cumberlidge. This then moved to the Bristol Industrial Museum, opposite to the Arnolfini Gallery at Harbourside, Bristol. I was so full of excitement to be involved in a world far removed from my daily work in surgery. The people involved were very different from my usual colleagues. Their conversation was so much more expansive and engaging. Although my dedication to surgery of the heart and lungs was undiminished, I found this entry into the world of the arts and the humanities in general fascinating and above all, simply put, FUN.

It was there that I met Ken Arnold (another Shropshire lad), the director of the Wellcome Trust in London. We sat chatting about the art world in general and how I had become involved. Gradually the conversation moved to the developments at the Wellcome. I knew of the Wellcome Collection, begun by Henry Wellcome. In 2006, the Wellcome Trust had more recently opened a new public building with temporary exhibition space as opposed to the vast permanent exhibition of objects collected by Sir Henry Solomon Wellcome (1853–1936). A gifted entrepreneur, he founded a large pharmaceutical company with his brother Silas in 1880. He endowed a large amount of money with which the Wellcome Trust was founded. He had a passion for collecting medical artefacts leading to a collection of 125,000 medical objects by the time of his death, including such oddities as Napoleon's toothbrush. Today the complete collection totals over one million objects.

Ken was looking for a subject as a theme for the first exhibition in the new space. I suggested that the only possible subject for the first exhibition was the heart. We discussed what it might look like, and he said that he would think about it. A short time later he contacted me to say that he was going to progress the idea and asked if I would like to be involved. I jumped at the chance and another exciting chapter in my life opened up.

It was huge fun. Essentially, as we were working for the Wellcome, the doors to many museums and galleries from which to choose exhibits were opened for us. Along the way, the Royal College of Physicians happened to be showing their collection of anatomy boards. These are dissected systems such as the blood vessels, the nerves and the lymphatics of human specimens displayed on wooden boards. They were made from dissections in Padua in the 1650s. They must have been made as teaching aids. The Earl of Winchelsea and Nottingham claimed that they were obtained from Dr William Harvey in the late seventeenth century. However, nowhere in Dr. Harvey's notes or letters does he refer to them. What Winchelsea overlooked was that his ancestor John Finch (1626-82) had been Professor of Anatomy, and was probably the previous owner. They were given to the college by a later Earl in 1823. He wrote the following to the Royal College of Physicians:

> Sir, I have in my possession some anatomical preparations which belonged to the late Dr. Harvey, which I have great pleasure in offering to the college of Physicians. These specimens of his scientific researches can be nowhere so well placed as in the hands of that learned body.

They reveal enormous skill in dissection and preservation and are extremely rare. The College of Surgeons also owns two of them. I was asked to be filmed in a commentary on them for the BBC and following this I was able to obtain an example to show in the Wellcome exhibition.

It was very important to me to include an example of the work of Leonardo in the exhibition. An approach by the Wellcome director was met sympathetically and as a result the Royal Collection were most generous in their support and lent two of Leonardo's priceless drawings of the heart.

Other exhibits included Jordan Baseman's movie which was housed in a black box like space which made for an extremely intense viewing experience for about fifteen people at a time. A selection of hearts from different species was on show, from the tiny field mouse to that of an elephant. As we were setting up the exhibition a whale beached on the Thames, near to Tower Bridge. Very sadly it could not be rescued. Frantic calls were made by us to the Thames river authorities and eventually, with the help of London Zoo and some adventurous vets, we were able to salvage the heart and to include that. At the other extreme, and visible only under a microscope, we had a Zebra fish heart, still only a heart tube, representing the earliest stage of evolutionary development.

A standout exhibit was the heart of Jennifer Sutton. Earlier that year Jennifer had undergone heart transplantation for restrictive cardiomyopathy, a life-threatening condition. She graciously allowed her explanted heart to be shown. Jennifer was able to attend the exhibition and to see her own heart in a pot. Her comment on first seeing it was stoical:

> Seeing my heart for the first time is an emotional and surreal experience. Finally, I can see this odd-looking lump of muscle that has given me so much upset. It gave me so much pain and turmoil when it was inside me.

In generously lending her old heart to the exhibition she said that she hoped to help increase the public awareness about organ donation and the disease that could have ended her life.

The exhibition was a huge success. During its run, several evening events were organised to enhance the experience of the public. One that I was responsible for was the first live television broadcast of an open-heart operation. In conjunction with Channel Four we staged the surgery so that it could be transmitted live by satellite from Papworth to the lecture theatre at the Wellcome and across the nation on the television network. Windfall Films were the company who organised the transmission. They were excellent to work with, kind, supportive and highly professional.

They completely understood the enormity of the undertaking and could not have been more accommodating. The set up was as follows.

First, I had to select a patient and then to gain careful informed consent from him and his family. I chose a patient with a severely leaky mitral valve. Most of these valves can be reconstructed leaving the patient with their own native valve, a happier outcome than prosthetic valve replacement. The patient and family graciously gave their consent without hesitation. Krishnan Guru-Murthy of Channel Four News was to be the interlocutor between my consultant surgical colleague and friend Samer Nashef and myself.

The environment in the operating theatre was similar to a normal operating session, with the addition of a camera man, a sound recordist and an editor supervising the filming. Outside the hospital was the large van with the transmission equipment for the satellite feed. I had my usual support with a surgical registrar Miss Betsy Evans (now an excellent consultant cardiac surgeon in her own right), a consultant anaesthetist with his support team of registrar and operating theatre department assistant. The nurse scrubbed in to help was Tracey Tritton with whom I had worked extensively before. Our brief was simple, the surgery would progress just as normal with the exception that I was wearing a head microphone and earpiece, so that my commentary could be heard by the viewers. The audience both in the lecture theatre and at large could ask questions whenever they wanted to, and they would be fielded by Krishnan and Sam. They would then rephrase if necessary and feed them to me. If it was a suitable moment I would respond. Questions could be asked via Twitter as it was then. As the evening progressed there were over one million hits on the site, closing it down at one stage. The report in *The Guardian* begins:

> There is an intake of breath in the auditorium as cardiac surgeon Francis Wells begins to slice through the fat of the grey hair-flecked chest.

Sam interjected reassuringly:

> ...the Wellcome does not want you to see the sternum (breastbone) being opened.

There was a relieved gush of laughter from the gathered crowd, a sell-out many times over. As the operation progressed, deep inside the heart there was pathology that had not been predicted by the pre-operative investigations. Sam and I had a word trigger to interrupt the questioning when I needed to concentrate hard and this we executed without the public realising it, returning to the previous interactions without a break. The operation went well, and the heart began to beat spontaneously at the end of the procedure and the relief could be heard from the audience.

It was such a success that we were asked to repeat the process two weeks later, which we did to another full house. The press response was mostly positive, as was that of the public. To my surprise, despite having kept the Royal College president John Black informed at every stage and having received his blessing, some in the Royal College of Surgeons objected and some months later I had to defend my position in front of a gathering of lay people and professionals.

The meeting was chaired by Lord Winston, with Krishnan and me along with Emily Roe, the head of specialist factual development, defending against some surgical opposition. Also in attendance were Lord Patel, the then chairman of the national patient safety agency, a medical ethicist and a legal representative. I am happy to report that the lay public were very supportive and expressed the opinion that the stance of some of the professionals was outdated. A follow up letter from the policy manager at the College stated how timely it had all been and how much the College had learned about current popular opinion for such things. A good ending if ever there was one.

Interestingly it didn't end there, and a rather backward view came out later from the United States of America when the American Association for Thoracic Surgery issued an absolute ban on surgeons taking part in live broadcasts of surgery to the general public. Of course there is a point to that. There are some surgeons who become more preoccupied with projecting themselves than with the absolute care of the patient. I contend that only very experienced surgeons should become involved in this form of public information exercise. Only surgeons who are prepared to interrupt the broadcast if necessary, and always to put the patient first should think of undertaking these events. Sam and I took every precaution with the two of us working together in hand in glove, supporting each other and knowing exactly what the other was experiencing.

There was no accompanying catalogue for the exhibition, but a book was published with chapters written by notable contributors. One such was Dr. Jonathon Miller, who qualified in medicine and was training as a neurologist when he decided on a life in the arts, as an actor, producer and director of plays and opera. It was a privilege to spend some time with him. His conversation was always interesting, but it was noticeable that he clearly held some regret at leaving the profession of medicine behind, despite such a glittering career in the arts.

Within the book, interspersed between chapters, there are interviews with medical colleagues conducted by Melissa Larner. When I suggested this format, I felt that it was a further chance to reveal to the public something of what it like to be a practicing surgeon or physician. The book, edited by James Peto, won first prize in the popular medicine category for the 2008 Medical Book Awards sponsored by the BMA.[11]

Mel Fraser

In 2002, I received a request from local Cambridge based sculptor Mel Fraser, asking if she could spend some time with me at Papworth. Mel was also supported by the Wysing Arts residency programme. I knew of her sensitive but bold sculptures, which are beautiful and unusual. We had an excellent working relationship. Mel made many drawings and eventually had decided on the form that she wanted to produce. I was invited to follow its progress and took the opportunity to see the other pieces of her work at her beautiful studio. The final piece is a wonderful amalgam of cubist form echoing the shape of the heart.

Following this, Mel graciously went on to tutor me in some early steps in sculpting.

We have remained in touch ever since and I am a great admirer of her work.

Marcus Woxneryd

In 2005 Marcus, a young artist based in Sweden, had obtained a significant grant from the Wellcome Trust. Marcus approached me with the idea of producing a piece about the sounds made by the body in health and disease. It was to be called Sonic Bodies.

Marcus described it as an interactive symphony of body noises. It would be staged in a large blacked-out box. The visitors would enter the box and be encouraged to initially gently, and then more forcefully, touch the various structures in the form of bodily viscera. The touching and squeezing of the objects would generate sounds from them. The gentle touching would produce the normal sounds and with stronger manipulation would generate pathological sounds. In addition, the presence of the visitors moving through the space would affect the sounds that they heard. Thus the orchestration came from the visitors, and it would never be the same twice. My part in this was to record sounds from the heart and lungs of people who volunteered to be a part of the project. Marcus approached specialists in other areas such as orthopaedics, obstetrics and ear, nose and throat medicine. The finished piece was enthralling and was travelled widely.

Katie Hughes

Katie is an accomplished young artist. Despite having cystic fibrosis with all that that entails, she extremely productive and is a very hard-working artist. Katie produced some wonderful drawings of hands at work in the operating theatre, There were also large-scale drawings of the scene in there. Katie wrote

> After graduating from CGLAS, I had the extraordinary opportunity to be artist in residence with heart surgeon Mr Francis Wells at Papworth Hospital. I was present with my sketchbooks at many open heart surgeries and made hundreds of drawings, The way that a large group of medical practitioners work seemingly symbiotically to correct one small point in the human body was a privilege to watch. As an artist my experience of life drawing set me up for understanding the way the bodies of the practitioners moved. Drawing people in motion means making quick decisions and is a practice full of energy that comes through in the drawings.

Mariléne Oliver

Mariléne had won fame for her family portrait which she had constructed in towers of glass from magnetic resonance scans. She had persuaded her mother, father and brother to undergo whole-body scans. Then taking each of the horizontal slices that the scanner creates of the body, she engraved the images onto glass with bronze. These were then stacked on top of each other so that each person could be seen in transparent three-dimensional life size. When she approached me for ideas, I suggested that we utilise this idea to render Leonardo's *Great Lady* in the same way.

Taking Leonardo's original drawing, Mariléne redrew every single line of Leonardo's drawing onto her computer with a complex grid so that the positions of each part could be recognised. Then I drew each organ out into its three-dimensional position just as it would appear on a section from a scan. Mariléne then etched them in bronze onto glass sheets as she had with her family portrait. The result was fascinating. As the light played on the sculpture, the three-dimensional form of Leonardo's image came and went as you moved around it, giving it an other-worldly quality. It was submitted to the Royal Academy for the Summer Exhibition in 2007 and was accepted. Six copies were made and all were sold, some to very prestigious museums. The collaboration was written up and published in the magazine *Leonardo*.[12] Mariléne has continued to develop a very distinguished career with many beautiful and intriguing art/science cross over projects.

Leonardo and Friends

In October of 2010, a conference was held in honour of Martin Kemp who was retiring from his post in Oxford. The conference was arranged to celebrate his life and work. It was held in St John's College and the Ashmolean Museum and sponsored by Mrs Gheri Sackler and the Leonardo da Vinci Society. It was an august gathering with important people from the world of Leonardo and the arts. History of Art luminaries including Frank Zöllner from the University of Leipzig, Professor Claire Farago from the University of Colorado, and Professor Francis Ames-Lewis of Birkbeck College London. Martin's long-time friend and associate David Hockney was honoured guest. In the lunch break we repaired to a pub on the high street and David decided to sit outside because of his desire to smoke. I didn't want to miss the opportunity of getting to know him a little better following the episode at the Royal Academy a few years earlier. Whilst we were chatting, his exploration of drawing on the iPad came up and he asked me if I had tried it. I responded that I had, and so he asked which programme I was using. I told him and he said, 'Well, you should try the one that I am using,' and he proceeded to load it onto my iPad and to draw, demonstrating what it could do. Soon after, his partner came out to join us and my iPad was put away. For some time, I was able to look at my 'original' Hockney until one day it was accidentally wiped. This made me reconsider what art is, and is it only worth anything if it can be preserved, and what would be the original, the drawn image on the screen, or a printed version?

Later that evening, whilst walking with Hockney to the reception at the Ashmolean, he suddenly stopped and turned to me and said, 'You are a doctor, aren't you?' 'Yes,' I replied, wondering what was coming next. He then began to recite a poem by W. H. Auden

> Give me a doctor partridge-plump, Short in the leg and broad in the rump.
> An endomorph with gentle hands, Who'll never make absurd demands,
> That I abandon all my vices,
> Nor pull a face in a crisis, But with a twinkle in his eye, Will tell me that I have to die.

He too had a twinkle in his eye and with a devilish smile he turned and we walked on. It amuses Hockney to see himself as an inveterate smoker confounding all of the anti-smoking medical advice and surviving well into old age. Perhaps it is his work ethic that helps him to survive. As a student apparently he wrote a sign in big letters, that he hung on his wardrobe door so that it was the first thing that he saw on waking up. It screamed, 'GET UP AND WORK.' He continues with that signage to this day and obeys it rigorously. His sense of humour continuously shines through. Largely in response to the lecturing that he has received over smoking, he has come up with the slogan, 'End bossiness soon'. Initially it was 'Stop bossiness now' but he thought that too bossy, and so he toned it down. He tells this story with his lovely Yorkshire accent and a chuckle in his voice.

Early in 2014, I received an email from Ali Rezaei Haddad who was director of Imaging the Future of Medicine. An afternoon of presentations was being arranged under the auspices of the Ted Talk organisation, this being a TEDMED event. The concept was to explore the multidisciplinary nature of medicine and to highlight the importance of the union of the arts and the sciences. It was to be held in the Royal Albert Hall, following a successful initial event the year before in South Kensington. The Royal Albert Hall had been chosen not just for its size and audience capacity but for the association of Prince Albert with both arts and sciences, which were so intertwined in the nineteenth century. A central theme was the multitude of scientific and medical discoveries that have come about through the ability of people to think outside of the box. Creativity is the essence of both disciplines and fostering that key ingredient in making discoveries and forward intellectual development is essential to the human condition.

My presentation at that TEDMED event was preceded by having to make a short 'selling' presentation to the director before going on stage. Once we had passed that hurdle the show got under way. The Albert Hall was packed. We were each introduced by Dara Ó Briain, a successful comedian and television star, who seemed to be slightly worse for wear, stumbling over his words, but he was entertaining. Walking out onto the vast stage in front of such a huge audience was extremely intimidating. In front of me on the ground was a large digital clock counting down the twenty minutes of the presentation. Spotlights directly on me meant that seeing the audience beyond the front row was exceedingly difficult, perhaps a good thing.

My presentation was titled 'Looking and Seeing'. Once I had started, the time flew by and all too soon it was over. Sadly, being single once again, only one person that I knew came to support me and that was Viv Kerr, whom I had known since medical school days. Viv remains a loyal friend.

Having been the first on stage, I could then relax and enjoy the other presentations, particularly that of trumpeter, Alison Balsom, 2013 Gramophone Artist of the Year, and three times winner of the Classic Brit and the Echo Klassik awards.

Coincidentally, we both had performed (if that is the right word for my appearance) on stage at the Latitude Festival. Me in 2012 and Alison in 2013.

I had been asked to do a gig in the Literary Arena. Things couldn't really become more bizarre, speaking about the life and times of Leonardo da Vinci with music of all kinds coming from every direction.

Earlier, I had been involved with Andrew Graham-Dixon, a popular media star and art historian in a BBC television series called *The Secret of Drawing*. We met at Papworth and in an empty operating theatre, suitably theatrically lit, we discussed the drawings of Leonardo, in particular those of the heart. Andrew asked me if Leonardo's work had influenced my own in any way. The conclusion was drawn, not by me, that Leonardo had in some way taught me how to do a better repair operation on the mitral valve than conventional teachers. The point that I tried to make was that, although the drawings are examples of perhaps the best draughtsmanship across the ages, the accompanying notes are edifying in a different way. Although much of his anatomical writing reflects the fanciful ideas of Galen, his approach to study was very forward-looking. Leonardo's dissection of a problem and his intense demands that anything under investigation must be tested from many points of view had impressed me greatly. This was in great contrast to the very didactic style of modern teaching. So, often he would lay out his observations as to why something was as it was. Then he would argue from the opposite perspective and then use this counterpoint to derive his final conclusions. He was clearly schooled in, or self-taught in the art of rhetoric.

I have spent a great deal of my time reconstructing valves inside the human heart. Cardiac surgery is a discipline where deviation from certain pathways can so easily lead to the death of the patient. As such, it is taught in a very didactic way to attempt to maintain safety. In medico-legal jargon there is a thing called the Bolam Test, whereby the duty of care can be shown to have been followed if a cohort of medical professional peers, often quoted as a minimum of ten percent, would have done the same thing. In other words, a doctor is not guilty of negligence if he/she has acted in accordance with a practice accepted as proper by a body of practitioners skilled in that art. Work that falls outside of those parameters can be judged negligent, the consequences of which are very serious for the medical professional under scrutiny. This leads surgeons and physicians to practice within established guidelines, and protocol driven medicine and surgery is now the order of the day. All well and good you may say, but this is also very restrictive in making developments. The point that I had been trying to make was that following Leonardo's questioning state of mind and lack of fear in challenging authority, led me to question some of the procedures that we were being taught as the only way to do things.

Learning to look intensely, and to really try to see the reality of what was in front of me, led me to other conclusions and to question the way that most surgeons were approaching the reconstruction of the mitral valve. This had come about because of a series of educational seminars organised by someone seen by many as the maestro of mitral reconstructive surgery Professor Alain Carpentier in Paris. Three times a year in L'Hôpital Brussais in Paris Le Club Mitral was held, with Alain declaiming the only way to go about repairing the valve. Whilst good results were generally obtained, and the techniques standardised in such a way as to be relatively easily and consistently taught, the natural physiology of valve and ventricle was being largely ignored. I wanted to follow a more physiological approach, and this was the message that I had gained from studying Leonardo and his writings. Never be afraid to think for yourself and to think outside of the box.

As a result, I went about reconstructing the valve rather differently and this I described in the programme. The next day several newspapers ran the headline, 'How Leonardo Gave Top Surgeon Change of Heart', and other such declamatory strap lines. Let me be clear: Leonardo, bless him, with all his handed down manuscripts did not teach me how to do mitral valve reconstruction, but he did emphasise the importance of independent thought based on sound knowledge, a different, but more important starting point.

In conjunction with all this interest around Leonardo I was asked to lecture in many different and prestigious venues. Speaking in front of a large audience in the lecture theatre at the National Gallery is a particularly wonderful memory. I enjoyed engaging with the interested public who were so keen to hear more about Leonardo's anatomical work, previously mainly the domain of the art history specialists. Perhaps my amateurish enthusiasm became infectious to others. Lectures at The Royal Institution, The Royal Society of Medicine and The London Medical Society followed. I was given honorary membership of the Harveian Society following a lecture to them at The Apothecaries Hall and I became an honorary member of the Medical Artists Society, something that gave me particular pleasure as I have always greatly admired the work of that group of artists.

A particularly happy association that developed from this work has been with the Getty Institute. Early in 2012 I was invited to lecture at the Getty on my work on Leonardo. The audience was a mix of art historians and local physicians and surgeons from the department of Cardiology and Cardiac surgery at UCLA. This was organised by Maite Alvarez, a senior curator at the Getty Institute. Also present was Massimo Ciavolella, Professor and Franklin Murphy Chair in Italian Renaissance studies in the Royce Hall on campus. Massimo had a very close friend and colleague Dr Rinaldo Canalis.

Nando, as he was affectionately called, was an outstanding professor of head and neck surgery and a wonderful teacher. He had a deep interest in, and knowledge of the history of medicine and the Renaissance. In partnership with Massimo he led a wonderful series of meetings on aspects of medicine, and the role of the arts and humanities in the Renaissance. These meetings attracted impressive speakers in these subjects from many centres around the world. I was honoured to become a regular contributor to this august body over the next several years. Books with summary essays on the topics followed.[12,13]

In 2017 I was approached by Maite asking if I would like to be part of another adventure at the Getty. This time the subject was Renaissance futurities. Futurities is a word that I had not encountered before and refers to future events, prospects or conditions; the quality of being in the future and in this case a discussion of science, art and invention. We were to hold a preparatory meeting in France at the Chateau de Bretesche in Misillac.

It was sponsored and funded by the Borchard foundation, the Getty Institute and UCLA. A few years earlier, through the auspices of Martin Kemp, I had the privilege of meeting Professor Morteza Gharib, Professor of Aeronautics and Medical Engineering at the California Institute of Technology (Caltech). Mory is a world leader in his field and has a wide range of interests. Our areas of interest once again overlapped in the world of Leonardo. He had beautifully shown how Leonardo had visualised gravity as a form of acceleration, this, 200 years before Isaac Newton's groundbreaking work.[14] We spent four happy days in and around the chateau, discussing the project and ideas. During that time, we visited the museum Les Machines de L'Île. A giant workshop where the most incredible functioning robotic forms of animals and man are made. Later we visited the municipal library where we were shown a fragment of notes by Leonardo that they held in their collection.

It had been a fascinating visit where I learnt so much from my colleagues, not least about Cyrano de Bergerac's wonderful book on an illusory trip to the moon and the sun. He describes a rocket powered by the heat of the sun vaporising a material that is emitted from the rear of the ship propelling it forwards into space.[15] A truly futuristic idea, now come to fruition.

I had travelled to Nantes by train, and although I had a return ticket a small group were travelling back to Paris by car, and I was invited to join them. In that group were Maite, Mory, Vanda Vitali, professional curator and Roger Malina, professor of art and technology and professor of physics at the University of Texas in Dallas. Roger was the long-time editor of the journal *Leonardo*. He is of Austro-Hungarian descent. His great grandfather Josef Malina was a butcher like my grandfather and father. His grandfather Frantisek decided to emigrate at the age of sixteen, settling in Brenham, Texas. There was a large Czech and Slovak émigré population in Texas at that time. Frank's father had shown interest in aeronautics and graduated from the California Institute of Technology. He had always had an overlapping interest in both the arts and science. He went on to found the Jet Propulsion Laboratory at Caltech, now the leading research innovator in space technology in the world today. Eventually, through shortcomings in the American government, he fell foul of them for fostering academic relationships with topflight Chinese engineers, whom the McCarthy regime prevented from working in the United States and deported. As a result, Malina resigned his position and took up life as an artist. One of his many important bridges between the arts and science was to begin the journal *Leonardo*. As can be imagined, the conversation flowed in a most interesting way.

The journey was undertaken in an apparently stolen car. Vanda had helped herself to the car of a friend who was away and had not had time to ask permission. She didn't seem at all concerned about the potentially criminal act and so we went on our merry way.

During the trip I raised the issue of the forthcoming 500th anniversary of the death of Leonardo coming up in 2019. I began to express ideas that I had spawned for an adventurous meeting to celebrate this auspicious event. Understandably, there were many meetings being organised celebrating his life and times in the Renaissance. Organising another rearward looking meeting seemed to me to be rather futile. Perhaps arrogantly, I wondered what sort of celebration Leonardo would have wanted to organise himself. It seemed to me, that being such an original thinker he wouldn't want to look backwards, but forwards and far into the future. A second futurities meeting.

We gave the meeting the title 'Leonardo da Vinci, Inventing the Future: Flight, Automata, Art, Anatomy and Bio Morphism'. To that end, I had planned an event running over three days with four major sessions. The first was on the evolution of flight, the second on his work on the heart and other anatomy, the third was on disruptive technologies, robotics and artificial intelligence, and the fourth on where art meets science. Everyone in that little car bought into the idea and was keen to help. It now just remained for me to organise it all, raise the money and book the speakers.

It was then that my friend and cardiology colleague in University College, Los Angeles, Noel Boyle, stepped in to help me. With Massimo, Mory Gharib, and Victoria Vesna, the professor of design and media arts, and the director of art and science at UCLA, I set about organising a look into the future through Leonardo's eyes, or at least my idea of what that might look like.

Whilst I was sourcing speakers, Noel was able to book the Nano-Science building, (UCLA California Nano Systems Institute) on the UCLA campus, in which we could stage the meeting. Holding the meeting in a building that houses some of the most advanced research in the world today seemed the appropriate place to celebrate the life and work of Leonardo. The topic ignited interest in many people and before we knew it, we had a stellar line up of speakers on a host of fascinating topics. In the section on flight, we began with lectures on Leonardo's studies of birds in flight and his attempts to build a flying machine by Leonardo experts Matthew Landrus and Domenico Laurenza. This was followed by a fascinating presentation by Maite Alvarez on Cyrano de Bergerac's very early science fiction novel *Voyages to the Moon and the Sun*, 1657. Later, we were treated to a presentation on the forthcoming mission to Mars by Charles Elachi, former director of the jet propulsion laboratory. This included a jaw-dropping presentation on the challenges that faced the engineers who were designing a Martian helicopter. This has since accomplished its mission to the red planet and performed beyond expectations. The leader of the Martian helicopter project was a young woman who exuded immense infectious excitement.

The session ended with a presentation by the Apollo astronaut Colonel Walter Cunningham. Walter flew on Apollo 7 with Walter Schirra, the commander of the mission, and Donn Eisele. Walter was the lunar module pilot and Donn Eisele the command module pilot. They were in space for eleven days from 11–22 October 1968, orbiting the earth 163 times. One of their main missions was to rehearse the docking and undocking of the lunar module in preparation for the lunar landings. The mission was made unpleasant for two of them as they developed quite severe head colds, the symptoms of which were exaggerated in zero gravity. Fortunately for him, Walter managed to avoid the infection. Their courage cannot be underestimated as they were the first manned mission following the tragic deaths of Gus Grissom, Ed White and Roger Chaffee in a capsule fire on the launch pad during practice for launch. All three died in appalling circumstances as their capsule was consumed by an explosive oxygen fire triggered by a spark from poor wiring in the atmosphere of pure oxygen. This could have halted the Apollo programme, but the staunch determination of the crews and the resolution of the problem by altering the cabin atmosphere from pure oxygen to an air/oxygen mixture allowed its continuation.

Tom Wolfe, the all-American author, immortalised the ego and heroism of the pilots on the space programme in his book *The Right Stuff*.[16] The book focussed on the daring deeds of Chuck Yeager but the courage shown and the high level of flying skills exhibited by them all is underpinned therein. It was a real pleasure to spend those days in the company of Walter and his lovely wife. Not at all the egoist that one might have expected, but a genial and quiet man who shared his experiences gladly. Sadly, he passed away in 2023.

The meeting ended with a wonderful piano recital by my friend and sometime piano teacher Patrick Hemmerlé. Late in the first day of the meeting, Patrick informed me that his encore at the end of the concert was to be a duet with me and then gave me the music to read and learn. Fortunately, there was a piano near the nanoscience building where I could quickly practice it. Patrick's playing of the Chopin Études was superlative, but the concert in the Schoenberg Hall on campus was tainted for me by my nerves at the thought of playing in front of such an audience. However, it went well, and I was filled with a feeling of exhilaration at the end of an exciting and successful event.

In conjunction with the meeting, I had shipped out the framed facsimiles of Leonardo's anatomical drawings and notes of the heart, that I had put together for the European Society for Thoracic Surgery which had immediately preceded the UCLA event in Lisbon. These were my own facsimiles of his drawings and notes accompanied by photographic prints of dissections that I and my colleagues Martin Goddard, consultant pathologist and Robert Anderson, professor of anatomy had made from the heart and lungs of an ox reproducing exactly Leonardo's work.

I had obtained the facsimiles many years before on a visit to the publishers Balliére, Tindall and Cassell, whose offices were around the corner from the old Charing Cross Hospital in Covent Garden. They were publishing my first book on thoracic surgical techniques that had been begun by my mentor Ben Milstein. He had generously passed on to me the text that he had started work on. At the same time Balliére, Tindall were in the process of publishing the collected anatomical works of Leonardo da Vinci held in the Royal Collection. As I was entering the office to pick up my first copy of our book, I noticed a pile of facsimile sheets of Leonardo's drawings and notes. I asked what they were doing there, and was told that they were to be destroyed, as some of the pages had printed badly. I was invited to take some. Naturally I chose the drawings of the heart. They are first class facsimiles but had lain dormant in my collection of oddities until I suggested to the president of the European Society for Thoracic Surgery that we could stage an exhibition in the annual meeting in Portugal. Exhibited in conjunction with our dissection photographs, they emphasise the importance of Leonardo's work, lost to the eyes of anatomists for over 250 years and they continue to astound new observers.

There have been many academic art history meetings that I have been involved with and through them I have met many fascinating people. In 2014, I was invited to present a paper comparing the anatomical works of Leonardo with those of Vesalius at a meeting titled the 2014 Vesalius Continuum. A bit of a tall order as Vesalius had published the greatest book on anatomy that the world had known to that date, and Leonardo's works amounted to unpublished manuscript pages. However, I accepted the challenge with relish and set off for the island of Zakynthos to celebrate the 500th anniversary of Vesalius' birth and the 450th anniversary of his death on that island (1564) after being ship-wrecked on returning from a pilgrimage to Jerusalem. Debating me on stage was a lovely Italian art historian and artist Roberta Ballestriero. She was there with her husband Owen and their beautiful black labrador. Roberta is a world expert in the history and restoration of ceroplastics, the art of wax modelling. I had heard of the extraordinary wax models of human dissection, among the finest collections in La Specola in Florence but knew very little about them. The conference passed interestingly, but I did feel something of an outcast amongst the Vesalius aficionados. Roberta, Owen and I struck up what has become a very close and lasting friendship. Together we visited several of the great collections of wax anatomies in Florence, Bologna, London (Guy's Hospital) and Vienna. For anyone interested in the history of anatomy they are objects that must be seen. In addition to the very high standards of accuracy, their execution is nothing short of incarnate beauty. A perfect example is the anatomical Venus, created by Clemente Susini, to be found in the anatomy museum of the Institute of Sciences in Palazzo Poggi in Bologna.

In that same museum is a posthumous portrait of the great anatomist and wax modeller Giovanni Manzolini, made by his even more skilled wife Anna Morandi Manzolini. In her husband's portrait his right hand is placed lovingly on a wax human heart, so accurately modelled that it is almost impossible to tell from a real dissected human heart. Following his death from tuberculosis in 1755, Anna modelled a self-portrait. In that portrait, she can be seen with her hands presenting a wax head opened to reveal the brain, possibly sending a message in defence of female abilities so played down for most of time and her affection for her husband.

There have been several other spin offs from my involvement in this world. For example, being asked to assist in important exhibitions of Leonardo and Michelangelo's anatomy at the British Library and the Queen's Gallery. It has been and continues to be a parallel career for me.

To be sure, surgery has been very rewarding for me; being able to help so many people over a fifty-year career is difficult to match in other spheres of life. Despite that, the pure joy that I have experienced in the world of the arts, and continue to do so, has been the factor that has made life exciting and stimulating.

Ballet and Opera

Irrespective of how busy I am at work I have always found time to enjoy music and theatre. When I moved from London to Cambridge, I initially thought that I would be cut off from the West End shows and so I made sure that I had booked to see something on a regular basis. In fact, I found that I could leave work at five in the afternoon and get to the West End in time for a quick meal and to be in my seat by 7.30. Afterwards the drive home was easy, and I would be in bed by midnight without much difficulty. Indeed, on several occasions I was home at a similar time to friends who lived in the suburbs of London. In fact, I attended more shows like this than when I had lived in London and it was all on my doorstep. Train journeys were to be avoided through their unpredictability and the late-night replacement buses are a nightmare.

Several performances stand out in my mind. The on-stage presence of Peter O'Toole is unforgettable. First, in Pirandello's great play *Henry IV*, and second in *Geoffrey Barnard is Unwell*. The hero, Geoffrey Barnard, was an alcoholic journalist in terminal decline, a part that O'Toole played to perfection and rapturous ovation. Theatre is an intimate experience unlike the remoteness of cinema, or these days, streaming on television. Sitting in anticipation of the rising curtain and the appearance of the players is magical. Not every performance is gripping but there is always something to discuss. I find it very sad that mediocre and shouty musicals are dominating over good plays well performed. I suspect that the degradation of teaching in schools has a great deal to do with it.

Ever since seeing Rudolph Nureyev and Margot Fonteyn in *Romeo and Juliet* I have been smitten by the ballet and go as often as I am able to. At one performance of *Giselle* when my daughter Joanna was five years old, we were strolling around between acts when suddenly, Joanna decided that she was going to run up the stairs between the old entrance and the newly converted floral hall. As I ran after her I saw her dash towards an elderly and elegant lady seated on a chair at the top of the steps. Joanna rushed towards her and leapt on to her lap. Shock and horror, it was Dame Ninette de Valois. I needn't have worried though as she was lovely to Joanna and struck up a conversation with her. It was at the same performance that during one of the acts, Joanna asked to sit on my lap so that she could see better. Completely entranced by the performance, I noticed that she was twisting the bouffant hair of an elderly lady in front of her. Luckily because of the distance of her hair from her scalp and the heavy fixative spray, I was able to disentangle Joanna's fingers from her beautifully coiffed locks without her noticing.

Joanna was a very sociable child. As well as jumping onto the lap of Dame Ninette, at an even earlier stage she ended up in the arms of a famous Hollywood actress. We were at the wonderful Getty villa when, aged about fifteen months (she had started to walk at eleven months), she bounced over to a lady sitting alone enjoying her coffee in the sunshine and began engaging with her. The lady swept her up onto her lap and began to fuss her. The lady was the Hollywood actress Shelley Winters.

Some years later, I was invited to a post-performance dinner in the opera house with members of the ballet and other staff. I took Joanna with me. I found myself sitting next to the Russian dancer Natalia Osipova. During conversation I mentioned that I was going to visit Moscow in two weeks' time. It transpired that the Royal Ballet were also going there and then on to St Petersburg on tour. I had booked tickets for the Bolshoi some time before and had forgotten that it would be the Royal Ballet performing there. As we chatted, the ballet mistress across the table from me suggested that I should join them in their last night party on stage after the performance. Of course I leapt at the chance. Once in Moscow, I had another pleasant surprise to find the Royal Ballet company staying at the same hotel as me. Consequentially, I had breakfast with the dancers each morning. The performance was stunning and the Russian audience, notably discerning of their ballet, gave them rapturous applause. The party was a lovely bonus.

Subsequently, I have visited St Petersburg and experienced wonderful performances at both the New and the Old Mariinsky Theatres. They are so different, the old theatre being of classical design and layout, with a classical baroque beauty inside. The new theatre is also beautiful. The foyer is a huge atrium with a huge wall of beautiful light brown and cream translucent marble reaching the full height of the building. Much of the outside walls are glass and the light just floods into the building from all sides.

The Bolshoi in Moscow is another classical masterpiece of theatre design, again in the classical baroque style. In keeping with its style is the Hotel Metropole just close by. It was a favourite watering hole of spies in the cold war and the place to be seen by the Muscovites prior to the revolution in 1917. That wonderful hotel is the central character in the book *A Gentleman in Moscow* by Amor Towles. The book is celebrated in the hotel and it was fascinating to read it whilst there.

The Kremlin is a short walk away from the Metropole. It is steeped in history. It has been a fortress for centuries and is a huge complex of palace, church and state rooms. The thing that surprised me the most in Moscow was finding a huge store, Gum, similar to Harrods, directly opposite the Kremlin, something that is not readily appreciated when Red Square is shown on television. When shown for the great military parades, the focus is on the outer walls of the Kremlin with the Russian leaders atop a very tall dais standing on the tomb of Lenin. The square filled with huge weapons of war and serried ranks of troops. The other surprise for me was the inside of St Basil's Cathedral. The outside is gloriously colourful with the exuberant onion domes. Inside, however, although beautifully adorned with mosaics, the chambers are small and quite claustrophobic, not at all what I was expecting. Outside the Kremlin walls are a series of low-lying memorials to the great battles of the past, Sebastopol, Leningrad and the Unknown Soldier. On one occasion, I saw Vladimir Putin laying a wreath at the Unknown Soldier memorial. Across the river from the Kremlin is the British embassy housed in a combination of some new and other more beautiful old buildings. Not far away is a tall apartment block or hotel in which so many artists, playwrights and political activists were held in the time of the Cold War, many being put to death by the regime. I was taken on a guided tour by a delightful plump late middle-aged lady whose husband had been a Trade and industrial attaché in the 1970s and 1980s. I asked her light heartedly if she had known any spies there in her time. With a glint in her eye, she replied:

> Darlink, we were all spies back then.

Being married briefly to a Russian woman allowed me to learn more about Russian art and music. Somewhat exciting was the fact that her mother had worked as a French translator for many years for the KGB. The sight of Lubyanka, the Russian base of the FSB and the KGB was somewhat spine chilling, knowing what had gone on there and probably still does. Despite all the horrors of the political regime, the Russian culture has always attracted me, the music of Tchaikovsky, Rachmaninov, Scriabin and Stravinsky being among my favourites.

The Hermitage in St Petersburg is among the greatest galleries of art in the world and the first stop of many visitors to that great city, and rightly so, but for me, the newly refurbished Hermitage XXI, in the General Staff building across the palace square is so much more exciting. It is the building from which the troops first took a stand against the Bolshevik revolution, but is now a modern masterpiece of interior design graced with beautiful works of art.

A must for me was to see two of the possible masterpieces by Leonardo da Vinci housed in the Hermitage. Therein is the *Madonna Litta* 1480–1490 and the earlier *Benois Madonna* 1478, named after the Benois family that owned it. The hand of Boltraffio, a pupil of Leonardo, is certainly possible in the *Madonna Litta*, but then it is a highly finished picture that doesn't have the usual halos that most Christian representations of the holy family have. The *Benois Madonna* I find very troubling with the ugliness of the Madonna and the presence of halos, however it is always interesting to see these famed pictures in the flesh as it were. As I approached the painting a mass of cruise ship tourists descended upon it and proceeded to have selfie after selfie taken with it, without appearing to study the painting at all. Even more sad was the fact that in the same room were some other outstanding paintings of real Renaissance significance, none of which caught the attention of the selfie brigade as they rushed onward to the next target, chasing the cruise ship flag held high by the guide on a mission.

Another wonderful gallery is the State Russian Museum, found in the Mikhailovsky Palace. It is packed to the gunnels with wonderful works by Russian artists, *The Ninth Wave* by Ivan Aivazovsky being among my favourites. For those not familiar with Russian nineteenth and twentieth century art, I heartily recommend correcting this omission.

St Petersburg is replete with wonderful galleries, museums and architecture. Referred to as the Venice of the north, it is criss-crossed with canals and bridges. A short boat trip down the Neva River outlet to the Baltic Sea is the wonderful Peterhof Grand Palace. Recently refurbished, it is resplendent in a yellow and white façade, dressed in gold plated sculptures adorning a sweeping cascade of waterfalls rising up ceramic steps. The influence of French and European culture in general can be seen reflected in the influence of Peter the Great, and later Catherine, Empress of Russia. Until the late nineteenth century French was the language of the aristocrats and native Russian kept for the working class. A wonderful book, 'To the Hermitage' by Malcolm Bradbury beautifully highlights the relationship between Denis Diderot, the French originator of the Encyclopaedia, and Catherine, whilst contrasting it with modern academics and their search for truth of the period.

There is so much to see and to learn in the old Russia and it is a tragedy of immense proportions that the state of war, cold or otherwise, that exists between the West and Russia denies the citizens of the world easy access to such immense treasures.

Opera has always captivated me. The combination of wonderful music, sung and played by masterful musicians accompanying often utterly ridiculous story lines is quite addictive. My father's favourite opera singer was Carlo Bergonzi. We had a long-playing record compilation of his performances. I knew little of opera then and was keen to experience it. Enter Bill, our medical school hall porter with a brother working in the Royal Opera House. He procured free, or much reduced-price tickets for some of us. Although mainly witnessed from the standing area in the gods, it allowed me to experience the wonder of opera for the first time.

I have been fortunate to have experienced many of the great operas both at the Royal Opera House and in the beautiful country setting of Glyndebourne. Whilst abroad at international meetings, rather than sit in the hotel bar until late at night, the favoured activity of many colleagues, I would seek out tickets to the great opera houses, concert halls or theatres of the world. When looking for single tickets at the last minute it is extraordinary the performances that one can get into. Opera houses in Vienna, Milan, San Francisco, New York and Los Angeles have all been visited. In 1992, in the space of three evenings in New York I was able to see the Tennessee Williams' *A Streetcar Named Desire*, with Jessica Lange as Blanche and Alec Baldwin as Stanley in the Ethel Barrymore theatre where it was first performed; Richard Dreyfus, Glen Close and Gene Hackman in the Ariel Dorfman thriller, *Death and the Maiden*; and the New York City Ballet with Michael Balanchine directing. What a few days that was. The meeting (AATS) was good also.

Perhaps the most dramatic evening that I experienced was at the Royal Opera House in October of 1992 at a performance of *Mayerling*. Sitting just two rows in front of us in the stalls was Kenneth MacMillan, the acclaimed choreographer. In the interval we all got up and left the auditorium for the second course of the meal we were enjoying in the restaurant. On returning to our seats the restart was delayed. Time passed and it was clear that there was a problem. We noticed that Kenneth MacMillan had not returned to his seat. After a considerable delay, Jeremy Isaacs, director of the ROH, appeared with a troubled look on his face. In the silent theatre he announced the shocking news that Kenneth MacMillan had passed away backstage. He asked us all to stand in respect . He informed us that the great man's last wish was that the performance should continue. The performance restarted but at the end, instead of the thunderous applause, the curtain was pulled back and once again everyone stood, many with tears in their eyes, before leaving the theatre in silence.

A few weeks before that, I had the good fortune to attend a solo performance by Luciano Pavarotti with the ROH orchestra. It was a very intimate concert which went long over the allotted time with Pavarotti singing may encores with personal reflections between.

There have been many memorable classical music performances that I have been fortunate to be present at. An early one that stands out for me is a superb evening with Dudley Moore, the comedian and accomplished jazz pianist with the London Symphony Orchestra at the Royal Albert Hall. Dudley interspersed jazz pieces with classical ones and comedy between them both. His finale was the Rachmaninov *Second Piano Concerto*, which he played with great gusto. I was also at one of Mitsuko Uchida's first performances at the Barbican in London. A master of Mozart's piano repertoire, she performed frequently with Jeffrey Tate. Miss Uchida is a flamboyant character. She walked onto the stage in a glittering sequined jacket which after sitting down and appearing to ready herself to play she jumped up and whisked off, tossing it across the stage and then sat again to begin her concert. Another great Asian pianist of the modern era is the Chinese pianist Yuja Wang. Her spectacular performance of *Rhapsody on a Theme* by Paganini at the 2023 Royal Albert Hall promenade concert brought the house down. Her encore of a jazz setting of *Tea for Two* was delicious.

I have been fortunate to be able to count Patrick Hemmerlé as a friend and part time piano teacher. A Parisian-grounded pianist who now lives in Cambridge, Patrick has an international following. Fortunately for us members and fellows of Clare Hall college in Cambridge he is the director of music and performs regularly in house. He continues to encourage me in my playing, which is more intermittent that it ought to be. Sitting at the piano and playing for an hour or more is very good at restoring equanimity in my life.

I do regard the arts as of equal importance as my career in medicine and it has made life much more meaningful. Perhaps I could have achieved more in the world of surgery if I had spent less time in the arts, but it would have been less enjoyable.

10

Motoring Adventures with Sir Stirling Moss and Friends

Movement is tranquillity.

Sir Stirling Moss

'Who do you think you are? Stirling Moss?' The face leaning in through my driver's side window boomed. 'No,' I replied, 'but he's here if you would like a word.' Raising his gaze across to the passenger side of my car, the man suddenly jumped to attention and stuttered 'Oh, sorry Mr Moss. I had no idea. Please come in.'

It was the evening of the opening of the Racing Car Show at the National Exhibition Centre in Birmingham, January 1994, and I was driving Stirling to the Autosport Dinner at a nearby hotel. I had been invited to the racing car show by another motor racing legend Caroll Shelby, of Shelby Cobra fame. Caroll had lived in England for almost fifteen years when racing in the 1950s and early 1960s. He had to retire early from racing because of a heart condition that ultimately led him to have a heart transplant in Stanford, California, carried out by Dr Norman Shumway, the true pioneer of human heart transplantation. As a result of his experiences and the kindness of the transplant team, he set up the Shelby Transplant Trust to fund heart transplantation in children in the U.S., raising money through motor sport events. As a result of the success of this, and his fondness for England where he had spent so much time, and with the advice of Dr Shumway, he decided to do the same thing in the U.K. The launch was to be in Cambridge. He brought Shelby Cobra Chassis Number 1 to the children's hospital in Cambridge and delighted the children present by doing wheelies in the car park. In the evening Professor Sir Keith Peters, the Regius Professor of Physic, had arranged a dinner at Christ's College, Cambridge to celebrate the event.

Only two of us present, had any enthusiasm for motor racing: Peter Friend, my gastroenterological surgery friend, and me. We made a beeline to sit next to him. I sat on his left and Peter on his right. It was a very entertaining evening with Caroll regaling us with tales of daring on the track in all sorts of cars throughout the 1950s and 1960s, and, of course, stories of his friendship and rivalry with, amongst other drivers, Sir Stirling Moss. Being involved in the heart transplant programme at Papworth, prior to his arrival, Dr Shumway had contacted me and asked me to look out for Caroll should any untoward event occur. The evening ended and we said our goodbyes and hoped we would meet again, little knowing how soon that would be.

In bed later that night, the phone rang at 1.30 a.m. I answered and heard a Texan drawl enquiring if he was speaking to Dr Wells. I said yes and instantly realised that the voice on the other end of the phone belonged to none other than Caroll. Instantly, I wondered if he was alright and didn't have developing symptoms of infection with his immunotherapy, or organ rejection. He replied that was not the problem and said

> ...just wanted to invite you to come with me on Thursday to Birmingham. I am opening the racing car show. Can you come as my guest?

Initially, I considered declining the offer because of the several patients booked into my clinic that afternoon. However, I rapidly realised the opportunity that was being offered to me and accepted his invitation.

I drove up early in the morning and, as arranged, met Caroll in the entrance to the N.E.C. He was ushered in as the motor sport royalty that he was, with me close behind him. We were met by two legends of motor sport Sir Jackie Stewart and Nigel Mansell, both world champions, and then escorted to the stage. I dropped back, knowing that I was not part of this central show, but on sensing this Caroll gently steered me with his hand on my arm, making it clear that I was very much with him. Before I knew it, I was standing on the main stage with Caroll, the sponsors and a small group of famous racing drivers, amongst them was Mr Motor Racing himself Stirling, later, Sir Stirling Moss.

Caroll was extremely attentive to me and made sure that I met all the colleagues that he had raced with, including the great American racers Mario Andretti and Phil Hill. At noon we were ushered into what today would be called the green room for an informal lunch. Stirling came over to join Caroll, who in turn introduced me. After hearing what I did for a living, Stirling began to show real interest in me and what I did. He was fascinated by the whole idea of heart surgery, and he eagerly began to ply me with questions, partly triggered by the experiences of his friend Caroll. I soon realised what a technophile he was. He was intrigued to learn how the patient was kept alive during the surgery and the workings of the heart-lung machine. As the conversation proceeded, he asked if it would be possible for him to visit Papworth to witness heart surgery. Thinking quickly, I replied, 'Yes, I am sure that could be arranged, but on one condition.' He asked what that was and I said, 'I will show you how to do open heart surgery if you show me how to drive around Silverstone,' the converted aerodrome that had become the famous home of English motor racing. To my great surprise he enthusiastically agreed. It was a deal.

During the afternoon, Caroll introduced me to several more greats of the motor racing world, some of whom would become friends as I grew to know Stirling more. As I was leaving the show at the end of a wonderful day, I bumped into Stirling standing alone at the exit, waiting for his driver. I somewhat nervously approached him and began to chat with him, after all here was my boyhood hero, whom only days before I had assumed was no longer alive, and just a mythic name from the mists of motor racing legend. Yet here he was, flesh and blood and brimming with energy. He was an absolute gentleman and, as I was to discover, a man who wore his fame lightly, never failing to sign an autograph, to allow selfie photos, and always answering his correspondence even though it came by the sack load. He insisted that his name remained freely accessible in the telephone book for anyone to find all of his life.

It soon became apparent that his driver was not coming, and so I offered to drive him to the venue where the dinner was being held, as we were going to the same event. It was below freezing that evening and frost was beginning to form on the grass and the windows. I set off in some trepidation to think that I was driving one of the world's greatest drivers and one I had idolised in childhood. As we approached the hotel where the dinner was being held there was a steep slope down to a barrier across the road with a porter's cabin next to it. As I braked to slow for the entrance the car began to slide on the freshly formed ice. Several images flashed through my mind of causing injury, or something worse, to a racing legend as we smashed through the barrier. Thankfully, we stopped with the barrier a hair's breadth from the windscreen. Stirling didn't utter a word, seemingly impervious to the incident. Perhaps years of driving at the limit had inured him to fear of risk. It was then that the porter emerged and uttered the immortal words, 'Who do you think you are, Stirling Moss?' That phrase has entered the lexicography of the English language in all parts of the world, such was the fame of the greatest driver never to have won a world championship.

I have found that motor racing people are warm hearted and extremely hospitable, and as a complete outsider that evening, I was made to feel most welcome and very much a part of the event, with Caroll and Stirling keen to ensure that all those present were aware of my own contributions to society. We were the guests of the editorship of the motor racing journal *Autosport*. Nigel Roebuck was hosting the event and was full of fascinating conversation.

To digress for a moment, and to emphasise the gentlemanly nature of Stirling, so rare in a highly competitive individual, here is a true story of his generosity of spirit. This unique and important act of charity by the man has gone down in the annals of motor racing history. It happened at the end of the 1958 world championship in the Portuguese Grand Prix. Stirling Moss was vying for the lead of the race and the championship with Mike Hawthorne, another leading British driver; Stirling being the quicker driver and Hawthorn the more careful. Hawthorn was accused of an illegal restart after a spin and stalling the car. Moss, lying second at that time, was able to overtake him and gain the lead. Once Hawthorn had restarted his car he was able to catch Moss, whose tyres were degrading, and to overtake him to regain the lead. After the end of the race, where Hawthorn crossed the line first, he was threatened with disqualification by the stewards for gaining an advantage by being push-started by a circuit marshal. In the absence of universal cameras as nowadays, the incident was reported to the stewards as an infringement of the rules, and they wanted to take the win away from Hawthorn and give it to Stirling. The difference in points as a result of this would also have given the world championship for that year to Stirling Moss. However, Stirling had seen what had happened and that Hawthorn had got the car going on his own. He reported this to the stewards, who promptly reinstated Hawthorn as the winner and thereby the new world champion.

Stirling's sporting attitude had cost him the world championship. Hawthorn became the first British World Champion and not Moss, whom everyone in the sport acknowledged as the best driver at that time. I asked Stirling if he had any regrets about his actions that day and he was unmoved from the fact that he had done the correct thing. Hawthorn died only a few months later in an accident on the A3 Guilford bypass in his Jaguar Road car, making Stirling's actions all the more poignant. He was twenty-nine years old. In the same year four drivers were killed on the track, amongst them, his great friend Peter Collins in the German Grand Prix and Stuart Lewis-Evans during the Moroccan Grand prix. The age in which Stirling was racing carried many fatalities each year.

My host for the day, Caroll, had raced in only eight Formula 1 races, of which he won none and scored no points, not exactly a stellar career in the Formula. However, he had, to use his own words, found a much nicer class of person at the back of the grid. Stirling Moss, his long-time friend, was at the front with other legends of the sport Tony Brooks, Roy Salvadori, and of course, perhaps the greatest of them all, Juan Manuel Fangio. The remarkable thing about Tony Brooks was that he was also a dental student at the time of his racing career and the one that Stirling rated alongside himself as the class of the field.

Not enjoying much success in that Formula, Caroll made his name and fame as a race and road car developer. He won the Le Mans 24-hour race in 1959 in an Aston Martin. His racing career blossomed in sports cars, winning the 1960 USA Road Racing Sports Car Championship in a Birdcage Maserati, also Stirling's favourite car.

His name will forever be attached with affection to the Shelby Cobra cars, both road going and racing, which he developed from the chassis of the English car maker AC. He rose to the challenge set by Henry Ford to beat Ferrari at Le Mans following a failed attempt by Ford to buy Ferrari, celebrated in the recent film *Ford vs Ferrari* (20th Century Fox 2019) with Matt Damon playing Shelby. With the help of British engineers, he built the classic Ford GT 40, named for its height of only forty inches from ground to roof top. This beautiful car went on to win Le Mans in various guises from 1966 to 1969.

During the following week, I followed up on Stirling's request to see some heart surgery and discussed it with Stephen Bridge, our very open-minded chief executive at Papworth. He was keen to support the idea and suggested that he would be an excellent person to open our new lecture theatre in the hospital. I contacted Stirling and suggested a date to which he readily agreed. It was important to have the permission of the prospective patients to see if they would allow such a non-medical person to observe their surgery. I approached the patients who had already been listed for that day and asked their permission. I was surprised by the excitement and enthusiasm with which they agreed, hoping that they might meet the great man himself. All was agreed and Stirling with his loyal and lovely wife Susie arrived early in the morning of the appointed day. First, I gave them a tour of the hospital, and then we got them changed into their theatre clothes. They were so gracious with everyone they met, who in turn were full of excitement with the experience. In the operating room, Stirling was thirsty to learn all that he could and was fascinated by the heart lung machine and the sight of the working human heart, at one point almost reaching over into the wound to point something out.

At the end of the operating list, we all got changed and retired to the lecture theatre for the official opening. There was a large turnout to meet them both and they stayed long after the expected departure time to ensure that they had spoken to everyone and given many autographs, at least one signed next to the patient's wound at his explicit request.

The following day, quite unexpectedly, large bunches of flowers arrived for all of the patients and the nurses that they had met on each of the wards and the operating theatres. Unbeknown to me, Susie had gone around them all collecting names and stations. The next day I received a lovely letter from them thanking me for arranging the visit and expressing the excitement that they had felt being allowed to witness such scenes of an emotional character.

Several weeks passed by and I had heard nothing further, when I received a telephone call from Stirling asking me if I could be at Silverstone for 6.00 a.m. the following weekend. The answer was, of course, an excited 'yes'. It was a fully marshalled track day with many exciting machines. I met Stirling and Susie behind the pits with his long-time mechanic Alf Francis. They walked me over to the car that had been prepared for the day. It was a two-seater racing Lotus that Stirling had raced in the mid-1950s. It was immaculately prepared and finished in a dark blue, the only colour, other than British racing Green, that Stirling, being such an anglophile, would be seen driving for most of his career.

When our time came to go out on track I went to the pit wall with Susie, whilst Alf got Stirling settled in the car. He beckoned me over, and above the scream of other racing engines warned me to be ready to jump in. He was going to do two warm-up sighting laps and then I had to leap in with no delay. As Stirling disappeared down the pit lane, I retired to the pit wall with Susie and Alf. I was warned once again that I must be ready for a rapid get away as Stirling did not like to be kept waiting once he was in racing mode. I counted the first time past the pit wall but when he didn't appear at the moment I expected, I saw him entering the pits one lap early, waving at me frantically to get in. I ran over, pulling on a crash helmet and fumbling with the straps as Alf passed the seat belt straps over my shoulders and between my legs. Heaving down on the straps he asked me if I could breathe. I said I could. Alf muttered 'not tight enough then' and pulled even harder pressing me very firmly into the racing seat. Before I could take a breath, we were off down the pit lane with Stirling yelling at me not to raise my hand from the well of the car when at full speed as it would yank it off in the slip stream.

Out onto the track we went, with the engine roaring gloriously and the wind accelerating past my face at rapidly increasing speed. We swept into Copse Corner, a right-hander, at great speed and with significant lateral

G-force throwing my head to the side violently. Accelerating out into Maggots, Becketts and through Chapel in a beautifully flowing movement, onto the high-speed Hanger Straight reaching a speed of 160 mph plus with ease. Down towards Stowe Corner, easy on the brakes as he drifted the car through the Vale and on to Club, hard on the throttle to Abbey Curve taken without lifting, swooping under Bridge and into the Luffield Complex. Braking hard again, my head thrown forwards and then to the right and left with immense lateral forces that I had not felt before, and finally through Woodcote at well over 140 mph before rejoining the pit straight. I glimpsed Susie and Alf holding the timing board aloft, which I could not read, but which Stirling had clearly clocked. 'Now. Old boy, we try a bit harder this lap' he said, indicating the gear that he was in nonchalantly with his left hand whilst clipping the apex of the corners and drifting out of them with consummate ease. I was clearly in the hands of a master of his trade, one that he revelled in and practiced to perfection, and loving it.

As we entered Stowe the next time around smoke began to pour up from under my seat alarmingly, only to abate as we reached the straights. At each corner the same thing happened and so we came back into the pits, where Alf diagnosed the problem as being my excessive weight. I was heavier than he had anticipated and the suspension on my side of the car was not sufficiently strong to prevent the wheel arches from rubbing on the tyres on my side as it became loaded on the right-hand corners. The problem was sorted and off we went for eight more glorious laps, the most exhilarating experience of my life thus far. Stirling, however, wasn't satisfied; he had wanted even more speed and went off with Alf to discuss what should be done about it.

I took the time to stroll down the pit lane to see what other formidable machinery was on show. At the far end was a particularly mean-looking Lamborghini sports car, guarded by very Italian Mafia-looking men with dark glasses, black suits, immaculate white shirts and pencil leather ties. I approached them and asked what one had to do to get a drive in their machine. They asked, 'Do you have a Super-Licence?' Something only world class racing drivers hold. Clearly the answer was no, but I rapidly pointed out that I knew someone who did, my new friend, Stirling Moss. This brought about an instant change in their demeanour, and they excitedly asked if 'Meester Moss' might like to drive their car. I said that I would ask him. I found Stirling with Susie and asked him if he would like to try the new Lamborghini stationed at the end of the pit lane. We sauntered over to the car, to the delight of my two Mafia acquaintances, and we were invited to try it out for a few laps. We strapped in and set off at high speed. After several laps, Stirling was getting into the groove. We came under Bridge at a very high speed, but as he turned into the first of the two tightening corners of Luffield 1 and 2, the car got away from him, and we spun across the infield through a full 720 degrees before being skilfully caught by Stirling, who carried on as though nothing had happened. After a few more laps, we came in and the 'Mafiosi' rushed up to enquire what the great man thought of their car. Without a sidewards glance he said, 'Load of old [manure], lots of power but no torque,' and walked away, leaving the two Italians dumbfounded in his wake. Another of Stirling's characteristics was not suffering fools gladly.

Thus began a strong and, as it turned out, life-long friendship with Sir Stirling and Susie. The next time we met they invited me to dinner in their Shepherd Market home in Mayfair. Stirling had acquired the site just after the war when it was a bombed-out building from damage incurred during the Second World War. He built it into an ultra-modern townhouse which starred in many magazines. It was on five floors connected by a spiral staircase and a lift. The lift had been constructed out of Kevlar by the Williams Formula 1 constructor's team. It was to play a significant role towards the end of his life. On calling the lift to the third floor, the door opened, and he stepped in, but there was no lift cabin, it had got stuck on the floor above. Stirling plunged the three floors, breaking both his legs and severely injuring his back. I was on a flight to Ethiopia about to take off when I received Susie's distressing call. As a result, Stirling was out of action for many weeks but being the determined character that he had been all his life, he was up and running sooner than any of us expected, although with a somewhat restricted gait.

This resilience was also in clear evidence after two major incidents whilst racing. The first, at Monza in 1958, was an accident that could easily have ended his life: his car was launched into the guardrail at the top of the steep banking as his steering sheared at 160 mph. Stirling always kept detailed newspaper cuttings and diary entries. His stoic note after that accident read, 'Broke legs, back, bugger!' Again, he was back in the driving seat quickly. However, he was not so fortunate at Goodwood in April 1962. In a still unexplained accident, he drove head on into the banking at high speed, sustaining multiple injuries and putting him into a coma for three months. Some months later, he had a trial run but failed to meet his own high expectations and decided to retire from front-line racing, perhaps prematurely.

At the dinner in Shepherd Market there were several household names. Amongst them was Norman Tebbit and his wife Margaret, both of whom had been seriously injured in the IRA Brighton bombing. The terrorists had attempted to kill Margaret Thatcher and her entire cabinet at the Grand Hotel during the 1984 Conservative party conference. Margaret Tebbit was rendered paraplegic.

When they arrived, Margaret in her wheelchair, they were confronted with Stirling's Kevlar lift. The wheelchair was too wide to fit. The dilemma of how to convey her up the three floors to the dining room presented itself. It was easily resolved, however, with Formula 1 team members present. At the entrance to the lift with Stirling holding the handles and Patrick Head, chief designer at Williams, on one side and me on the other, the wheels were swiftly removed to allow the chair to enter the lift. We rushed up stairs, and Susie, stopwatch in hand, timed us as they arrived and we replaced the wheels in record time. The Moss' strong sense of humour was in full view as was that of the Tebbits, who took it all in good part.

As conversation flowed round the dinner table, it became clear that Patrick Head was an excellent mimic. He began by taking off Nigel Mansell's Birmingham accent perfectly. Norman Tebbit also had a great sense of humour. He had starred as the most memorable puppet in the satirical television show *Spitting Image*. Known for his direct and sometimes aggressive demeanour, he was portrayed as a leather jacketed, skin-head type. When asked if he had minded this portrayal his response was quite surprising. 'Not at all. Didn't you notice I always won any encounter?' Indeed, he had. He went on to recount a story of when travelling from Merseyside to London, he had encountered a group of Millwall supporters. Cries of 'Where's your bike Norm?' went up. On arrival at Euston station, he was surrounded by the Millwall fans who insisted on escorting him to his taxicab, at one point carrying him shoulder high. They even made up a song, 'In Praise of Norm'.[1] Having spent his early life as a pilot in the Royal Airforce, flying early jets such as the Meteor and Javelin there was a common steely sense of purpose between the two men. What is little known about Tebbit is that he had to bail out of a burning jet, smashing his way through the canopy and breaking his back in the process. He went on to a career in commercial jets before entering the House of Commons. It was a memorable evening in many ways.

At that time, my marriage to Helen was deteriorating and Stirling and Susie showed me great kindness offering me their house as a refuge at any time. Stirling had suffered similarly during the breakdown of his first marriage and taken refuge with Innes Ireland for several months. He had married Katie Molson, heir to the Canadian brewing fortune, but she found the strain of watching her new husband risk his life every weekend too much and they parted to Stirling's great sadness. For us, the criminally long working hours and the pressure that I felt early in my consultant career led to circumstances that were difficult for wives to deal with, even for the ever-patient Helen, who supported me through some very difficult times over the following several years.

Stirling was a regular guest at many Formula 1 races and took me along with him, usually as his driver in my car. He was also known for being a somewhat miserly character, conserving money wherever he could, but I didn't mind at all. Being swept into the heartland of Formula 1 with Stirling was a great adventure. As a passenger he was always chiding me to 'go for the gap old boy, don't hang around'. He held little regard for speed limits and had been caught speeding in Chetwynd in Shropshire testing a Mini Cooper for a motoring magazine. I have experienced going around Hyde Park corner on two wheels with him in a smart car and many hair-brained journeys in powerful courtesy Mercedes that he was loaned wherever he travelled. Travelling with Stirling was always exciting. His adventurous driving even extended to two wheels. However, he was not infallible. In 2003, he crashed his 250 Piaggio scooter on a wet road in south London. Despite a broken hip and torn muscles in his shoulder, he rode home on the scooter before collapsing and being taken to hospital.

During British Grand Prix weekends I would stay overnight with them in Shepherd Market before rising early to drive them to Silverstone. Sometimes their son Elliott would accompany us. As we approached the track we were diverted into evermore privileged lines until, on entering Silverstone, we would find ourselves only one of two cars parked outside the British Racing Drivers' Club – the other being the Bugatti Veyron of Bernie Ecclestone. The days spent with Stirling were huge fun, especially on one occasion when my son and daughter Joanna and Nicholas were with me. Joanna was whisked off by Stirling on the back of his scooter on an autograph signing trip around the paddock. The 'crumpet' as he regularly referred to all good-looking women of any age, would request signatures on bare thighs, arms and, the more adventurous, even on their breasts. He always obliged with a broad smile.

Being able to enter the paddock and the pits with him on race day was a special thrill. We would meet many of the drivers and characters such as Lewis Hamilton's father Anthony, the team owner Frank Williams and Michael Schumacher to name a few. After one race we had a memorable champagne tea with the Pampas Bull, Jackie Ickx, Jackie Oliver and Juan Manuel II's nephew, of the same name. The champagne flowed and the stories became more and more race-y. I heard wonderful stories of the great Juan Manuel

Fangio directly from his nephew, who was attending the British Racing Drivers' Association dinner to accept an honorary lifetime achievement award for his uncle who was too unwell to travel at that time. Finally, at the great man's funeral in 2003, Stirling was one of the guests of honour and a pall bearer along with Sir Jackie Stewart, Jose Froilan Gonzalez (the Pampas Bull), Carlos Reutemann, 'Toto' Fangio, Fangio's younger brother and the then president of Mercedes-Benz Argentina. For Stirling, Fangio was the greatest driver of them all and the one that he set as his own benchmark for performance.

Stirling continued to race in more minor series and latterly in classic cars, especially at the revitalised Goodwood track owned by Lord March. At one of them in the mid-1990s he was racing a Maserati 250F in a field of drivers that contained Martin Brundle and Damon Hill, both much more recent Formula 1 drivers, Hill a world champion. He had failed to do the practice runs required for a place on the grid and hence was forced to start at the back. It was a rainy day and, as those who know motor racing are aware, it is in those conditions that the truly great shine. I was in the main start-finish line grandstand with Susie. Every lap Stirling had made up places and on every lap there was a great cheer from the grandstand as he passed, acknowledging the crowd as he went with a flourishing wave of his left hand, whilst at full chat. As the race progressed, he moved up to third place with only the two recent Formula 1 drivers Brundle and Hill ahead of him. Swooping through the famed St Mary's Bend he overtook both on the outside to gain the lead which he never lost, taking the chequered flag to the absolute delight of the crowd. After it was over Susie and I met him in the tea tent to enjoy a restoring cup with the hero returned, when Brundle and Hill strolled up asking him what he thought he was doing out there? Stirling jauntily replied with a broad smile on his face, 'You boys want to learn how to drive', to great hilarity all around.

Stirling's favourite statement about driving at ten-tenths on a racetrack will live as a testament to his sublime skills. 'Movement is tranquillity,' he said, when describing his emotions when in tune with a thoroughbred racing car. Amongst his many wins in so many different types of car, perhaps the most memorable was his win of the 1955 Mille Miglia in Mercedes 722 at an unbeatable speed, averaging just under 100 mph for the 1,000 miles of open road on which the race took place. He had taken his friend, motoring journalist Dennis Jenkinson, with him. They had reconnoitred the route with Jenkinson recording each twist and turn on a roll of paper, which was then incorporated into a toilet roll like container, which Jenks, as Stirling referred to him, scrolled through as they went. The trust shown by Jenks in Stirling's driving prowess was enormous as they launched off bridges at 150 mph and more with no view or knowledge of what lay on the other side other than the notes. Eventually the race was terminated as there had been so many deaths of drivers and spectators. It is still regarded as the greatest racing drive of all time. Next to this, must come his victory in the 1961 Monaco Grand Prix when he saw off the factory Ferraris in what was really a Formula 2 Lotus Climax car entered by Rob Walker Racing. Driving for much of the race with no cover on the gear lever and making many hundreds of changes per lap he wore a hole in the palm of his hand, something he only noticed at the end of the race. This put him in the eye of Enzo Ferrari who had wanted Moss to drive for him for a while. Negotiations followed but Stirling being the anglophile that he was demanded that Ferrari do the impossible and paint the car in British racing green. Whilst denying him this, Ferrari did agree to paint it blue, which he accepted. Sadly, Moss never got to drive it because of the career ending accident at Goodwood. The car remains in the Ferrari Museum in Modena having never turned a wheel in anger out of respect to the legend that was Stirling Moss.

I saw that car on two later occasions. The first came about through a friend, who is head of cardiac surgery in the University of Verona, Giuseppe Faggian. We had known each other for a while professionally, and he had invited me to Verona to share some surgical experiences with the mitral valve, a subject that we were both interested in. When the science/surgery was done, Giuseppe slowly unveiled a secret tour that he had planned for me. Previously the owner of the restaurant opposite the Ferrari factory in Modena had been his patient. He had negotiated a visit to the factory to see the Ferraris being made and to the Ferrari Museum. I was not told where we were going but as we approached the signs to Modena the truth dawned on me. We arrived and drove through the famous gates to be met by his delightful friend and then introduced to the senior staff. A full tour of the plant was next, followed by the museum tour and there it was, Stirling's Blue Ferrari. The next time that I saw the car was at the design museum exhibition of Ferrari's designs and beautiful cars.

Following the factory and museum tour, we all repaired to the restaurant opposite the factory for lunch in the room that Enzo had dined in when not at the races. I noticed that others were being given wine with their meal but not me. I was soon to find out why. As soon as lunch was over, we were whisked off to the Ferrari test track at Fiorano where I was treated to several laps by the chief Ferrari test driver in one of their high-performance cars. It had been a very special day indeed. The weekend did not end there, however. Giuseppe then whisked us off to Alba in Piedmont for the opening of the truffle season the next day. I was treated to a wonderful large white truffle to take home with me. It had been a unique experience. The truffles were being weighed and graded in a small smoky back room screened off from the narrow front of the shop by a heavy Indian carpet suspended from the rafters. Standing behind the truffle grader was an armed gendarme, such was the value of the fare on display. The village was shrouded in early autumn mist with moisture hanging in the air. It was a magical and indeed somewhat mystical experience. Both Guiseppe and I enjoyed all aspects of motor sports and many a long conversation ensued. He was the proud owner of a beautifully maintained Aston Martin DB4 handed down to him by his father who had bought it as new from the factory. Every year they journeyed over to the factory for its annual maintenance.

On a more serious note, it was at the 2000 British Grand Prix that Stirling introduced me to a new business acquaintance Tom Cressman, with whom he was marketing car cleaning products amongst other things. His girlfriend was Jane Andrews. They were there together and seemed a delightful couple. In fact, we got on so well that they invited me to dinner with them to be arranged later in the year. I though no more of it until one day late in September I received a telephone call from the Metropolitan Police asking to interview me in relation to a recent murder. I was shocked. Apparently, Andrews had been expecting Cressman to propose marriage to her on a recent holiday and he had failed to do so. On returning home, an argument ensued during which, fearing violence, Cressman called the police to ask for protection but none came. Later that night, whilst he was asleep, Andrews hit him with a cricket bat, rendering him unconscious. She then stabbed him to death, before running away and disappearing for several days. She was found semi-comatose in her car, having taken an overdose of drugs in a failed suicide attempt. She was sentenced to life imprisonment but escaped after nine years only to be recaptured after three days in a hotel room with her family. Apparently, my name and address were the last entries in the pair's diary. Thankfully, it was just a fact checking interview and that was the last of my involvement. The story was all the more sensational as Jane Andrews was the dresser for Sarah, Duchess of York. Andrews was imprisoned for eighteen years.

February 2000 saw my fiftieth birthday. Stirling and Susie had arranged a special day for me. I was to report to the Aston Martin factory in Milton Keynes at 10.00 a.m. I was met by Walter Hayes who had been in charge of Ford Motor sport for many years, overseeing the Ford GT project and the World Rally Championship cars, in which Ford had been dominant, as well as being key in the development of the Ford Cosworth engine that was so dominant in Formula 1 in the 1960s. He was also responsible for signing Sir Jackie Stewart who went on become world champion several times. He had begun life as a journalist. He became associate editor of the *Daily Mail* newspaper at the tender age of 32, and was the last editor of the *Sunday Dispatch* newspaper. He found his way into motorsport through the auspices of Colin Chapman who headed Lotus cars. His pedigree in motorsport of all types is unassailable and it was a huge honour to be shown around the Aston Martin Factory by him. We had lunch together and then I was informed that we had to be in London for late afternoon.

I was greeted by Susie and ushered into the drawing room where Walter and his wife had already arrived and were sitting with Stirling with big grins on their faces and open Champagne and fancy cakes. Following present opening and hearty conversation I was ushered over to the Park Lane Hilton, which stood just behind Stirling's house, for an excellent dinner. All in all, a very memorable birthday with wonderfully entertaining people.

Walter had remained close friends with Henry Ford II who by then had moved to live in London by the Thames; they used to meet for cocktails every Saturday afternoon. On one such occasion, Ford asked Walter what he thought that they should do that week. Walter replied, 'Let's buy Aston Martin. They are in some trouble and we can turn them around.' And so they did.

Another story that Walter told me was that at one stage, when he was a newspaper editor, he and his wife were going through a short but rather turbulent time. His wife Elizabeth, a retired state registered nurse, was in thrall to horoscopes. Walter went to the editor of the daily horoscope in the paper and asked him to publish one that he had written especially for his wife's star sign. In it he suggested that all those under her sign should think carefully about their relationships and behave more considerately towards their partners or bad things would befall them. Apparently, it worked, and quietude descended once more on the Hayes household. A warning for all those who follow their horologists too assiduously.

There were no bounds to Stirling and Susie's hospitality towards me. On one occasion when I was in the United States at a meeting, they invited me to their Florida home. Still not knowing them that well at that time and feeling I should take them a present I was flummoxed by what to buy. There was a bookstore at the airport and I found a handsomely illustrated volume on historic cars. It seemed appropriate and so armed with that tome and a bottle or two of good red wine, I set off satisfied with my purchases. I was met at the airport by Stirling in the top-of-the-line Mercedes saloon car, loaned to him in his capacity as life-long world ambassador for Mercedes-Benz.

The journey to their house on the water was no less interesting than every other trip with Stirling driving. 'Out of the way, twit. Look at that idiot.' Every corner apexed and the racing line followed the whole route.

On arrival, I proffered my gifts, but as I did so I saw the very same book that I had bought for him on the coffee table. Apparently, Stirling was sent practically every newly published motoring book for review. I was to discover that the top floor bedroom of their house in London, had almost every major book on cars and motor racing ever produced as well as the significant number that Stirling had produced himself. Not a great start I thought, but Stirling was gracious in accepting it. I then produced the wine only to be told that his only tipple was the white wine version of Wolf Blass Yellow Label. He drank nothing else. My double embarrassment was smoothed over with good humour and effusive gratitude for my generosity, which of course they stated was completely unnecessary.

In 2005, they celebrated their twenty-fifth wedding anniversary at the Windows restaurant in the Park Lane Hilton. It was a very grand affair with many guests and a dance band. I was sat between David and Vicki Mason, old friends of the Mosses. David had earned an OBE for the work that he did in gaining compensation for the families with children that had been so badly affected by the drug Thalidomide. It had been given to pregnant women to overcome the nausea that is so common in pregnancy. A powerful side effect of the drug is to impair blood vessel growth and this in turn halted the growth of the limbs. It had been an extremely tough battle well told in his book on the subject.[2] I had clearly been seated next to them in Stirling's attempt to get help for Vicki, who had suffered renal failure. She had undergone a kidney transplant which was then failing. They had been told by renal specialists in London that nothing further could be done, other than lifelong dialysis, something that was consuming their lives. David is a significant dealer in the world of high-class art. He has a major gallery in the west end of London. He also was a racer himself and had been in Formula 1 in the 1950s, but not in the class of Stirling. Until very recently he was still racing successfully in the Ferrari Challenge series. The conversation drifted towards Vicki and the dilemma that she faced. They explained that they had been told that further transplantation was out of the question. I knew that that was not necessarily so and offered to make enquiries for them of my close friend Peter Friend, who is Professor and Director of the Oxford Transplant Centre.

The evening came to a close and we agreed to talk again when I had found out useful information. In short, I was able to introduce him to Peter, who in turn successfully re-transplanted Vicky, removing the burden of thrice weekly dialysis. Following that we struck up a friendship which endures. David is a very generous man and knowing of mine and Peter's interest in motor racing, he arranged several track days for us in his beautiful race prepared Ferraris, under the tutelage of a professional driver Callum Lockie. Many exciting hours have been spent on track with him and his wonderful group of supporters in F.F. Corse. My best lap time for the Grand Prix course being two minutes and twelve seconds. To put that in perspective, the Ferrari challenge lap record is two minutes and four seconds with the Formula 1 drivers easily lapping in one minute and twenty-eight seconds or so. Not good enough for me to give up my day job, but reasonably respectable.

In the late 1990s, I was referred Lord Renton, a peer of the realm and the then Father of the House of Lords, for surgery. At the time he was in his mid-nineties. Despite his advanced age, he was keen that I should operate on him so that he could get back to the thing that sustained him. 'Rather too much garden and not enough help, old boy,' he proclaimed when I asked him to what he attributed his activeness at such an advanced age. He was keen that I should use his case as an example and gave me full permission to use his name in that context. He wanted to inform people of his situation to give others hope in infirmity. During his recovery period the subject of motor racing came up, and he told me that he had taken his driving test for the first time just short of his 95th birthday at the insistence of his lawyer daughter.

Having started to drive in the 1930s when no licence was needed, he had never sat a test. She was concerned by the ever-increasing number of dents appearing in the family Rolls Royce. At her insistence he approached the head of the traffic police in Westminster and the sergeant at arms in the House of Lords and I suspect against their better judgement persuaded them to give him a test, by driving to the east coast and back with the police chief in the passenger seat. This was done and Lord Renton was given a clean bill of health to continue driving despite his daughter's trepidation. He went on to take and pass the driving test, the oldest person in the UK at that time to achieve this.[3] Whilst talking about this, the subject of Stirling Moss came up and he expressed his long-standing admiration for him. I raised the fact that with all of the sporting heroes in the United Kingdom who had received a knighthood, Stirling wasn't one of them. He confessed that he hadn't noticed that and perhaps something should be done about it. Whether this had anything to do with the subsequent events I shall never know, but within six months Stirling became Sir Stirling and Susie, very deservedly, Lady Moss.

I enjoyed many happy times with Stirling and Susie. They were always kind and supportive through good times and bad. Susie was an extraordinary host and the most loyal wife imaginable. She controlled Stirling's diary, making sure that he was always where he needed to be, on time and smartly turned out. His racing overalls were always clean and freshly pressed. Susie was a wonderful cook, with nothing being too much trouble for her. One Saturday afternoon, whilst Susie was relaxing in the bath, Stirling came home and casually announced that he had invited someone to dinner. That someone turned out to be the famous Michelin starred chef Anton Mossiman, head chef at the Dorchester. Totally surprised but unfazed, Susie rose from the bath, dressed and left to shop in one easy movement. For most, the thought of cooking for a world-famous chef would be prohibitively daunting but Susie took it all in her stride. During the meal he announced that her home cooking was better than that which could be found in any restaurant of any class. Stirling's son Elliot trained with Mossiman and is now an extremely skilled chef himself.

Sadly, one day at a function at the R.A.C. club on Pall Mall, Susie lost her balance and fell backwards on some stone stairs and fractured the base of her skull. The lasting effect of this was to deprive her of her sense of taste, essential for fine cooking. From that time onwards, her delight in cooking was lost.

Misfortune was to strike the Moss household again in 2016, when on a trip to Singapore Stirling was taken seriously ill and admitted to hospital as an emergency, rapidly needing intensive care. He never recovered from this and died peacefully at home under the care of Susie in April 2020 aged ninety-four. Susie died of a broken heart not long afterwards.

The final chapter in our relationship came when Elliot, Stirling and Susie's son, invited us to the memorial service that he had arranged at Westminster Abbey, a fitting venue for a British icon who had brought so much pleasure to people around the world. His Royal Highness the Duke of Kent represented His Majesty the King. Eulogies were spoken movingly by Elliot, Sir Jackie Stewart and Simon Taylor, respected motoring journalist and long-time friend of Stirling. It was an intensely moving affair. As we walked out of the Abbey, before the tomb of the unknown soldier was a table placed in the centre of the aisle with Stirling's pith helmet that became his trademark and next to it his ten British Racing Driver's Gold Stars, something that no other driver has achieved.

In the courtyard outside the Abbey, several of the cars that Stirling had raced so successfully were on display. Mercedes was extremely generous with their support and sent over the famous Mille Miglia winning car number 722. It was the last time that the car would be allowed out from its Mercedes Museum home. After the service in the packed cathedral we were invited to the R.A.C. club on Pall Mall for refreshments. In the entrance lobby were two more of Stirling's race winning Mercedes beautifully presented, and in the reception room were some of his many trophies. It had been a grand send off for one of Britain's great sporting heroes. Let us hope that Stirling's trip to the next world was 'speedy and tranquil'.

In 1996, Peter Friend (another car crazy surgeon) and I decided that we were going to do the Racing Drivers' Course at Donnington Park Racetrack. We booked our places and waited for the time to pass with mounting excitement. The trip didn't have an auspicious start for me. First, I took the wrong turning on the motorway during an excited conversation with Peter, which added forty minutes or so the journey. Then when we arrived the hotel had a squash court and we decided to have a game. During it I fell onto the vertical handle of the racket and managed to displace my third and fourth costo-chondral junctions, a particularly awkward and painful injury. It was to interfere with my driving in the tight cockpit of the singe seater car. That was my excuse at least.

The following morning, we were at the track for 6.00 a.m. to sign on. When we arrived, we immediately realised that we were likely to be outclassed. We were surrounded by karting champions from all over the globe. All were 'wannabe' Formula 1 drivers, aged between fifteen and eighteen. Here we were, in our forties, looking very aged against these fit young men. Amongst them was Marino Franchitti; his brother Dario was an Indy car champion of the first order, winning the championship four times and the Indianapolis 500 three times. Mario went on to be a class driver himself competing in the Le Mans series. Our saving grace was that most of them had forgotten to have medical checks before arrival. We just happened to have blood pressure monitors in the back of the car and set up a small medical clinic in the paddock to allow them to carry on. Of course, we were an instant hit and accepted into the group somewhat like father figures. The week began with lectures and time on track, first in saloon cars and later in the week in singe seaters. All track work was regulated with rev. counter speed limits gradually increasing as we progressed. Work on skid pans and essentials of high-speed control were taught. The week culminated in a full race day on the Sunday, with outside entrants, and the opportunity to gain our racing licences. It had been dry and sunny all week, but as we gathered at race control at 6.00 a.m. for the day's briefing, the rain began to fall heavily. Not what we had hoped for. Mild panic began to set in.

First, we had to qualify for our places on the grid over several timed laps. This we did, and although we were not at the back of the grid we were, as Caroll Shelby had told me, amongst a better class of person, my friend Peter being one of them. I remember leaving the pit lane for my last timed lap and as I did another car came past at full chat and a shower of water from his wheels poured over me, partially filling the foot well around the pedals with a small lake.

The time came for the race. We were strapped in and set off on the warm-up lap with the rain still falling. At the end of the start and finish straight there is a right-handed slightly adverse camber corner, Redgate, which I wasn't too comfortable with, followed by the Craner Curves downhill and very fast. We lined up for the grid and waited for the red lights to go out trying to keep the perfect revs on the engine before letting out the clutch and launching off the grid. The red lights went out. I released the clutch. Nothing happened! I was standing still with wheels spinning as the remaining cars on the grid shot past. Up ahead I could see an almighty accident happening as cars piled into each other whilst trying to brake for the first corner. By then, I was off and running and steered my way around the others to find myself in second place. Up ahead was Peter who had succeeded in getting away somewhat better. As the race progressed several of the other cars with the more skilled drivers overtook us, but we had our own race to enjoy. Trying to pass Peter on the entrance to the chicane at the start finish straight, I lost control and spun out but managed to keep going. The rules were that if you had a spin you had to come into the pits for the car to be checked. This I did and although not finishing last it put me further behind. I wasn't last but neither would I trouble Michael Shumaker any time soon, but we had got through the week unscathed and we had had a lot of fun and were now in proud possession of our racing licences.

Dad had shared my enthusiasm for motor sport, making his own hot rod as a young man, whilst working in the local garage in Clun before entering the butchery business. However, as 'the shop' came to dominate everything, the times that we had to experience some enjoyment in the sport were extremely limited. On 30 July 1967, I had persuaded Dad to take me and my schoolfriend Roger Bradbury to the BOAC 1,000 km sportscar race at Brands Hatch. Roger's father was also a butcher in the prosperous town of Malpas, Cheshire. The attraction of that particular race was Jim Clark, arguably the best, or certainly among the best, race drivers of all time. He was supposed to be sharing a car with my personal favourite Graham Hill, along with many other great names who were also taking part. Back then the journey from Clun was a long one. The M1 motorway was open for a large part but the rest of the journey was on A roads. We set off very early in the morning, arriving shortly before midday. It turned out to be an extremely fateful occasion. During the lead up to the race it was announced, to the disappointment of all present, that Jim Clark would not be taking part as he had been ordered by Colin Chapman to race in a Formula 2 race at Hockenheim. Not long after the race had started an announcement came over the tannoy that Jim Clark had had a fatal accident. An eerie hush descended over the crowd as all enthusiasm for the event evaporated. It had been extremely disappointing not to see him race at Brands, something that had drawn most of the crowd that day. This news was disastrous and soon after people began to drift away and wend their way home. The only other fatality that seemed to have the same impact on the world of motor racing in an age of fatal accidents was to occur twenty-six years later, when the great Ayrton Senna was killed in the San Marino Grand Prix. Both deaths were predicted by some to be the end of Formula 1 as a sport, but despite these tragedies it survives.

More recently, I have enjoyed watching Claudia derive similar thrills from the racecourse at Castle Combe. Although she holds a driver's licence, most of her driving has been on right-hand-drive roads. So when I took her to Castle Combe for a day on track with some powerful cars, she was initially somewhat daunted. I think the instructor in the car with her was a bit concerned when she told him that she had not driven a car with a stick shift for many years. However, once she was up and running some respectable times were put in with no damage done to pride or car, and she had a suitably impressed tutor.

I have enjoyed and experienced many interesting and exhilarating times at Grand Prix since, and maintain an avid interest, fuelled to greater heights by my friendship with Sir Stirling. I have survived getting lost in the hills around the track in Barcelona, attending the Spanish Grand Prix with my long-time friend from medical school Andy Davidson (the mimic!), got stuck in the mud with the Papworth transplant van at Silverstone and weathered the rain with my son Nicholas in the Ardennes hills at Spa. I hope that there will be many more to enjoy in the coming years.

In 2015, I was contacted by my friend David Mason, who told me that he was going to see a Ferrari in the Staines area and wondered whether I would like to go with him. When we arrived, there was a beautiful Daytona, a 355 and a 348TB all in Ferrari red. Whilst David negotiated the price of the much more expensive Daytona, I was taken by the little 348, somewhat more in my price range. David noticed my interest and with his dealer's skills negotiated a very good price. I fell for it and bought it. It is more a piece of automotive art than a really good car, and in truth I struggled to get my 6 feet plus frame in and out of it. However, it had always been a secret ambition of mine to own such a piece of automotive history and so I closed the deal.

After I bought it, I read a quote from Luca di Montezemolo who had taken over Ferrari just as the car was launched. He declared that the 348 was the worst car that Ferrari had ever produced. Was he correct? History has disproven him as it is a strong car which has performed well and continues to carry favour. Not long after I had bought it I was in Milan for a surgical meeting. I came across an artist sitting in the Piazza della Republica. He was painting famous cars. I approached him to ask him if he would consider producing a watercolour of my 348. He asked me where it was and I told him that it was in England. He laughed and asked how he was going to do that. I produced a photograph and asked if that would do? He agreed and I asked if he could complete it in 48 hours as I was leaving for England. He laughed once again making it clear that it would take a week or more. I asked him whether he would accept the commission if I were to pay him in advance. He laughed once again at my perceived naivete in giving him money and leaving the country, I said that I thought that I could trust him, and we made the transaction. Six weeks later a carefully wrapped parcel arrived with the painting and a lovely note thanking me for trusting him and saying how rare that trust is nowadays. Soon it will be the only memory that I will have of that lovely car, as it has to be sold with the advancement of retirement.

Although seen by many as a somewhat childish pursuit, motor racing has given me a huge amount of pleasure and my friendship with one of the greatest ever has been an enduring privilege.

11

'New' Home Alabama

> Sweet home Alabama, Where the skies are so blue, Sweet home Alabama, I'm comin' home to you
>
> Here I come Alabama.[1]

We left home in East Sheen on Friday 30 December at 9.15 a.m. It had been a chaotic departure. As we were driven away in a taxi bound for the airport, we left behind a plumber in the toilet and a man on the roof managing problems before our tenants moved in. Some nursing friends were renting the house for the year.

The first stage of our journey, the Delta flight from Gatwick to Atlanta, was uneventful and Joanna, only three months old at that time, managed well although she didn't sleep. As we disembarked from the connecting flight to Birmingham, the snow began to fall, lightly at first. Expecting Alabama sunshine, we were dressed for sunny climes and so this was a big surprise. The hotel room that I had booked in the Birmingham Hilton, close to the university campus, was extremely cold. So cold that we had to move rooms in the middle of the night to be able to sleep. New Year's Eve was spent hiring a car and visiting our apartment where we had something of a surprise, but more of that later. Compared to the society that we had left in England, the simple accessibility of everything needed for daily living was extraordinary to us. We found supermarkets, superstores for cars, furniture and household goods open all night. Compared with the UK, where everything was closed by five in the afternoon, this was extraordinary. After only a short time I was able to buy a car at midnight, a second-hand Datsun Sentra. My desire for a gas-guzzling American leviathan had to be tempered by common sense. I was informed that the reliability of the Japanese cars compared with the

American built ones was much superior and made them more desirable. It was a good choice and ran faultlessly all year. I was even able to sell it for the same price that I paid for it when we left.

The year was packed with exciting new experiences. I found that the contrasts between life at home in England and in the deep south of America were so great that they could occupy a book of their own.

Recently, I have rediscovered several letters that I had written home to my parents. At that time of course, there was no email, or any form of social media and the i-phone was long into the future. It was expensive to phone home and so I restricted that to once a month at most. I had been brought up to write letters and wrote home regularly. My parents had kept most of my letters and passed them back to me some years later. Therefore, rather than relying on my memory I have reproduced some of them here as a contemporary narrative. They convey a flavour of the time spent in the deep south, and those cultural differences that we experienced. Here are a few from across the year of 1984:

Saturday 7 January
1853A Arboretum Circle Alabama 35216

Dear Mum, Dad, Charmian and Gran,
Well, we're here! It's been a pretty hectic week. We flew into Atlanta at 4.20 pm local time (10.20 for you), where we had to change planes. We left there at 7.30 pm local time (1.30 pm for you) and because we crossed another time zone, arrived in Birmingham at 7.20 pm (1.30 am UK). We got to the hotel at 3.15 am UK time. Dressed in summer clothes and shocked to find light snow when the aircraft doors opened! Apparently, it hadn't snowed there for several years. Must have brought it along.

Total travel time 15 ½ hours! Joanna was marvellous. Slept only short periods but smiled and laughed throughout! The first room they put us in at the Hotel (Downtown Hilton) was v. cold, so I asked to be moved and that was o.k.

Saturday a.m. I hired a Dodge Charger and set off to look for our house (apartment). We called in at some supermarkets and got some basic food & then on to the apartment. It is very nice and clean, - BUT NO FURNITURE other than a bed for us, a crib for Joanna and a chest of drawers! Saturday afternoon (New Year's Eve), we were whisked off by Harold (He knew of our dilemma from the condominium manager) to his showroom to pick out some hired furniture, cutlery and other essentials. This we did but couldn't have it delivered until Tuesday pm as it was Bank Holiday. Now that it is installed it looks nice. Will send photos.

We then had to buy basic utensils and bedding. The kitchen has a large fridge/freezer, washing-up machine for plates etc (never seen one before) a double oven and cupboards but no washing machine. There is a laundrette on site as well as a swimming pool. The weather now is beautiful. Freezing at night but was 61 degrees yesterday during the afternoon. Clear blue skies and sunny. Sunday and Monday were spent getting ourselves kitted out and finding our way around. You need a car to get everywhere and so my next main task was to acquire one.

I had to obtain a social security number, a bank account and get the phones connected and the power. We bought our telephone at the local store $30! By now my head was in overdrive, but we were winning. Jet lag was a slight problem as I kept waking at 3.00 am.

Tuesday, am I went to work and had a whole load of things to sign and do. Thursday to the Am South bank to open accounts. Had to acquire a short-term loan of $6,000 to buy a car.

Thursday spent looking intensely for car. Depressing! They are the same price as in UK. Japanese cars said to be the best, so bought a 1982 Datsun Sentra coupe with 22,000 miles on the clock for $6,580. Not bad. Hope it runs ok.

Everyone is very kind and helpful with a lovely 'Suuuthern Acceeent'! I was invited to lunch at the Rotary club on Wednesday and was the guest of honour. Had lunch with the president of an air-conditioning company and the president of my new bank, Am South! Not a bad start.

Through all of this Joanna remained bright, healthy and cheerful.

This afternoon into work for the first time properly. Meetings all morning – very interesting but next week work begins in earnest. They want to turn me into "the world's expert in Pulmonary damage during cardio-pulmonary bypass." We'll see!

The girl running the condominium where we live, is the granddaughter of William Temple, Archbishop of Canterbury during the second war. She has a real southern accent. A strange juxtaposition! What a coincidence.

Miss you but won't be long until I am back

All my love

Francis

The car was bought at midnight along a strip of car showrooms and giant stores that were open all night. Another new experience for me. The kindness shown to us as a family was extraordinary and the term southern hospitality became real to me.

Sunday January 15

Dear all,

Last Sunday we were whisked off to Church by the president of the air-conditioning company, Mr Stegalls. I get the impression that they are multi-millionaires (I suppose he would have to be, running the largest air-conditioning company in this climate).

Mr Stegalls was a long-established member of the Birmingham city Rotary Club. He invited me to lunch at the club to welcome me to Birmingham. During the lunch, the origin of the name of the U.A.B. research building, the Quarterback Tower, arose. Apparently, early after John Kirklin had moved from the Mayo clinic he had been invited to present a topic of interest to the Rotarians. The then relatively new operation of coronary artery bypass surgery for coronary artery disease, was his topic. Afflicting well fed and sedentary middle-aged men, it was something many of them were suffering through a somewhat hedonistic lifestyle. Dr Kirklin began to present in the only way that he knew, with projected slides heavy with data. After a few minutes the "winningest college football coach of all time, 'Big Bear Bryant', coach of the 'Crimson Tide', the Alabama college football team asked the question, "Dr Kirklin, what d'ya need?" He was referring to a fund raiser for a research building. John answered with a significant dollar amount. Big Bear glanced around the room, took a head count and said, "Dr. Kirklin, you have got it, now sit down and let's see the plays!". And that was it. The money was given, and the research tower built and gained the name of the Quarter-back Tower. Church is not quite what we are used to! It is Presbyterian, very modern and huge! It is an extremely sociable event, and everything starts at 9.30 a.m. with a Medical Ethical meeting would you believe. Followed by Children's Sunday school which everyone including the parents attend. Then the real service begins at 11.00 am and is on closed circuit television as well.

It's just as you can imagine with the preacher in ordinary lounge suit and a massed choir standing in a raised stage at the back. No Altar as such. Everything is done from the bible (hence the term the bible belt of America). Everyone has their own bible heavily underscored on every page. Tithing is practised throughout the whole community and the warning of God's wrath was wrought upon the whole congregation if anyone failed to pay and start praying right now! America is of course the centre of the known and unknown Universe, and everyone else (except the English, I might add, who according to the preacher are 300 years ahead!) are heathens. We were not Presbyterian or southern Baptist followers and so didn't attend the church again. One Monday morning about six weeks later, I was surprised to find the preacher waiting for me outside the theatres in U.A.B. He had come to enquire how we were and whether we would be attending his church soon. Clearly worried for his errant potential flock. It was done in a very caring way but somewhat overbearing. I explained that we were Church of England in the softest way that I could, and he accepted that gracefully, but offered ongoing support and help if any were needed.

Afterwards we were taken to the Vestavia Country Club for lunch. A grand large house with large swimming pool and many tennis courts. There was a black woman playing the piano with white gloves on! Lunch was very American – roast beef with muffins! We were taken to the Stegall's house on the way to church to freshen up. It is a huge pinewood home set in 20 acres of forest with its own road up to it! Not a bad little place. Work was interesting this week, but I miss the clinical responsibility. Money seems no object in the department. I have been given virtually a free hand to get my project off the ground as it is the main project of Dr. Kirklin's department this year. I hope that I can make a success of it. The regular Saturday morning meetings worry me a little, as we are expected to give frequent, in depth talks in front of the whole faculty. We get heavily criticised by Kirklin and the others if not up to standard. There are always serious out-of-town luminaries present, such as Dr's Denton Cooley, Norman Shumway and Michael DeBakey to name a few. My first talk is in two weeks' time, so I had better get cracking with that. I found out yesterday that I can hire a piano for twenty-five dollars a month so I think I will arrange that next week.

Do write soon and fill it with British news as that doesn't penetrate this far.

All love,

Francis

On 22 January I wrote:

Dear Mum, Dad, Gran and Charmian,

Last week was an interesting one getting my research up and running. I hope to begin the experimental work next week. On Saturday I have to give my first presentation on Saturday morning. I am not looking forward to it as they are expected to be of an extremely high standard. I suppose another way of looking at it is that it is a good chance to show what I am capable of.

We have got a piano! $25 per month. I bought a short-wave radio to get news from home as there is none here.

It has been surprisingly cold here. 10–20 degrees below freezing. The mornings are sunny with blue skies, however. Joanna has had unremitting diarrhoea, and I have taken her to the paediatrician. Luckily, he is treating her for free as I am part of UAB, otherwise the cost would be huge. I think the system is iniquitous. If you haven't got the money or insurance, you don't get treated! I have seen patients turned away already. It makes me realise how lucky we are to have the NHS. Don't let people knock it.

It's virtually impossible to get any English newspapers here. There is one shop (The Little Professor), but they are usually 2-3 weeks old. Living here is very expensive. Food is dearer and electricity is hugely expensive, around $150 per month. Car insurance is approx. £280 per year.

I got into the operating theatre a bit last week. Things aren't very different. In fact, I thought that there were some things that we do a little better.

Please write back

Love to everyone

Sadly, letters from home were few and far between, probably because of my mother's illness and Dad so busy with the shop and looking after her. Hence the audible mild pleading in the letters.

The piano shop was on the north side of the main east west thoroughfare, in the more run-down part of town. It had a huge floor area with many pianos of all types. Downstairs was a large sheet music department and upstairs there was a small concert hall with a Bösendorfer full concert grand with the extra octave underneath a wooden flip up cover. It always seemed to be empty. Once I got to know the owner, I was invited to visit whenever I wanted, to pick out some sheet music and to play the wonderful concert grand upstairs. It became a regular lunch-time event for me.

Sunday 12 February

Dear Mum and Dad and Gran

It was lovely to speak to you on the phone today. I hope I didn't worry you too much over Joanna. She is better in herself despite the continuing diarrhoea. I rang the paediatrician again this morning and expressed my concern. We are going to take her down again tomorrow to get her urine and motions cultured.

The weather here is very changeable at the moment. Yesterday it was about 65 degrees but humid and grey except for a short time in the afternoon when the sun came out. Then it was just like a summer's day at home.

Earlier in the week it was below freezing point. Today it is windy and warm with sunny skies. No wonder everyone is going down with infections. Apparently as the spring comes on it becomes more and more windy with occasional tornadoes! In the summer it's just hot! Give me British weather any day.

As you say in your letter, it's nice to have a piano around again. They do tune it as part of the agreement. It was tuned before we took delivery of it, so I don't think it will need perhaps more than once again during the year.

The car is going quite well. There are a couple of problems..... I am going to take it back to get them fixed under the warranty. Driving on the right is becoming natural now although occasionally at some complicated junctions I have to think a bit! The American drivers are even worse than the French! All the American cars indicator lights are the same as their brake lights and flash red, so that when they are braking and it is a bright day you often cannot tell if they are braking or indicating, apart from which, they usually don't!

Their driving test is not very taxing I believe. They have a 20-minute multiple choice questionnaire on the highway code and then drive once around the building, with a highway patrol man! We are not going to bother taking it. We are driving on an international drivers' licence. Petrol is very cheap here. Shopping is very different from at home. You don't walk down the street as you would in Shrewsbury or Birmingham etc., you have to drive to the shopping malls which are essentially shopping centres. There are no Butcher's shops that we can find. It is all sold pre-packed in the supermarkets. Their requirements from food are quite different to ours. They are more interested in adding vitamins and subtracting caffeine etc. The milk is sold in large plastic containers, rather than being delivered in bottles as at home, It doesn't taste very nice. It has so much added Vitamin D.

With lots of love

Francis

The changes in lifestyle that we all live with today and that the Americans were already experiencing were yet to arrive in the UK and so much of it felt very foreign to us.

February 19 1984

Dear Mum and Dad and Gran,

My talk went very well. Dr. Kirklin even went so far to say that he thought it was a beautiful presentation. So, I felt quite satisfied with my performance. I now have to keep it up!

How did Mum get on at Mr Mark's house in Cheshire when you went to look at the decompression chamber? Do you think that you will try it?

At that time my mother's multiple sclerosis was taking a great hold on her abilities to move around and to do anything for herself. She was willing to try anything at that time. Anecdotal information suggested that decompression chambers could help, something that was discredited soon after. Multiple sclerosis was very ill-understood at the time.

> Yesterday after I had finished at work, we went out for a drive to the Tannehill state park. It was about 20 miles through the countryside. It was fascinating to see. There are no areas of cultivation as there are in England, it is 80% woodland with some pasture.
>
> The majority of people seem to be very poor. They live in the typical old wooden shacks raised from the ground on wooden or brick pedestals. Just as I imagined it would be after reading Huckleberry Finn.
>
> At the State Park they had a collection of the original wood and log cabins of the pioneers. One was built and owned by an English Methodist minister who came over in the early 1800's and walked from his landfall in the Carolinas, through the empty country until he reached that spot where he built it with his own hands. It is amazing to think what those people endured to make a new home for themselves.
>
> This area was the heart of the Confederacy in the Civil war and suffered severe losses both in property and manpower. It was interesting to note that Birmingham city simply did not exist 100 years ago. There was just a large, wooded valley occupied by the Creek and Chickasaw Indians.
>
> They have built the city around a large Iron and Steel industry as the area stands on iron ore and coal. It was called the 'Magic City' because of this combination and later Steel City for obvious reasons.
>
> In 1979 the Steel works closed and as you can imagine unemployment was huge, especially among the black people who made up 60% of the population at that time. The steel mills are just reopening, and so unemployment is falling. The black population is now around 50%. They all live on the north side of the city so there is little mixing. They have been very kind to us. I find it very distasteful the way they are treated. It is as bad as South Africa in that respect.
>
> Joanna is putting on weight again and is now 16lbs 11ozs.
>
> All my love
> Francis

With respect to the black population, I witnessed some awful incidents such as the husband of my laboratory technician, a local sheriff, trying to force a teenage boy to cross the road rather than allowing me to make way for him whilst walking down the street towards us. I refused to comply and let him pass me, but my actions were not liked. The same lab technician was emptying out her large handbag in her office looking for her car keys when I was standing next to her. Out tumbled a handgun, a cannister of Mace spray and an alarm for calling for help. I asked her if she knew how to handle the gun and she told me that she went to target practice every Friday evening. On persisting with my questions, I asked if she had ever had cause to use it in anger. Her reply: 'Oh yes, but sadly I missed. I won't let that happen again.' Clearly, we were in new territory here.

Sunday March 4 1984

Dear Mum, Dad and Gran,

It was lovely to hear from you and thanks for the material on Clun and environs. It is such a fascinating history. It seems to have played such an important part in the borders between Wales and England throughout history. I like the idea of 'Clunites' banding together and fighting against both sides in the Civil war. I think that the Americans would love this history. To them ancient history began in 1780 or so. In fact, I am reading a history of the US at the moment, and they refer to anything prior to 1700 as prehistory. They seem to ignore their native Indian ancestry. On my birthday I had a phone call in the office at work from our bank (AmSouth) from the chief cashier, to wish me a happy birthday. And then all the tellers lifted up an extension and about 10 girls sang Happy Birthday down the telephone. Can you imagine Mr Marshall [the manager of the Midland bank in Clun] doing that? It was very nice of them.

We had snow this week. Snow in March in Alabama! We woke on Wednesday morning to find it white over outside! It remained below freezing all day with snow flurries. There was never more than a light covering but it literally brought the city to a standstill! All the schools were closed, and many people didn't go to work. There are two steepish hills on the way to work and when we set off at seven am we got to the top of the first hill to find the police with their highway patrol cars sealing off the road. We found another way around. The following day it had all gone.

The rest of northern America and the central planes area has had a huge amount of snow, and I think is still suffering a blizzard in some parts. We had a tornado warning a few nights ago. There are low pitched bleeps from the TV followed by a printed message. We are in the lea of a hill here and so should be well protected.

Later in the year at the height of the tornado season, a large one ripped through the southern edge of the city. We were driving home from the university and were guided under a large overpass to shelter until it had passed.

On Sunday we were invited to an afternoon tea-party with a middle-aged woman who is the secretary for the Rotary club. It was pleasant but a very strange gathering. There was an American chap about my age who was a behavioural psychologist (archetypal male nouveau intellectual) and with him his Peruvian dentist girlfriend. Then there was a woman who kept donkeys and the chief of police for Birmingham who recently came down from New York and is involved in all sorts of scandals over removal expenses. With him was his wife, a peroxide blond from Brooklyn and us with Joanna! Weird. The policeman kept telling us how Birmingham was known as John Wayne city in the rest of America because the police have a tendency to just "blow you away" with their 45 Magnums prior to asking any questions. One of the police in his command had 12 guns in his patrol car, including sawn-off shotguns, a 45 magnum and a sub-machine gun! I ask you, isn't it stupid? But that seems to be so like the Americans in general. They go overboard with almost everything they do and live their lives in mass hysteria. When they speak every sentence is so full of superlatives that they have nothing left to describe something really good.

On Monday we had tickets to go to the civic centre in Birmingham where Isaac Stern was performing two violin concertos, one by Mendelssohn and one by Mozart. He was excellent but the Alabama Symphony was not spectacular. On one occasion he had to slow down to let them catch up! It was the first time that Stern has performed here, and I suspect it may be the last. However, it was good fun, and we enjoyed it.

I have discovered that some of the airlines here offer a ticket called "See America plan", where you can buy one for $380 and travel to 20 cities or have 10 return trips to and from Birmingham. The offer expires on May 30th but if I can get one it will cover my trips to Boston, New York and Miami which I will have to do in that period of time. The department will pay for it for me, so I will just have to buy one for Helen, Joanna goes free. That will leave us with 7 return trips. We could go to the Grand Canyon for a weekend or go to the West Coast. It is a great opportunity. All you need is proof that you are returning to the UK at the end of the year which of course I have on my visa.

On Friday we had two other English couples to dinner, David and Daphne Farquharson who are over from Edinburgh. He is an obstetrician. Eamon and Philippa Breathnach, the other two, are over from London,

> but he has elected to stay. I think that his wife would like to go home. I think that by the end of the year we will have had more than enough as well. However, life has been interesting so far.
>
> This coming week I begin my pig experiments. Anaesthetising them is going to be fun. The next challenge is to operate on them and put them on bypass. I could do with your help Dad. Perhaps we could pay your flight over as a visiting Professor of Pig Anatomy.
>
> The following week I must give a talk on the results, and I thought that I would preface it with a slide of the advertisement of the shop – High Class Butcher, purveyor of Pork etc! I will let you know how I get on.
>
> Love to everyone.

The gun culture was an anathema to me and still is. Not long after our arrival, there was a news item where a man had woken up in the middle of the night to find a person at the end of the bed. Naturally he shot the person dead. It was his wife. One of my predecessors, a well-known cardiac surgeon with something of a hyperbolic personality, declared that his first purchase on arrival in Birmingham was a Colt 45 handgun. Of those who knew him, none were surprised.

> April 12, 1984
>
> Dear Mum and Dad and Gran.,
>
> We got back from Boston and Toronto last night at about 9 o'clock. We both had an interesting time. We flew out together on Friday at 10.30 am from Birmingham via Atlanta where we changed aircraft and then flew to Detroit together. At Detroit Helen had to catch another plane with Joanna, but it was at the same arrival lounge. So, when the aircraft stopped at the gate, I got off with them and made sure that everything was o.k. before reboarding the plane to fly to Boston. They then caught the next flight to Toronto (to stay with Sarah [Cox] and family. They managed perfectly well, and Joanna was as good as gold. She really is very well-travelled now.
>
> When I got to Logan airport in Boston, I got a taxi into Boston to meet the Ash's at their gallery in Newbury street. They run a private Art gallery selling mainly 18th Century English and American watercolours.

I had first met the Ashes in Cambridge (UK), where they had opened a sister gallery and lived for two years. Mr Ash had won the award as the best insurance salesman in the whole of the continental US for several successive years. They lived in an old house near Bourne when in Cambridge, and I met with them quite often. They were a gallery which represented Dennis

Flanders, an English watercolourist who had followed in Turner's footsteps, painting towns and the countryside of England. He also made drawings of all the great twelve livery companies of the City of London, including my own the Haberdashers. Flanders had made a painting of the old Charing Cross Hospital, which hung in the main lobby of the new hospital, but one day it disappeared. On enquiring, I discovered that the hospital management had sold it to Mr Arnott, the eye surgeon that I had worked with in training. As in the American saying, what goes around comes around: one day in their gallery in Cambridge, Mr Flanders came in and we were introduced by Mr Ash. I asked him about the Charing Cross picture, and he was shocked to hear that they had sold it as he had given it to the hospital as a gift to celebrate the move. I asked him if he still had the sketches for it and he said that he did. I asked him if he would consider doing the painting again just for me, and to my surprise, he said that he would. A month later he appeared with the new picture for me. The Ash family were delightful, and we remained friends for many years. The letter continues,

> Boston is an interesting city with a mixture of old and new. It is of course part of our British history, and all the towns, villages and counties are named after English places from whence the settlers had come. For example, there was Essex County, Sussex County and Gloucester and the towns were named Andover, Tewksbury, Gloucester, Norwich and so on.
>
> The housing though, is quite different. 90% are timber framed but quite pleasant. Walking around Boston was fun. I saw the 'old meeting house' where the Boston tea party was planned. The original ship on which it took place (the Beaver) is still there.
>
> I saw Bunker Hill where the British Redcoats beat the Massachusetts Militiamen at great cost. In the centre of town is a small cemetery where some of the famous founders of Boston are buried – all English of course! It is remarkable to think what they must have endured all that time ago. On Sunday we drove out into New England. It is very wooded and slightly hilly. The impression is of great space everywhere, as each house has lots of ground around it.
>
> They were just getting over the severe storms they had last week with 100 mph winds and 14 inches of snow in one night. The bark was stripped off the trees and many had been blown over. This was the tail end of the tornadoes which had hit Carolina.
>
> On Monday and Tuesday, I went to the [thoracic surgery] course, the reason for my visit. It was excellent and very worthwhile. On Wednesday, I walked over the Charles bridge to Harvard. It is interesting but nowhere

near as nice as Cambridge (England). I went to morning prayers in Harvard chapel. That was very pleasant. My flight left Boston at 1.30 for Detroit where I met Helen and Joanna again. We then flew the remaining journey home together and got back to the apartment at 9.00 pm. Helen and Joanna had had a nice time with Sarah and her family in Toronto. In ten days' time we are flying down to Panama City for a long weekend with another couple and their daughter. That is on the Gulf of Mexico and should be really nice.

Love from us all

Francis, Helen and Joanna.

My meeting with Dr Hermes Grillo was very profitable. He was a most delightful and true gentleman, who had world fame for his work on the trachea, being considered the father of tracheal surgery. His seminal paper on that subject stands today on the same plane as Professor Alain Carpentier's paper on the mitral valve. We formed a strong friendship, and his mentorship was very valuable for me for many years to come. Sadly, he lost his life in a taxi that suffered a car accident in Ravena, Italy, at the age of eighty-three.

May 11, 1984

Dear Mum and Dad

We have just got back from a week in New York. Joanna seemed to enjoy herself a great deal. She was the centre of attention everywhere we went. We left Birmingham on Friday on the ten'o'clock flight to Atlanta. Our connection was about an hour later to New York's La Guardia airport. The flight was comfortable, and we got in about 3.15 pm. local time. We then got a yellow taxicab to Manhattan where we were staying. We were initially put into the Shoreham hotel but that was so awful we moved around the corner to the New York Hilton.

That was a lot better.

On Saturday we went sight-seeing to the World's Trade Centre. The twin towers were the largest building in the world until the one in Chicago was built. From there the view was incredible. It is like being up in an aircraft. When we came down from there (the lift travels at 160 feet per minute) we walked over to the South pier and got on the Staten Island Ferry and went over to Staten Island. The view of the skyscrapers on Manhattan from there is magnificent. When we got back we took a bus from the ferry terminal through Greenwich village and up to Macey's store, under the Empire State building. Macey's was a bit of a let-down. Advertised as the

World's biggest department store, I didn't think it was anything like as nice as Harrods. On Sunday we went for a walk in Central Park with John and Lizzy Wallwork who were visiting for a surgical meeting. We then went to the Metropolitan Art Museum in the centre of Central Park. This was superb. It is the finest gallery and museum I have ever been into. On Monday and Tuesday, I attended the Association of Thoracic Surgeons, my reason for being there. On Monday night I had dinner with Terence English at an Italian Restaurant.

With love

Francis

The year flew by in a whirl of laboratory work, clinical experience, travel and new friends. To begin with, as the research involved animal studies, I had to get an animal license and learn laboratory techniques. I was quickly enrolled on the appropriate courses within the University. All of this was efficiently arranged by the support staff in the department. All so very different from experiences in the UK. My research studies involved operating on rats at first and then pigs for a major part of the protocol. The animal laboratory facilities were excellent, and the animals treated extremely well with lots of space in clean conditions with good food and regular veterinary inspections. At that time the animal rights supporters were very active in England, with many cases of abuse to laboratory staff. This was not the situation in Alabama where tolerance was high and the need for laboratory work to further the ability to treat patients seemed very well understood. Dear Bill Tracey was a key person in the organisation and management of this side of things within the department.

Being used to the miserly financing at home, I had begun to plan the experimental work with my thrifty English approach. I spent a lot of time trying to acquire the necessary apparatus for the least expenditure. An important part of the study was to measure radioactive emissions from radio-labelled material in the lungs of the pig. I had worked out a cheap way of doing this using columnated probes. The results were adequate but relatively crude. When I presented the protocol that I had worked up to Dr Kirklin and the department, he was appreciative of my attempts to save money but asked me if the method that I was proposing was state of the art. Of course it was not and so he asked what was. My reply was to use a gamma camera but that they were very expensive. His reply astounded me, 'Whatever the cost, get one.'

I muttered that a new one was over a quarter of a million dollars, but he was unwavering in his insistence. In the end, I found a reconditioned one for just over $60,000 and acquired it. I noted three years later, when I returned to the department for a visit, it was sitting in the corridor outside the laboratory suite with a dust sheet over it. Gentle enquiries revealed that it had not been used since my departure. Such was the availability of funding for research in some wealthy American research labs.

During the experiment we needed to move the anaesthetised animals to the radiology department in the next-door Veterans' Administration Hospital. This entailed a journey through several corridors and then a sprint through a patient waiting area to our destination. The shocked faces on the visitors can only be imagined as we ran through with the pig on its back under a sheet and its little legs in the air, and Bill leading the way whilst squeezing the ventilator bag, each of us in our laboratory operating garb.

Catching the pig in the morning for the day's experiments was quite a circus. Bill had great fun watching me trying, until he stepped in, and masterfully and gently took hold of the animal and lovingly looked after it until it was safely asleep.

The process involved some careful surgery, instituting cardiopulmonary bypass. During the first week, in my initial attempt I had trouble in placing the cannulas into the right atrial appendage of the heart, which tore, and I lost the poor pig. Later that day, walking down the corridor from the operating theatres to the offices I met Dr Kirklin, who in a jocular fashion asked me how thigs were going and had I got the Nobel Prize yet? I confessed my difficulties that morning, explaining that the tissues were very weak and had torn. He stopped in his tracks and engaged me with a paralysing stare, saying, 'That is just bad surgery. I do not want to hear that again.' Needless to say, I didn't lose another pig in the entire year in Birmingham. The animals were treated extremely well and were very precious.

I left for work at 5.30 a.m. most days to catch the early morning ICU rounds. At that time the drive from Arboretum Circle to the University was a pleasant twenty to thirty minutes in our little Datsun Sentra. The highway had six lanes in each direction. The result was little traffic congestion. From early April, the temperature and humidity began to rise sharply so that being outside became quite uncomfortable for us Brits from colder climes. In the peak of the summer, it became a dash from one air-conditioned area to another. The University library was about a twenty-minute walk from the Quarterback Tower and not something I enjoyed in the middle of July. The reward, however, was a very cool, almost cold library interior, with wonderfully friendly and helpful library staff. The feeling of immense relief as the cold dry air washed over me was wonderful. It felt like plunging into a cool stream on a blisteringly hot and humid day. I did most of my planning and writing there.

I was intent on not just finishing my research project whilst in Birmingham, but also, on having my thesis written and ready to go to the printers on my return to the UK. It remains an all too common occurrence that surgical trainees would leave the writing up until the end of their sabbatical from clinical surgery, and then as the surgical training took over their lives once again, the thesis would end up as a dust-laden pile of paper on a shelf somewhere with the higher degree abandoned. I didn't want this to happen to me after all the hard work that I had put in, with 12- to14-hour days and the toll that took on the family in a far-away place. To achieve this, I made sure that every section was written up before moving on to the next stage. A big help with this was winning an early word processing computer in a lottery in my local AmSouth bank. For each attendance at the bank, the teller issued a slip with one's name and contact details.

The 'Southern Belles' seemed to love my English accent and, knowing my role as a lowly research clinician, each time I went in every teller submitted a slip for me. The draw was made late on a Friday afternoon when I was in the operating theatre. I asked one of my American friends to go over to find out who had won. When he returned, he told me that it wasn't me, but someone called Walls! I was suspicious of the Southern accent mis-pronouncing my name, so I went to check the following morning, and sure enough it was me. Until then one of Dr Kirklin's several secretaries Stephen had very kindly typed each section for me. He was delighted to learn that now I could do all of the typing myself. When I left, instead of taking it with me, I gave it to Stephen in gratitude for all his hard work.

The days consisted of ward rounds of the patients at 6.00 a.m., then into the operating theatre on three days a week for a morning case with Dr Kirklin or Pacifico. This was usually done by mid-morning and then the rest of the day was spent in the laboratory or in the library writing or researching the project. The environment was quite ruthless and on one occasion the senior resident had to admit to Dr Kirklin that he had not responded to calls to the paediatric ICU bedside of a child who had developed serious complications. After a dressing down in front of all of the nurses and junior staff he was instructed to go to his office, to clear his things and not to return. As far as I was aware that was the end of his career in cardiac surgery.

The surgical department was very well organised, with everyone geared up to get on with the job. Quite unlike the NHS, if extra cases became necessary, there was no argument as to when they could be done. As soon as a theatre became available the patient was sent for, a function of well-paid and looked after staff. The short-sightedness of the UK system with poor pay and conditions for non-medical staff is the root of almost all of the problems that we suffer today.

Dr Pacifico (we referred to him as 'Al Terrifico' as his surgery was among the best I had ever seen) was so efficient that he would take all six theatres on each day he was operating and line patients up one after the other with a team of operatives which included junior surgical staff and operating theatre department technicians setting up the cases for him. His surgery was slick and executed with minimal moves. He would regularly complete ten to twelve cases each day. I had seen nothing like it before or since. During his career he operated on more than 30,000 cases. He was equally as adept at congenital and acquired heart lesions. Despite being a cardiac specialist, he would dart into the surgeon's room for a cigarette and a shot of black coffee between each case. I can still envisage his tanned and sallow face, eyes half-closed through the rising cigarette smoke and with his head on one side as he spoke to us in his clipped New York accent in deep concentration. Brooklyn born, he had a wonderfully strong identifiable voice. He seemed restless and always moved swiftly. Conversations with him were as efficient as his working style. His entire career was spent at the University of Alabama.

One day I was walking from the operating suite with Dr. Kirklin when we met Al walking swiftly in the opposite direction. John stopped him, saying, 'I'm sorry to hear about your Dad Al.' He had been admitted with an evolving heart attack and needed urgent surgery. Al informed him that surgery was indicated soon. JK asked who was going to do it. Al replied, 'the best surgeon', and before anything further could he said, 'I'm doing it', and strode on.

He did operate on his father and, as we all knew it would be, he was fine and recovered well, so typical of the man. Dr Kirklin was a pioneer of the specialty, but his surgery could be pedestrian at times. Al 'Terrifico' reminded me so much of John Pendower, the general surgeon at Charing Cross for whom I had worked; pragmatic, decisive and accomplished, with great skill and timing. They were of similar build, stance and presence and walked determinedly and briskly with a slight forward stoop

Everything that I needed for my research study was made easily available. If I wanted up-to-date information from other departments, one call from Dr Kirklin fixed everything. Superoxide radicals were becoming a big thing and the world authority at that time worked in the Ochsner clinic in New Orleans. I had met him briefly at a conference on Super-Oxide radicals in Miami, that the department funded for me. On informing Dr Kirklin of this he said, 'Well, go talk to them, just tell them that I asked you to call.' I did and was instantly invited down for a couple of days to learn all about it. Such was the power of the name Dr. Kirklin.

One of the most important medical statisticians of international standing was Dr Eugene Blackstone. Currently, Dr Blackstone is full time head of clinical investigation at the Sydell and Arnold Miller Family Heart, Vascular and Thoracic Institute at the Cleveland Clinic in Cleveland Ohio. He had worked alongside Dr Kirklin in the department, having been appointed to an endowed chair at UAB as cardiovascular research professor of surgery in1980. As my project was the lead investigation in the department, I was not trusted with the statistical analysis. It had to be done by Gene and his able assistant David Naftel. That left me with some free time, and I used both it and my clutch of plane tickets to travel widely.

Born into a family of active musicians, Gene was an organist and pianist of considerable skill and was very knowledgeable about the inner mechanism of the pipe organ. His father was an organist, who agreed to teach Gene if he spent three-quarters of his time learning the piano and the remainder on the organ. Later in life, he had an organ installed into his house in Birmingham. He said that whenever his children visited, all of them accomplished musicians, they had to bring with them their instruments and a tuxedo, as a Blackstone family concert would be the order of the day. Recalling his story made me think of the brilliant Nottingham based Kanneh-Mason family of today. More recently Gene was head hunted to move to the Cleveland Clinic. He agreed on the grounds that he could build a house on the banks of Lake Erie, which he then proceeded to do. It was designed as a sound box for an Aeolian-Skinner 7,406-pipe organ. A gargantuan instrument that has become an international standard in home organ design featured in many international architectural and music magazines.

During my time at UAB Gene, Dr. Kirklin and Brian Barrett-Boyes were writing the seminal text on paediatric and adult cardiac surgery. Gene was crunching all the data from the vast patient data bank in U.A.B. and the other two were writing the text. We fellows contributed by researching specific topics that we presented at the Saturday morning meetings and refined for sections of the book. Each time I finished a block of experiments, he would take the data and do the statistics.

Wonderful trips for short break holidays to California, Seattle and Florida were possible because of the special deal on flight coupons, enabling me to travel widely. In addition, I was able to visit several other units to gain experience in them. A three week visit to Toronto General hospital to work with the thoracic surgeons was arranged. It was a huge privilege to spend time with Griff Pearson, Joel Cooper, Alex Patterson and Tom Todd, perhaps the most powerful and influential thoracic surgical group in the world at that time. They welcomed me into their midst and involved me in all of the programme's work. They became long-term friends. At the same time Dr Clem Hiebert was on sabbatical following retirement from Boston. Another true gentleman, Clem and his wife Pam (a British Airways hostess in her earlier life) looked after me on a daily basis. Clem was a wonderful teacher with a vast experience. Through these experiences I learnt a huge amount, including several surgical techniques that I was able to implement in my clinical work in Cambridge.

I was introduced to Professor Tirone David, cardiac surgeon at Toronto General. Tirone was equally generous with his time showing me many surgical techniques that he had developed. We have maintained a career long friendship. At Stanford I was hosted by Craig Miller, a Stetson sporting cardiac surgical entrepreneur with a wry sense of humour. At that time, Craig was doing early work on intra-luminal stenting of aortic aneurysms. Craig contributed outstanding work on the physiology of the mitral valve which framed my thoughts on the functional assessment of the valve in health and disease. Along with Bud Frasier in Texas and Randy Chitwood in Carolina, Craig is a strong student of history, something that I share as of great importance.

A measure of the importance of those characters is the fact that Griff, Joel, Alex, Tirone and Craig all became presidents of the American Society for Thoracic Surgery. Griff received the first lifetime achievement award from the AATS in 2004 and was described in an article celebrating his life as a legend in thoracic surgery. He is recognised by many as the founder of thoracic surgery as a specialty unto itself, rather than a branch of general surgery.

During those weeks in Toronto, I was able to stay with an old medical school friend Sarah Cox and her family. Sarah moved to Toronto early after graduation from Charing Cross and became an important physician in oncology there and was very much loved by patients and staff with whom she worked. Tragedy of immense proportions befell Sarah. Her mother and sister died of breast cancer and her father had taken his own life, a fate that was to befall Sarah as well.

Whilst in U.A.B. the use of the internal thoracic artery was gaining significance as the conduit of choice in coronary artery surgery, still in its relative infancy. It was first described by Vasili Kolessov[2] and developed by Frank Spencer in New York in the mid-1960s. It's very positive impact on surgical outcome was not appreciated until the early 1980s. None of the surgeons at U.A.B. were using it. Dr Kirklin asked me to visit the Cleveland Clinic, where Dr Bruce Lytle, an excellent coronary surgeon was pioneering it's use, and to learn their techniques to bring back to Birmingham. Bruce was another legend of the specialty and an adventurous motorcyclist to boot. Sporting a large white handle-bar moustache and a shock of Einsteinian white hair, he was one of the most recognisable surgeons on the world stage. A story illustrating his grit and determination recounts his falling from his Harley Davidson in the middle of Nowheresville Ohio, alone and sustaining a broken leg. With no help he put his shoulder under the bike lifting it upright and brushed himself off to ride home and to the hospital. He welcomed me into his practice and on the first day of my arrival took me through the procedure of internal mammary (thoracic) artery take down. The American surgeons were all so very hospitable and the visit included a tequila-soaked dinner in a local diner with the firm of colleagues.

Visits to Baltimore's John Hopkins Hospital, Washington, Stanford and New York followed. I remember so clearly walking along the corridor at Hopkins looking in awe at the roll call of famous names starting with William Osler and William Halsted, the first surgeon in chief there. Alfred Blalock and Helen Taussig were also there, and latterly, and belatedly, the celebrated technician, Vivien Thomas who devised and conducted the first inter-arterial shunt for Tetralogy of Fallot in the 1940s. Called the Blalock-Taussig shunt, it connected the pulmonary artery to the subclavian artery increasing blood flow to the lungs. It is used in the blue baby syndrome of Fallot's Tetralogy, where the pulmonary artery was narrowed and a hole in the heart shunted blood away from the lungs across the heart. Vivien had carried out all the laboratory work and was present at the insistence of Dr Blalock at the first procedure in a patient. It is now widely recognised that Vivien did the important parts of the surgery. Not only had he worked out the surgical procedure but also modified laboratory instruments to be used in the operating theatre as none that were suitable had existed prior to that operation. Because of his lowly position in the medical hierarchy and the colour of his skin, his vital and pivotal role was swept under the carpet for decades. Finally, in 1976 he was awarded an Honorary Doctorate by Johns Hopkins University, and his portrait sits next to that of Dr Blalock on that wall of fame in Hopkins.

My visit to Hopkins began inauspiciously. I arrived relatively late in the evening and after checking in to the hotel on site I realised that I had forgotten to bring several items, including toothbrush and toothpaste. I had noticed a small five and dime store at the far end of a large car park outside the hospital and so decided to visit to make my purchases. Inside, it was quite busy and after collecting together the things I needed I went to the check-out. The queue was long and so I joined the back of it to wait patiently for my turn. After a short while a loud voice emanated from a somewhat large black lady at the front of the queue. She bellowed, 'Hey! White boy! You come here now!' and ushered me to the front of the queue. I thought that was charming, but as I turned to pay, she said, 'You pay fast, boy, then get out. The last white boy here got his head blowed clean off.'

Needless to say, I didn't hesitate but paid and left quickly. The next morning at the early morning ICU round the attendant asked me what I had done when I got in the night before. I told him the story, and he reinforced what I had been told and said I was lucky to get away with it.

In New York, I was invited to the local multi-disciplinary team working together for the better management of patients with lung cancer. The format at Mount Sinai was similar to the ones that I had attended with Peter Goldstraw at the Royal Marsden, next door to Royal Brompton Hospital. My host was Bob Ginsberg, an outstanding pioneer in the treatment of lung cancer and a wonderful teacher. The staging of lung cancer has been the biggest advance in the management of this dreadful condition, and I was exposed to the finer elements of it at that time. As seems so often to be the case that medical men die of the diseases they treat, so it was with Bob. He succumbed to lung cancer being a long-time smoker. In his obituary in the journal *Lung Cancer*, a former trainee recalled that he taught his trainees to think outside the box and to practice evidence-based medicine, also to have a healthy scepticism of one's own accomplishments and always to strive for quality and not credit. He was another rather blunt character, and what you saw was what you got, and in being so he was a delight to be around. It was such a privilege to have had the opportunity to see such giants of our specialty at work and to be befriended by them.

A highlight of the year was being able to witness a total eclipse of the sun. On 30 May from around 1.00 until 3.00 p.m., the sun moved to cause a complete eclipse. As a result of the relative distances of sun and moon from the earth at that time, what we witnessed was the solar flare from an annular eclipse, where the moon covers all but the periphery of the sun, revealing the peripheral flare. Standing on the roof of the nearby car park the event was dramatic. As the sky darkened the birds did indeed become quiet and the street lights came on. We had managed to get our hands on darkened glass so that we could observe it safely. The temperature fell noticeably. It lasted several minutes but it seemed a lot longer. The next similar event in North America would not be witnessed for another seven years.

Shortly after my return to Cambridge, an American travelling research group called the Thoracic Surgery Club was formed with a relatively few members, all of whom were characters such as just described. To my amazement I was invited to join them and attended one of the first meetings on Sanibel Island off the west coast of Florida. It proved to be a memorable time for several reasons, two of which were as follows. On the evening of arrival, a category two hurricane came through the island forcing us to lock ourselves inside. The following morning, we emerged to see that there was extensive storm damage to trees and some buildings. However, the meeting proceeded and was great fun as well as being very instructive. On my return, I joined a British Airways flight from Miami to London, which became headline news. Sitting not far in front of me was Sarah Ferguson, Duchess of York. She was surrounded by journalists. Not long after take-off, they began to annoy her and in response, she threw some bread rolls at them. Of course, the following day it became front-page news.

Evening socialising in Birmingham began very early as did the whole working day. Dr. Kirklin was up and exercising his horses at 5.00 a.m. and on the wards by 7.00. I discovered the early to bed phenomenon to my cost when invited to a dinner party at Dr. Kirklin's home. I assumed that it would be a social event with a timing similar to that which I was used to at home in England; to arrive at 7.00 p.m. for dinner at 7.30. Arriving there at what I thought was a slightly early time of 6.45 p.m., we found many people about to leave. The whole event had begun at 5.00 p.m. My stumbled apologies were accepted, and I didn't make that mistake again. On another evening, after dinner with a lovely Mexican anaesthesiologist at our more acceptable UK timing, I was being driven home after dark and saw the shocking sight of a burning cross of the Klu Klux Klan on a distant hillside. The Klan was still very much in action and terrorising black people across Shelby County.

A complication happened whilst I was in Alabama, which almost caused me to return to Cambridge prematurely. On the same day in July, with Terence English on leave in South Africa, John Wallwork was on a heart donor run in Birmingham. He was in a police car travelling at high speed when an elderly couple in a Morris Minor car pulled out in front of them. The police car was unable to avoid them and slammed into the side of the car. There were no fatalities, but the elderly couple were injured quite badly, and John had suffered a significant whiplash injury, but was otherwise unhurt. At almost exactly the same time, Terence and his family were driving into Cape Town in a large S.U.V. Suddenly, a man ran across the road in front of Terence's vehicle. He had just broken into and burgled the house of a judge. Terence could not avoid him, and the man was killed. Fortunately, Terence and family were unhurt. His only somewhat acerbic comment was that 'all of a sudden everything went black'. I had been within a hair's breadth of rapid recall to replace both colleagues.

As surgical fellows we were not strictly allowed to do any independent operating. However, one day I had found myself assisting Dr. Kirklin in the operating theatre with an acute aortic dissection [a life-threatening event where the main artery in the body splits its wall under pressure]. It became a long and difficult procedure and wasn't going so well. Towards the end there was quite a lot of bleeding from the back of the aorta. Dr Kirklin, by then in his seventies, was becoming very tired and I offered to look after the patient whilst he had a rest. Gratefully, he accepted and left the room. Not having a licence to operate by myself then, what I did next was a bit risky, but the patient's life was in the balance. I knew where the bleeding was coming from and quickly set about stopping it. With the compliance and help of the assisting nurse, we quickly placed the cannulas back into the heart and restored cardiopulmonary bypass. I was then able to get access to the back of the decompressed aorta, from where the bleeding was arising, and with a couple of well-placed sutures was able to stop the bleeding, close the aorta and wean the patient from bypass, now no longer bleeding. A while later Dr Kirklin returned to the room and I was able to say with a white lie, that the bleeding had seemed to stop. He thanked me and asked me if I would close and left the room.

All too soon the year end began to loom over us, and I had to wrap up my thesis. With everything analysed and written up I made an appointment with Dr Kirklin to receive his approval for submission. The only time that he could offer me was 11.00 a.m. on Christmas morning! All went well and I received his blessing for submission. I had achieved my goal, and it was ready to go to the printer on my return to Cambridge.

Not long after I had returned to my post in Cambridge, he was awarded the honorary fellowship of the Royal College of Surgeons in London. A few days before his arrival he called me to ask if I could arrange for him to visit the gallops at Newmarket. As mentioned already, he was a huge equestrian fan with his own string of horses. Every year he travelled to Big Sky in Montana for the wild horses round up. He had ridden all of his life and was extremely knowledgeable.

I had recently operated upon a jockey from one of the big stables in Newmarket. I called him and put the problem to him. He immediately offered to meet him and to look after him. I rang Dr Kirklin back and told him the good news. I informed him that we needed to be waiting beneath the clock tower in the middle of Newmarket at 5.30 a.m. I asked the stupid question, 'Is that a problem?' The answer does not need repeating. I picked him up at 5.00 a.m. from the Garden House Hotel in central Cambridge and we set off for Newmarket. Exactly on time, the jockey was there and ushered us out onto the gallops. There, emerging through the mist, steam emanating from their nostrils, came hundreds of beautiful racehorses. Dr Kirklin was in his element. He immediately began to engage with the trainers and the jockeys in a very animated and knowledgeable fashion. Before long a problem began to emerge as Dr Kirklin was supposed to be giving an honoured guest lecture at Brompton Hospital mid-morning and the time was rapidly approaching that we had to leave but I could not tear him away. There was only one thing for it, and I telephoned my old mentor Chris Lincoln, his host in London, to say that Dr Kirklin would give the lecture that afternoon as he was enjoying the gallops so much.

Following a grand round of complicated cases at Brompton, we all departed for the Royal College of Surgeons in Lincoln's Inn Fields, where he delivered a guest lecture, and had an honorary fellowship bestowed upon him. This was followed by a dinner with the president, the council and guests, of whom I was one. Towards the end of the dinner Dr Kirklin, rose and strode down the long table to where I was sitting. Smiling, he reached down and picked up my menu card and took it back to his place at the head of the table. I could see him writing, and as we all left the room, he came over to me, shook my hand warmly, thanking me for all that I had done whilst with him in his department and handed the menu card back to me. On it he had written:

> Dear Frank, between pigs, aortas & Newmarket, my memories and thanks are very deep. John K.

Clearly, he knew everything that went on around him. A truly great man.

To prevent being taxed in the USA it was necessary to be there for a year and a day, as it had been with my flight arrangements, to take advantage of the cheap extra tickets. We therefore left Birmingham on 2 January 1985. On 3 January, I began my new life as a junior consultant surgeon at Papworth Hospital.

Soon after my return to Cambridge, I was able to take the manuscript and all of the illustrations to Stoakley and Son, book binders in Trinity Street, in existence since the eighteenth century; there was a real sense of Dickensian tradition within the old walls. Five copies were required. The thesis had been submitted to London University as my alma mater. I remember going to the senate offices with pride with the finished books to deposit them. I was expecting a grand room with a bit of pomp but was confronted with a tiny dusty and dishevelled office with theses piled so high around the secretary, that I could hardly see her. Indeed, it was such a shambles, that I asked for repeated assurances that my thesis would not be lost in the veritable jungle of books piled high with seemingly no order to be seen. I left with a significant degree of trepidation as to their destiny. Afterwards I awaited the outcome and hopefully the viva.

This followed with an old friend and already distinguished cardiac surgeon and researcher Tom Treasure, who himself had been research fellow with Dr Kirklin in UAB. Indeed, before I left, he and his lovely consultant psychiatrist wife entertained me to dinner to give me some tips about the forthcoming adventure. The viva was interesting, and the questioning quite deep, but the outcome was successful. My thesis was submitted for the Rogers Prize for theses submitted to the university in that year. I also applied for an annual Hunterian Professorship of the Royal College of Surgeons. The title of my thesis is 'The Effects of Cardio-pulmonary Bypass on Alveolar Barrier Function with Particular Emphasis on Alveolar Epithelial and Endothelial permeability.'

I was successful and was awarded the professorship, which demanded a lecture at the Royal College of Surgeons. The great day arrived on the 15 April 1987. I had been warned by others, notably Professor Roy Calne, to expect a small audience. He recounted the fact that for his lecture, other than family and the president and court of the college, there was only one other attendee. He had processed into the lecture room behind the president and his entourage. Following the introductions, a small door, high up, at the back of the lecture theatre opened slowly and noisily. An Indian gentleman crept in and sat quietly on the back row. After the lecture was over Roy rushed up to the gentleman whom he saw quietly leaving the hall, to thank him for coming to his lecture. After breathlessly thanking him, the gentleman shyly apologised profusely, stating that he had entered the wrong room but somewhat embarrassed, seeing all of the college dignitaries in their finery, had neither the heart, nor the courage to leave until the end.

Determined to see that the same fate did not befall me, I invited lots of colleagues and friends from Cambridge and hired a bus to take them all down to London. With my mother not able to attend, my father came alone. He, however, was made very welcome and Matt Paneth who had come along with others from Brompton, soon renewed his friendship with him. I went one stage further and arranged a dinner for everyone at the college that night. This time I was at the top of the table feeling immensely proud of my achievements which was a complete change for me. Now, as my father was an M.B. (Master Butcher), I was now an M.S. [Master of Surgery]. I had squared the family circle.

12

So, This is What It is all About

> As a day well spent brings happy sleep, so a life well used brings happy death.
>
> Leonardo da Vinci, Codex Trivulzi. 27r.

Just nine years after qualifying, one year ahead of my projected time scale, there I was, about to begin as a fully-fledged consultant cardiovascular and thoracic surgeon at the now prestigious Papworth hospital. My colleagues included Sir Terence English, although yet to be knighted. As described before he had successfully set himself up as a transplant guru. He was a true South African gentleman and something of a disciplinarian with enormous strength of character. Sadly he passed away in November 2025. He had restarted heart transplantation in the United Kingdom, and in many ways, led the United Kingdom into a fresh start with meaningful success, although the contribution of Sir Magdi Yacoub at Harefield should not be underestimated. Surfing that success (man of the year in several national publications) Terence went on to be first a member of the Council of the Royal College of Surgeons of England, and then perhaps, the most successful president of that august body in the last thirty years. President of the BMA and Master of St Catharine's College, Cambridge followed, and other awards and distinctions flowed thick and fast. Terence was the one at Papworth who was always supportive of me in developing thoracic surgery and the mitral valve programme.

My other new colleague was John Wallwork who some might say is a rather brash but highly entertaining fellow. To many he was a breath of fresh air in an otherwise somewhat stodgy atmosphere. He had recently returned from the chief resident's post at Stanford, California, via St Bartholomew's, London. He had been in post at Papworth for just over two years. The dynamics between John and Terence were interesting and not always comfortable. Two triple A personalities with significant egos were always going to be a challenging. Prior to Stanford, John had been registrar to Philip Caves in Glasgow, a rising star of transplantation, who whilst working with Norman Shumway in Stanford had developed the technique of right ventricular biopsy to assess the grade of cardiac rejection following transplantation. This was a game changing development which enabled much closer control of immunosuppression in the balancing act between infection through over suppression, and rejection from under suppression.

Dr Shumway had encouraged a somewhat 'Wild West' approach to the practice and development of cardiac surgery in all its aspects, and by all accounts his department was great fun to work in. John had brought that infectious humour back with him. In fact, the Stanford technique pervades Papworth to this day. Several sayings resound in the unit. For example, 'If you're not having fun, then it's not worth it.' When things are going badly and all hope seems to be lost, the canto would ring out, 'Keep on operating, just keep on operating', in other words, never give up. I can recall several patients that have been saved at Papworth by that persistence, allied to sensible thought, and a ready availability of colleague support.

Never a fan of coronary bypass surgery, nor was it ever a mainstay of Stanford's work, Shumway could be heard to say, 'Never miss an opportunity not to do a graft', and whilst that sounds cynical the examples of surgeons trying to graft every little coronary branch on the heart are legion. They seem to forget that coronary artery disease causes significant collateral blood flow to develop and introducing a significant increase in blood flow into the general pool of blood flowing to the heart, will suffice. The smaller vessel grafts are likely to close down soon after surgery and thus add nothing to the operation. Keeping things simple is another attitude celebrated by the Stanford team. A frequent call was, 'One graft in each corner is all you need.'

To preserve heart function whilst perfusion has ceased during procedures on the heart there are two principal requirements: a still heart and a cold heart. Shumway devised a system of a cold circuit in the pericardial sac around the heart which, if used properly, will keep the heart at around 12 degrees centigrade, thus hugely reducing the metabolic demand. Stopping the heart with a high dose of potassium ensured its arrest in the relaxed state, further reducing metabolic activity. This accompanied by moderate systemic hypothermia, cooling the rest of the body to thirty-two degrees, gives optimal conditions. Infusing the coronary arteries with the patient's own blood at that temperature, with the added potassium, ensures that any lactic acid produced at a low level, is neutralised by the natural buffering system of the blood. Food and oxygen are present in the blood to jolly the myocardial cells along at the much reduced level of metabolism that continues at those low temperatures. This 'Stanford technique' has stood the test of time and as judged by clinical outcome, is the equal of any other more complex protection method that is more expensive in time and administration.

As mentioned before, the third colleague at that time was Richard Cory-Pearce. He had been on the staff as a senior lecturer and research fellow and was a great antidote to both of the others. He came to work in an old pick-up truck, often with chain saw in the back, and wearing cowboy boots, sporting a James Robertson Justice beard and a 'corpulence' to match. He was soon to move to Sheffield as senior lecturer in the department of surgery with a view to taking up the post of professor but sadly that did not work out.

In all, it was a lively group of contrasting personalities into which I had to find a way to function. Barely the age of most senior registrars, and with much less experience than many, I found myself somewhat less than comfortably ensconced in this group of pleasant, interesting, but quite egotistical personalities.

However, I could not have started life as a consultant, in this, the most demanding of specialties, in a more supportive and professional environment. I owe John, or JW as he was affectionately called, a great deal of thanks for he was extremely supportive and a great confidence builder. For that I will always be grateful. Another Stamford quote that he had brought with him was 'don't worry, there isn't a problem that you can get yourself into that I cannot get you out of'. Ready to stand across the table from you for hours to take you through an operation with a lot of joviality decompressed the stress wonderfully well. He has quite small and podgy hands, his 'paddy pads', but with which he was amazingly dextrous. He was probably the finest coronary surgeon of his generation. Bold and caring where and when necessary, he was extremely well-liked by nursing staff and patients. Cardiac surgery has had the reputation over the years of evolving arrogant and angry surgeons. Certainly, this has been true in more units than has been healthy for British cardiac surgery, but I found in Papworth the very opposite. Despite the strength of personality of those around me, everyone was focussed on the best possible care for the patients and in doing so were intent on supporting each other. Help was always at hand and generously given. To all trainees John's mantra was always, 'The only instrument you need to know how to use is the telephone.' In other words, the biggest crime was not asking a colleague if unsure of what to do. He was true to his word and whatever the time of day or night would always be there to support and to help in a humorous and pleasant way. I will always be grateful for that, especially in my early years. For his first couple of years after appointment to Papworth, John lived 'en famille' on site at Papworth, whilst they looked for an appropriate house in Cambridge. I do remember being conned into cleaning his car on a Sunday afternoon if the wards were quiet, as do several of his other trainees. Living on site he was readily available, day or night, which was taken advantage of by some of the staff. I was to discover the effect of this availability also, as when I started, I was living in the same hospital house that the Wallwork family had vacated. Being so close at hand, the nurses would call us in preference to the junior staff, to get a definitive management decision.

It was John who arranged my first operating list at Papworth with his usual sense of humour, but also practicality. It consisted of the removal of sternal wires from the chest of a previous patient, and the drainage of a cervical (neck) abscess in a patient who had undergone oesophagectomy, by a colleague. He even hovered around to make sure I was alright, and when I was timidly finding it difficult to break through into the abscess cavity in the neck, donned a pair of gloves and with one deft movement of his rather stubby index finger, broke through, allowing large amounts of pus to flow from the wound. Laughingly he left me to finish off extolling the virtue of experience and a bit of confidence. His exuberant personality was on show for everyone, when on one occasion we he had been asked to give an opinion on a very sick patient on the Intensive Care at Addenbrooke's hospital.

Relishing the prospect of discovering some catastrophic and incompetent management he grabbed me by the arm and said: 'Come on, let's have some fun.' Bursting through the doors into the ICU, mimicking the actor Elliot Gould in *M.A.S.H.*, he cried out, 'The pros from Dover have arrived. Where's the patient?' Those familiar with the movie will know the sequence from which he was quoting. The only thing that was missing were the golfing spikes and the plus-fours. Whatever the appearance, the attitude was intoxicating. Sure enough the patient was being mishandled, and he was whisked out of that setting into the old Papworth and restored with urgent surgery, executed by John with me assisting. He was an excellent and fearless surgeon throughout his career.

Having spent the last year in research with no real operating experience I was certainly very rusty. I had only done one mitral valve replacement on my own. The procedure of mitral valve repair seemed safer to me, retaining all of the mitral apparatus as it does. Hence my early interest in developing it, allied to my experience of hearing Professor Carpentier give the AATS guest lecture, summarising his work eighteen months before. This was the start of one of my main interests for the years to come.

For my first few years, each night I would go to bed and rehearse the next day's procedures in my mind's eye, over and over again. This helped me ensure that no mistakes were made. Although I found surgery exhilarating and rewarding, I always retained a slight anxiety which would manifest itself as a pounding heart as I approached the hospital in the morning. This was particularly the case on surgical days. Not so with the thoracic cases, perhaps because of my extensive general surgery experience with great mentors.

Transplantation and Artificial Hearts

In the time since the first heart transplant of the new era, (January 1979), Terence English had firmly established the transplant programme as a sound therapeutic option in advanced heart failure with strong evidence, both in survivorship and quality of life. Along with Professor Sir Magdi Yacoub, he had championed it to government and attained full NHS funding for the project. This had taken tenacity, careful planning and good organisation with great attention to detail, all of which were Terence's strengths. John was more relaxed in approach but no less rigorous in the careful and thoughtful management of the patient. Whilst Terence had to be very bold to make the procedure work and to work well, John's more liberal approach encouraged a little more lateral thinking, as was seen in the introduction of the immunosuppressant cyclosporin A, established in liver transplantation by Sir Roy Calne. Although a drug with great potential, there was not much knowledge of how to control dose response in the transplant patients. John with Roy worked out a method of assessing maximum dose levels through monitoring kidney function. Its adoption in the unit had to wait until Terence's retirement from the transplant programme.

It was a thrilling time on that programme, progressing into not just heart transplantation but also combined heart and lung, and single and double lung transplantation. It really was the most 'in' place to be in heart surgery at that time. Although Sir Magdi Yacoub had an equivalent developing programme, it was more a one-man band at Harefield where he was based. At Papworth it really was a team effort. Quickly, I was brought up to speed in the removal of organs for donation and the implantation procedures as well. In truth, once the awe of seeing an empty open chest has been assimilated, the actual procedure of sewing in a new heart is quite simple and straight-forward. The key to a successful transplant can be summarised in four points, 'good donor, good donor and good recipient good recipient', another of Shumway's mantras reproduced by John. Of course, there are individual challenges in some difficult patients but generally that is true.

The real art form comes in the post-operative maintenance of walking the tight rope of immunosuppression and rejection, something that fell more into the hands of the transplant physicians as time passed. Heart and lung transplantation was the next step up, and John had championed that bringing the concept with him from Stanford and having the courage and chutzpah to make it work. Always keen to teach, it wasn't long before I was taken through my first heart and lung transplant. All went well and on completion in the early hours, in celebration, the two of us moved to the Bridge Hotel in nearby Huntingdon for a Champagne breakfast. Although we had been up all night, breakfast was followed by a full day in the operating theatre, no European working time directive compensatory rest in those days. Cardiac surgery demanded the 'right stuff', as popularised by Tom Wolfe in the book of the same name, recounting the lives of the first astronauts. At one point in the book he describes the egos of the potential astronauts being interviewed, as not being able to fit into the Astrodome, never mind the small room in which they sat. There can be no doubt that the elements of that ethos pervaded our specialty. We were pushing back boundaries and innovating at a rapid rate. There can be no more exciting a time in cardiac surgery than that time and I was in the thick of it with a front row ticket surrounded by pioneers at home and abroad.

The only problem for me was, that as my experience grew, I found transplantation less interesting. It was a repetitive process of two or three surgical procedures, usually carried out in the dead of night after many false starts. Let there be no doubt, I was in awe of the potential for it to change lives for the better, and for patients it was their last hope. As such it was and remains highly commendable, but the number of people in terminal heart failure that could be helped was and is small in comparison with the vast number of deserving patients at large. The necessary investment in time, money and personnel was huge in comparison with more conventional surgery. It is a continuing anathema that, because of the severe shortage of donors, precedence is always given to a transplant operation over, often very deserving, patients needing conventional surgical solutions, either in hospital or waiting to come in. In the financially restricted world of the NHS, it seems that there is no way around this problem. I threw myself into the work with as much energy as I could muster but always had that nagging doubt in the back of my mind regarding the pressure it caused on the conventional services.

Truthfully, I was more interested in the cut and thrust of complex non-transplant surgery of all of the organs in the chest and those in proximity. My interest in thoracic surgery wasn't really shared by my colleagues and although very competent surgeons in all aspects of heart and lung surgery they were very happy to leave all of the non-cardiac surgery to me to deal with. That is not to say that my cardiac involvement was in any way diminished. It wasn't and I carried out equal amounts of heart operations as the others, but I had daily surgical lists with mixed thoracic and cardiac cases. Lung, oesophageal, thymic, tracheal and chest wall surgery, as well as the other minutiae around the edges of thoracic surgery were a large part of my work. Ben Milstein and Peter Goldstraw had schooled me in all aspects of thoracic and vascular surgery, and I relished the variety of challenges.

Putting previous comments to one side, there were many amusing and occasionally exciting moments in transplantation, on donor runs especially. On one occasion accompanying Terence on a donor run in a helicopter, our pilot became lost whilst trying to find Brighton in dense fog. For what felt like an interminable time, we were flying at as low an altitude as was safely possible going up and down the coastline trying to recognise landmarks to guide us in. On another occasion we flew to a small airport in Southampton in a small fixed-wing aircraft. The pilot came in very low over the hedge on final approach and banged the twin engine turbo-prop aircraft hard onto the runway. A waiting police car dashed off with us to the hospital. On our return with the heart safely on ice in a box, we couldn't see the aeroplane. Then we saw a member of the ground staff standing at the entrance to a hangar at the far end of the runway with its door open and the lights on. He was waving his orange light sticks at us, calling us over to the hangar. Inside was our aircraft with engine running and props. turning with chocks under the wheels. The pilot beckoned us into the aircraft. As we strapped ourselves in, he told us that the runway was a bit short for that type of plane but not to worry. With engines roaring, the chocks were pulled away and we launched forward onto the tarmac and away over the perimeter hedge. Everyone breathed a sigh of relief.

On yet another occasion we were flying to Cardiff from Marshall's Airport in Cambridge. The pilot, a British Airways captain was waiting for us and informed us that the conditions in Cardiff were difficult with quite dense fog. Did we still want to go? My reply, as senior person on the mission was, 'You decide, I will sort out the heart when we get there but flying is your business.' We took off and all seemed fine until the last few miles when, as predicted, the fog was very dense on the ground. As we came into land, I noticed that the grass at the edge of the runway was flashing past the left-wing tip, but the other wing tip was still way up in the air. A lightening quick adjustment by the pilot corrected the aeroplane's attitude and we landed with a firm bump and hopped up and down to a standstill. On getting out and taking the equipment from the nose cone, I noticed that the pilot was lighting a cigarette with shaking hands. I asked him what the matter was. He just pointed casually to the front of the aircraft, which had come to a stop a few feet from the perimeter fence.

There were other forms of excitement. On British Grand Prix day, Silverstone becomes the busiest airport in the country with endless helicopter flights ferrying visitors, drivers and the press in and out of the circuit. As a consequence, it is hard to find a helicopter for a donor run. On one such occasion we were offered an excellent set of heart and lungs from north Wales. We couldn't find a free commercial helicopter. However, the armed forces sprang to our help. There was an S.A.S. helicopter leaving for a training mission in the Snowdon area and they offered to take our team with them. On that occasion, one of our very experienced surgical trainees Jo McGoldrick was going to pick up the organs. True to their word the heavily camouflaged Wessex helicopter arrived and landed on the cricket pitch at Papworth and whisked them away. Donor retrieval completed, the same team picked them up and flew them back to Papworth. For added spice, the pilot made them rappel out of the helicopter at the hover of 50 feet, rapidly disappearing into the night as soon as the team was safely on the ground. Of course they loved it.

In 1986, we began the programme of isolated lung transplantation at Papworth. This was a more challenging project than the heart programme because of the problems associated with healing of the junction between the airway. The lung has a dual blood supply, first described by Leonardo da Vinci in 1512. Leonardo dissected the heart and lung block of an ox and made a detailed and correct description of the separate blood supply to the airways arising from the aorta, distinguishing it from the blood going to the air spaces from the pulmonary artery for gas transfer. If the blood supply to the bronchial anastomosis is inadequate it will not heal, and bronchial disruption will result. Very careful surgery was needed to accomplish the safest possible join in the airways. Others tried joining the internal mammary artery to the bronchial artery of the recipient, but it was not a reproducible and creditable addition to the procedure. Keeping the airways as short as possible and wrapping the join with local tissue was the safest and most reproducible way to support healing.

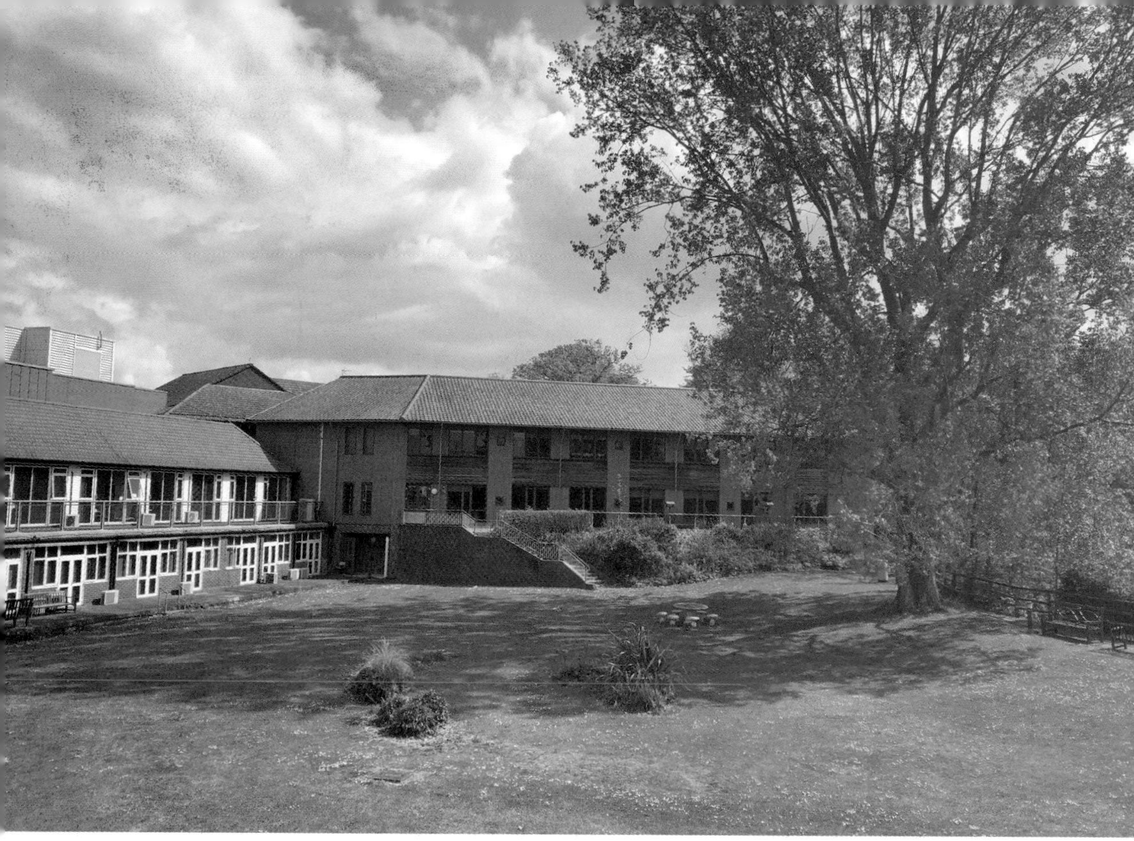

Above: The original Papworth Hospital. The new surgical unit extension can be seen to the right of the picture. (*Author's collection*)

Right: The Duchess of Kent visiting Papworth Hospital with the author as guide. (*Author's collection*)

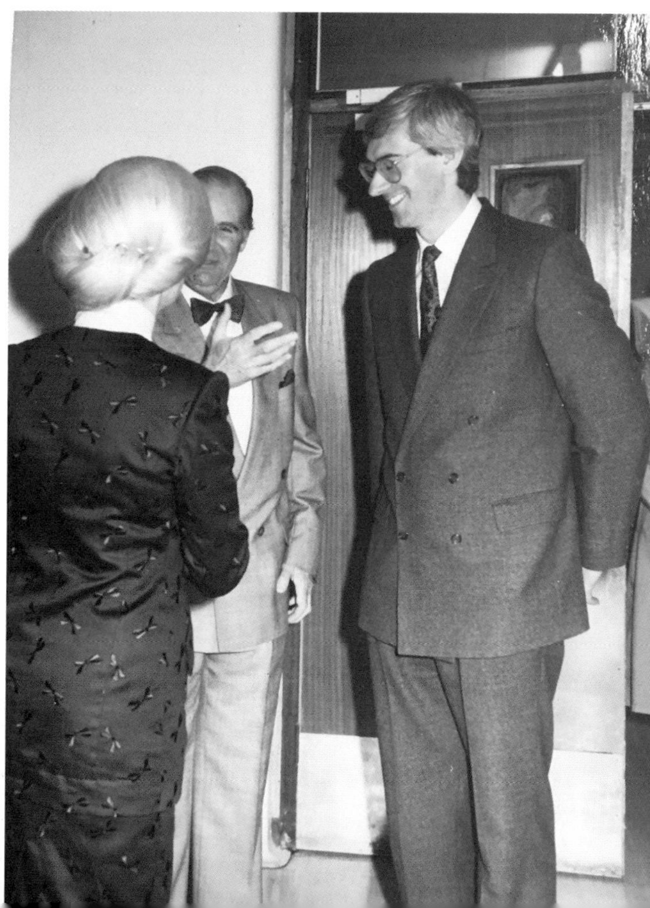

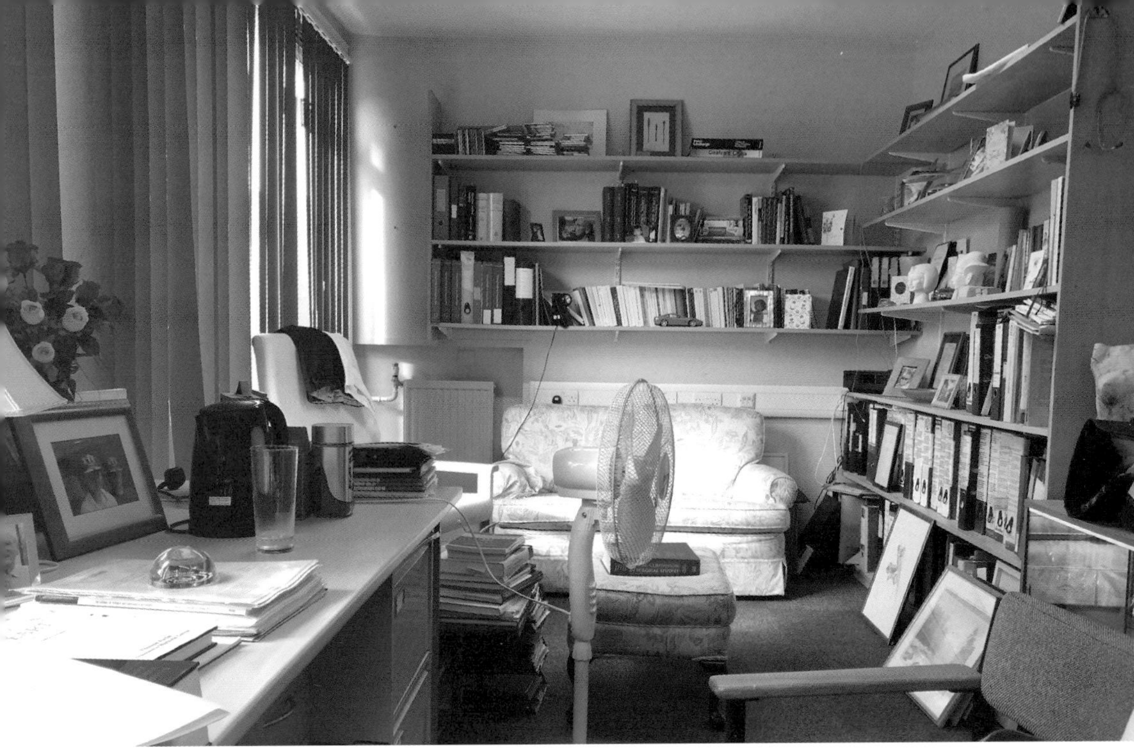

Above: My office in the old hospital. Now we are reduced to 'hot desks' in the new hospital. (*Author's collection*)

Below: Press announcement of the first total artificial heart implantation outside the United States of America. (*Newspaper cutting from* The Daily Telegraph, *4 November 1986*)

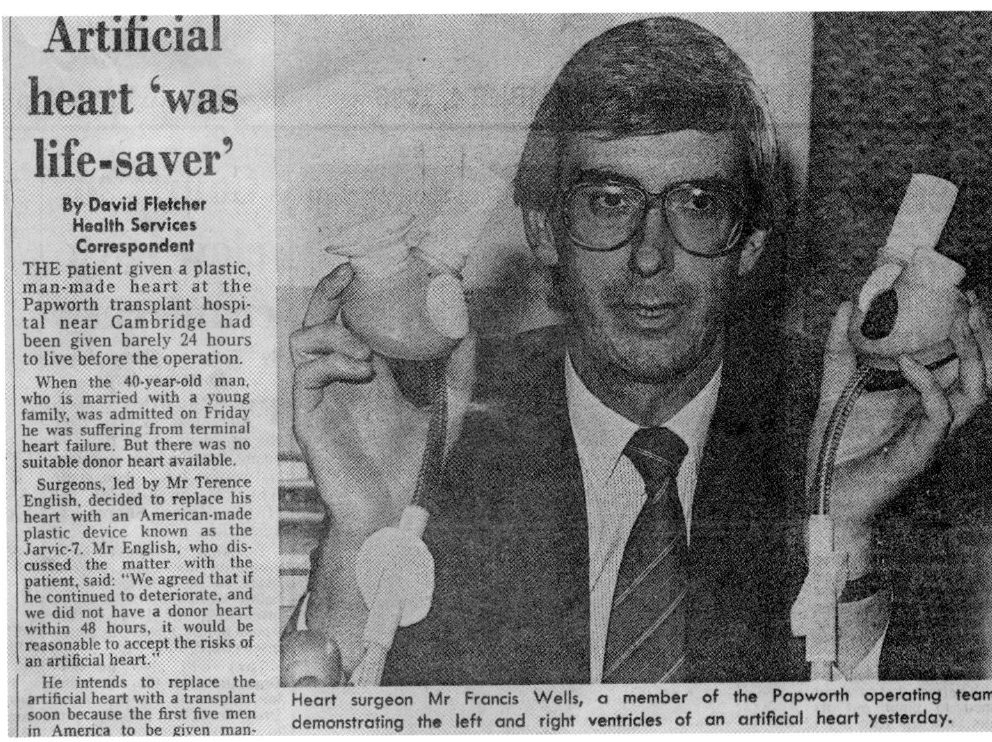

Artificial heart 'was life-saver'

By David Fletcher
Health Services Correspondent

THE patient given a plastic, man-made heart at the Papworth transplant hospital near Cambridge had been given barely 24 hours to live before the operation.

When the 40-year-old man, who is married with a young family, was admitted on Friday he was suffering from terminal heart failure. But there was no suitable donor heart available.

Surgeons, led by Mr Terence English, decided to replace his heart with an American-made plastic device known as the Jarvic-7. Mr English, who discussed the matter with the patient, said: "We agreed that if he continued to deteriorate, and we did not have a donor heart within 48 hours, it would be reasonable to accept the risks of an artificial heart."

He intends to replace the artificial heart with a transplant soon because the first five men in America to be given man-

Heart surgeon Mr Francis Wells, a member of the Papworth operating team, demonstrating the left and right ventricles of an artificial heart yesterday.

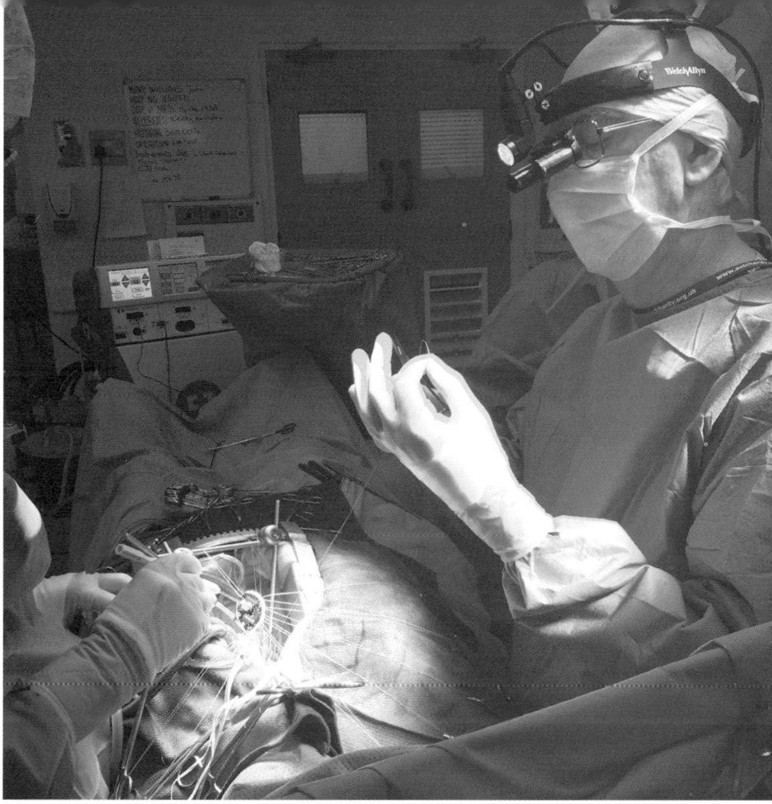

Right: The author doing his favourite thing, repairing a mitral valve. *(Author's collection)*

Below: A wet lab teaching session with trainee surgeons. (*Author's collection*)

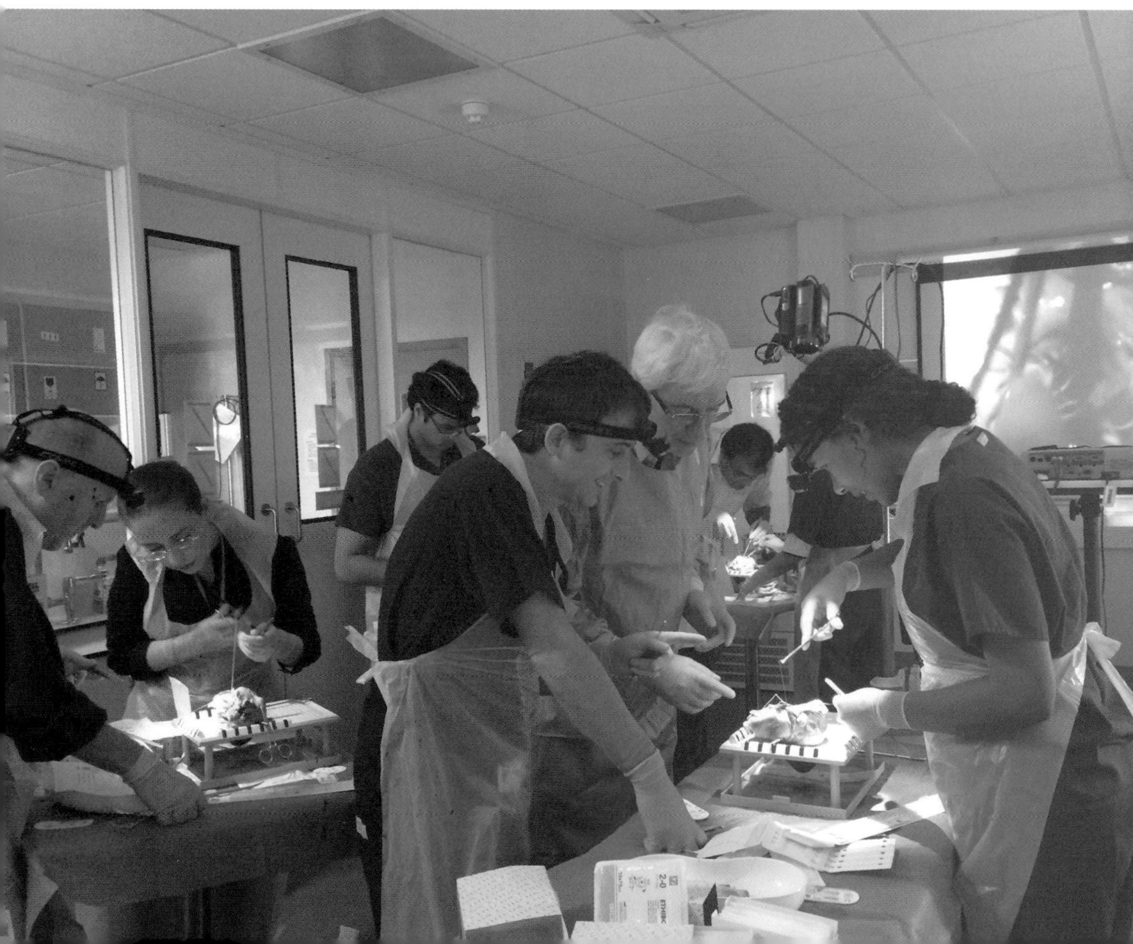

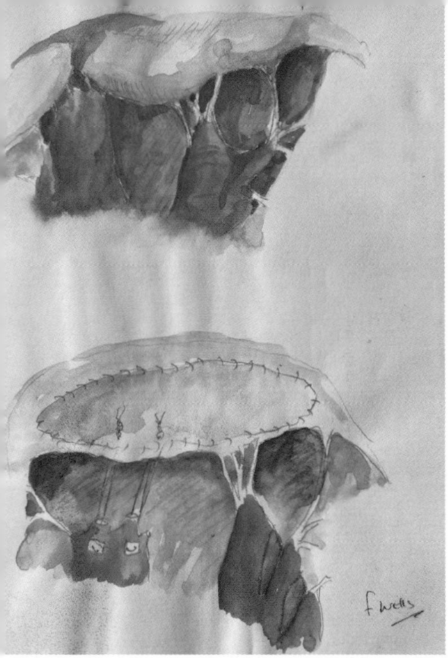

A post-operative sketch of a valve reconstruction from an operation note. (*Author's collection*)

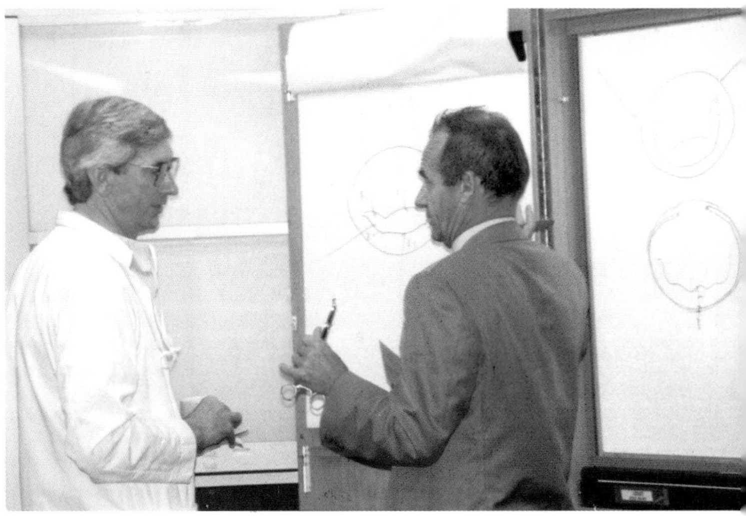

Professor Alain Carpentier and the author discussing the minutiae of mitral valve repair during the first mitral valve repair meeting at Papworth Hospital. (*Author's collection*)

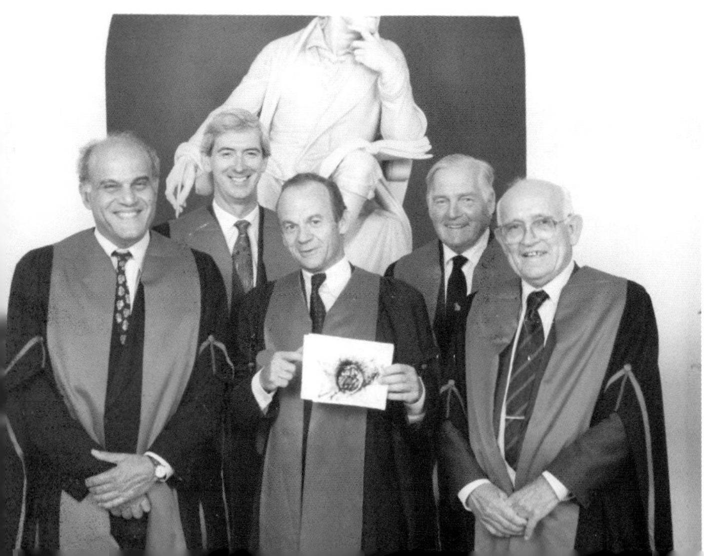

Presenting images of Napoleon's stomach and post-mortem details to Professor Alain Carpentier in front of the statue of John Hunter in the vestibule of the Royal College of Surgeons, London. From the left, Professor Sir Magdi Yacoub, the author, Professor Alain Carpentier, Sir Keith Ross and Donald Ross. (*Author's collection*)

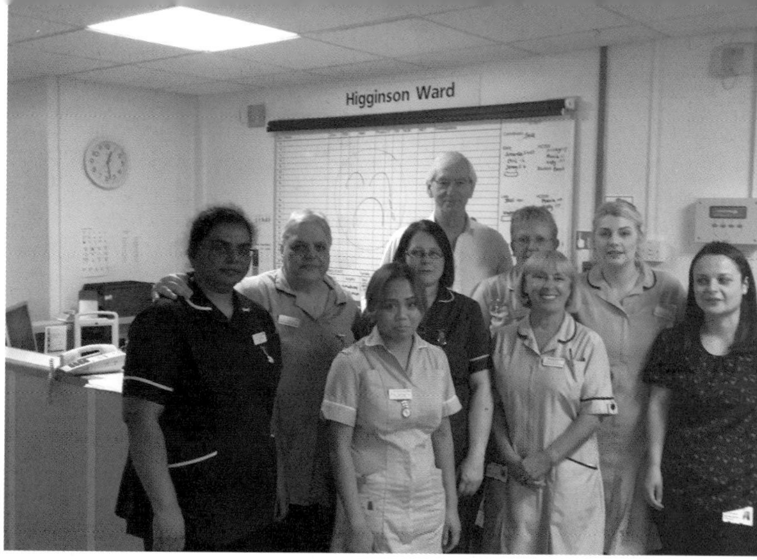

Staff of Ground Floor Ward at the old Papworth Hospital during the last week of work before closure forever. (*Author's collection*)

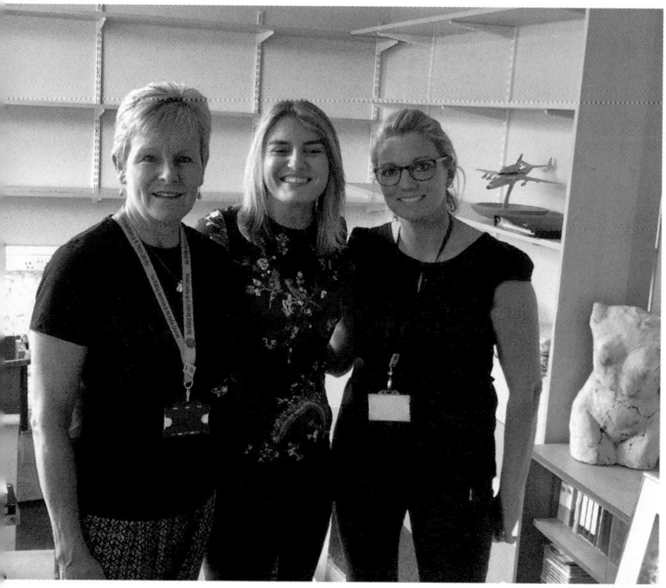

My secretary Joanna Aveling to the right and colleagues Sue Kidling on the left and Abi Bardell in the centre, helping me to finally clear my office. (*Author's collection*)

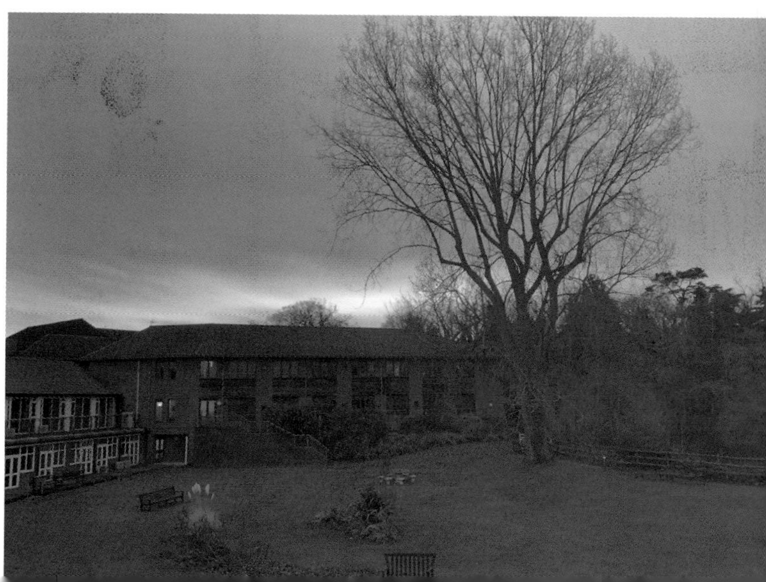

The sun sets on the old Papworth Hospital. (*Author's collection*)

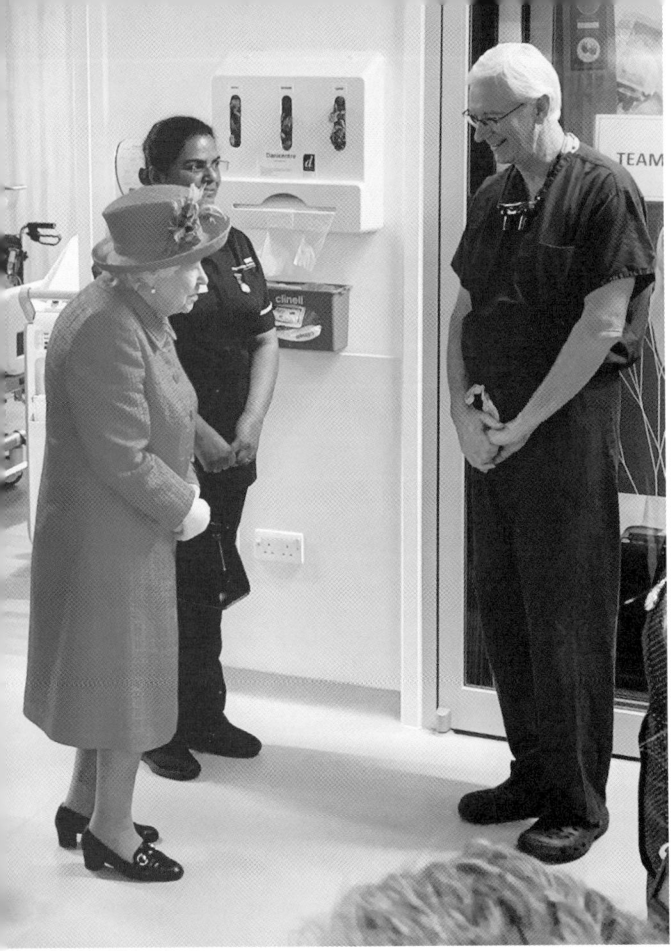

Left: The author meeting Her Royal Highness Queen Elizabeth II at the opening of the newly titled Royal Papworth Hospital, which had just received royal ascent. (*Author's collection*)

Below: The local team in the children's hospital in Addis Ababa. (*Author's collection*)

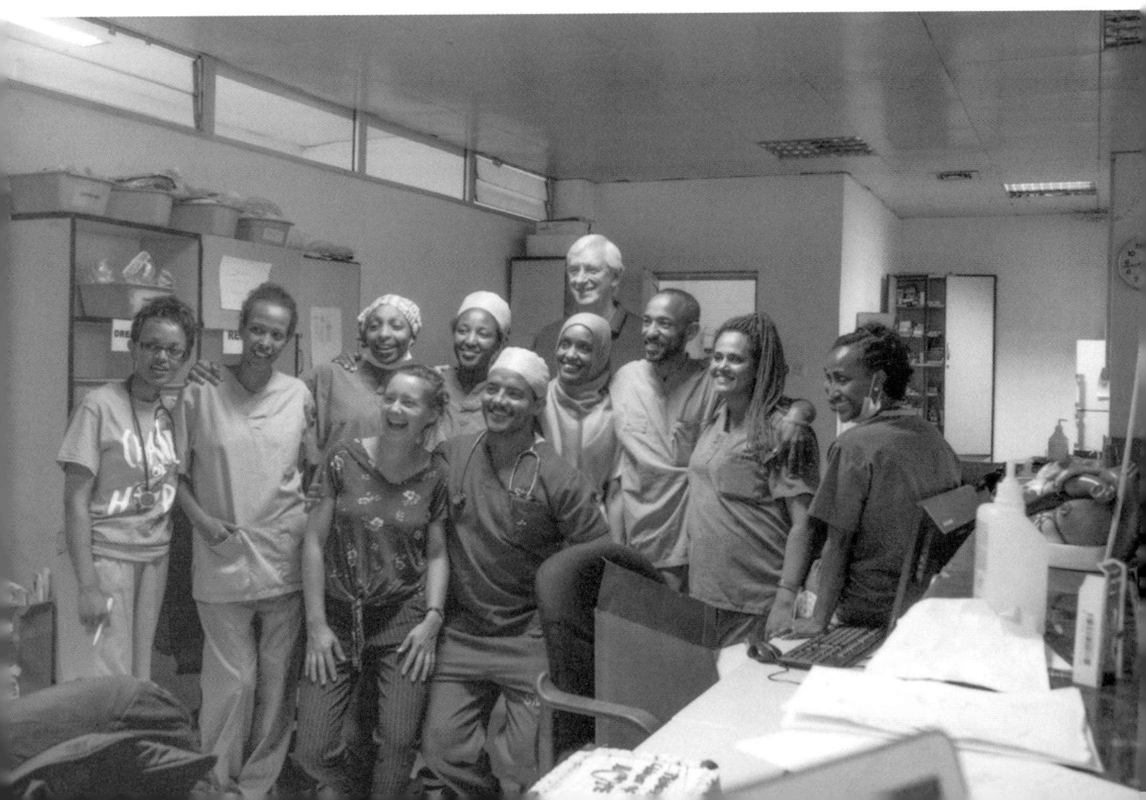

A young patient just awake five hours following intra-cardiac repair. As with so many of the children, smiling almost immediately on recovery. (*Author's collection*)

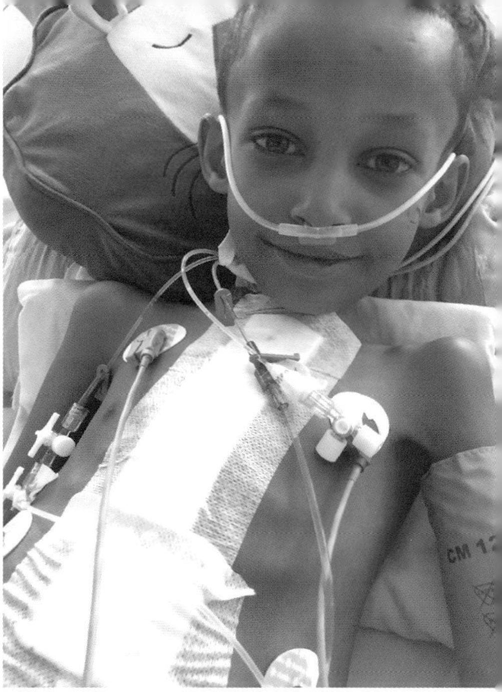

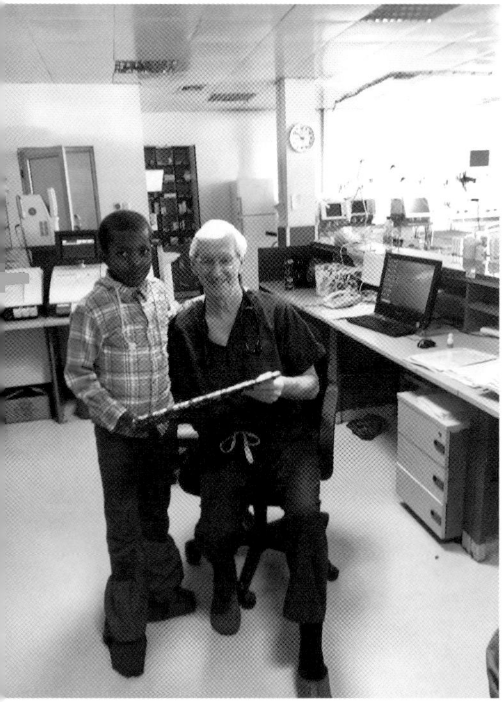

The author with a recovered patient one year after operation. He had brought me a lovely present of a portrait with his father. Just before I operated upon him, he had been deemed inoperable by another team. (*Author's collection*)

Abinet, my first patient whom I had operated upon fifteen years earlier. Abinet at her marriage. She now has a child of her own. (*Author's collection. Permission for reproduction given by Abinet*)

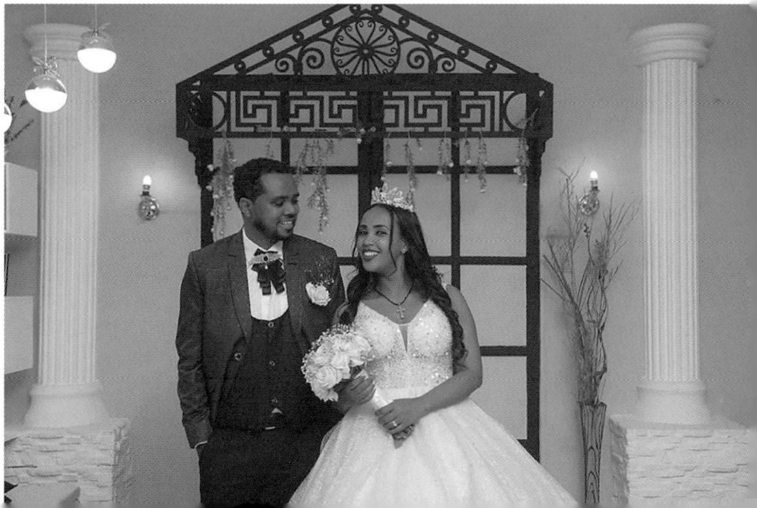

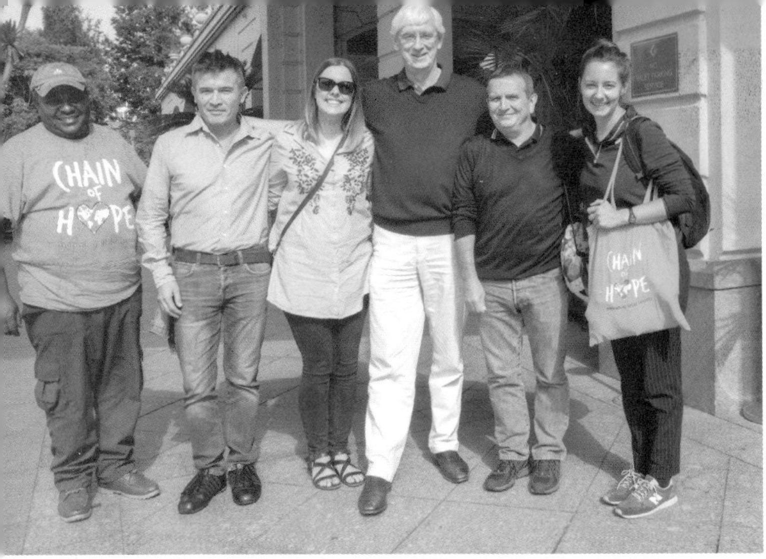

The author with the team of wonderful nurses and our driver in Ethiopia.

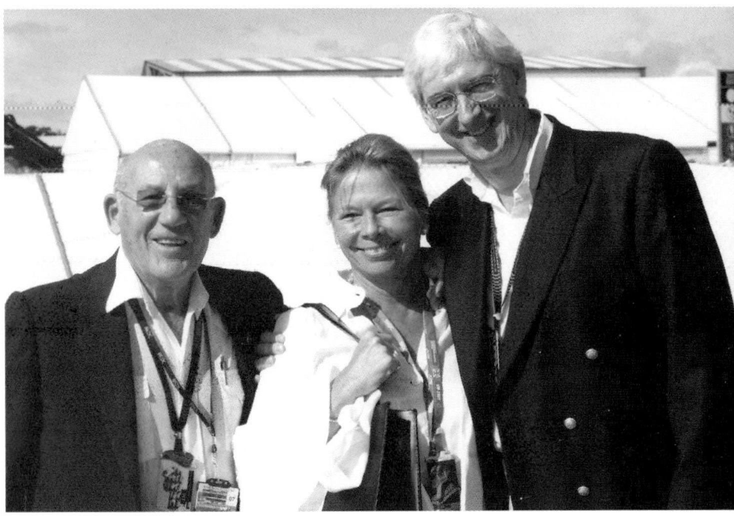

The author with Sir Stirling and Lady Moss at a British Grand Prix, Silverstone. (*Author's collection*)

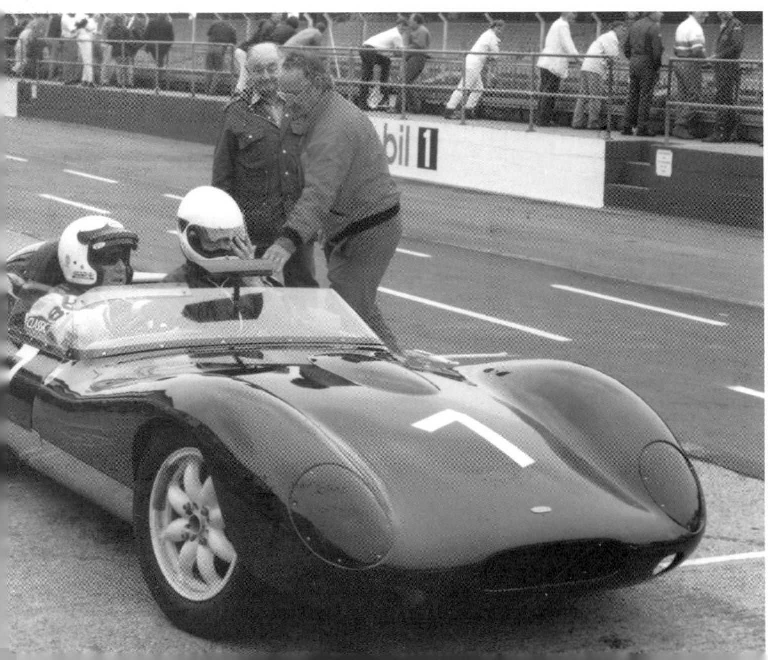

The author as passenger with Sir Stirling Moss about to embark on hot laps of Silverstone Grand Prix circuit. (*Author's collection*)

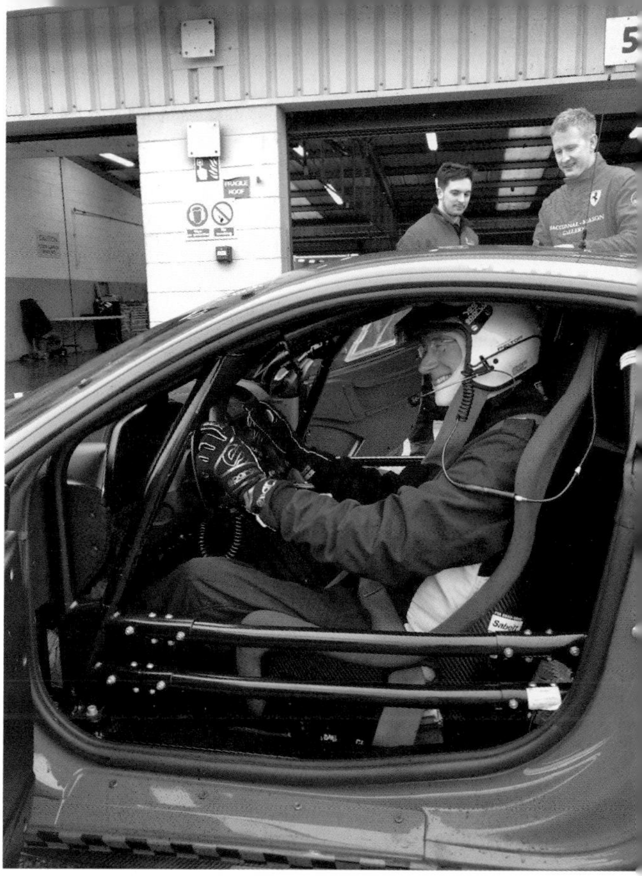

Right: The author just about to embark on hot laps in the fully race-prepared Ferrari F 458 belonging to David Mason OBE, in the pits at Silverstone, under the guidance of professional racing driver Ross Wylie. (*Author's collection*)

Below: Two of Sir Stirling Moss's racing Mercedes at the R.A.C. Club on Pall Mall at the memorial to the greatest racing driver, Sir Stirling Moss. (*Author's collection*)

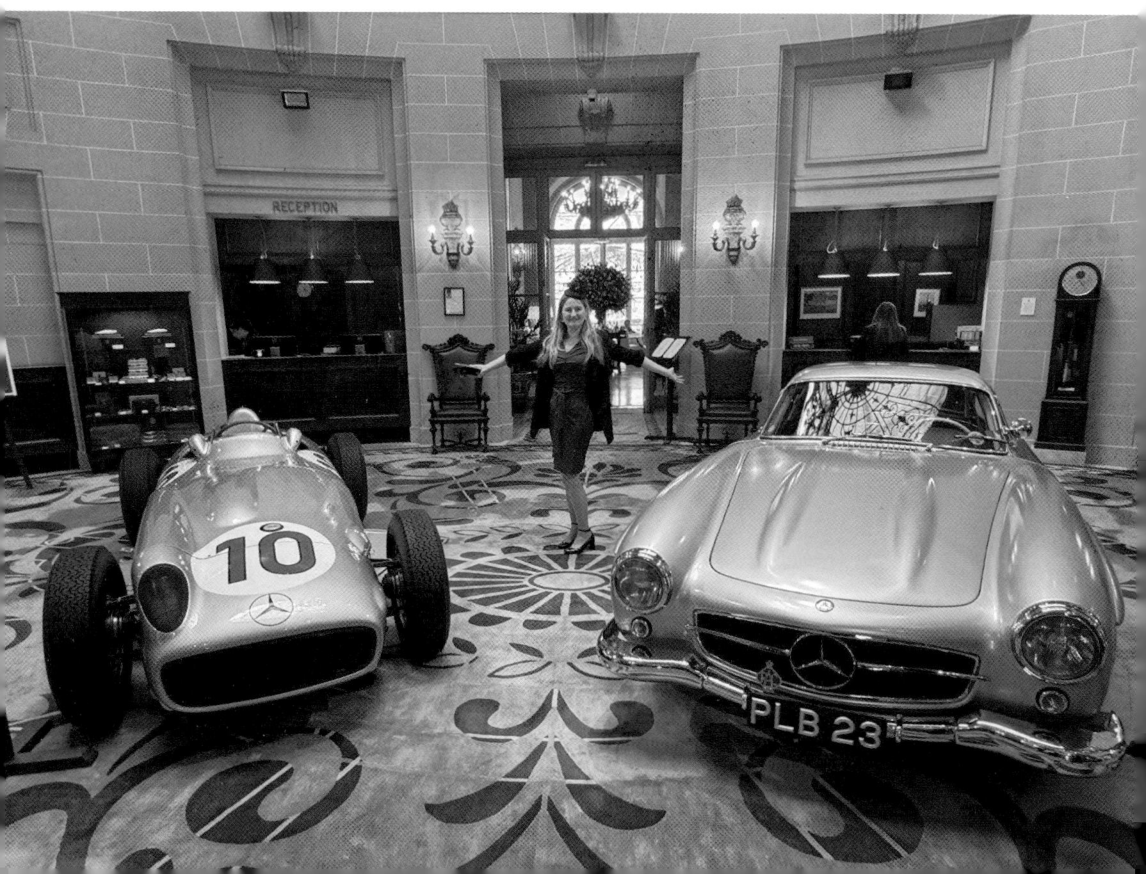

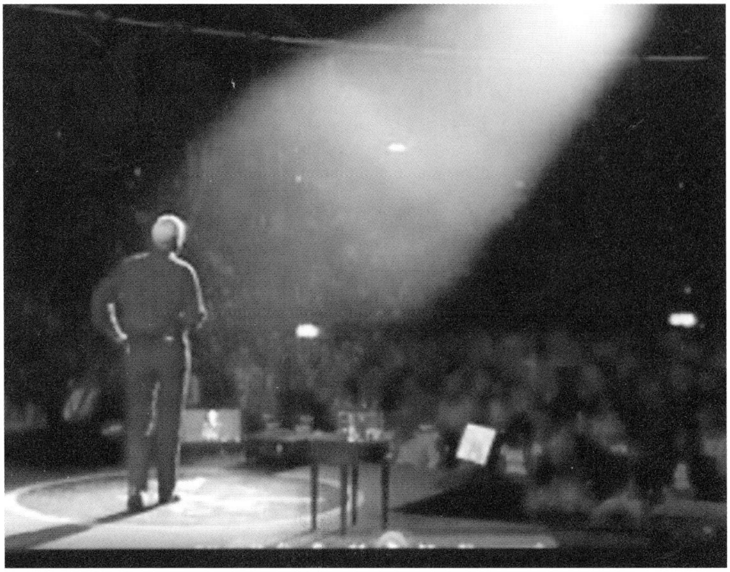

The author on stage at the Royal Albert Hall nervously delivering a TED MED talk. (*Author's collection*)

Below: Mel Fraser's heart sculpture and the author's hands cast in bronze by artist Eleanor Crook. (*Author's collection*)

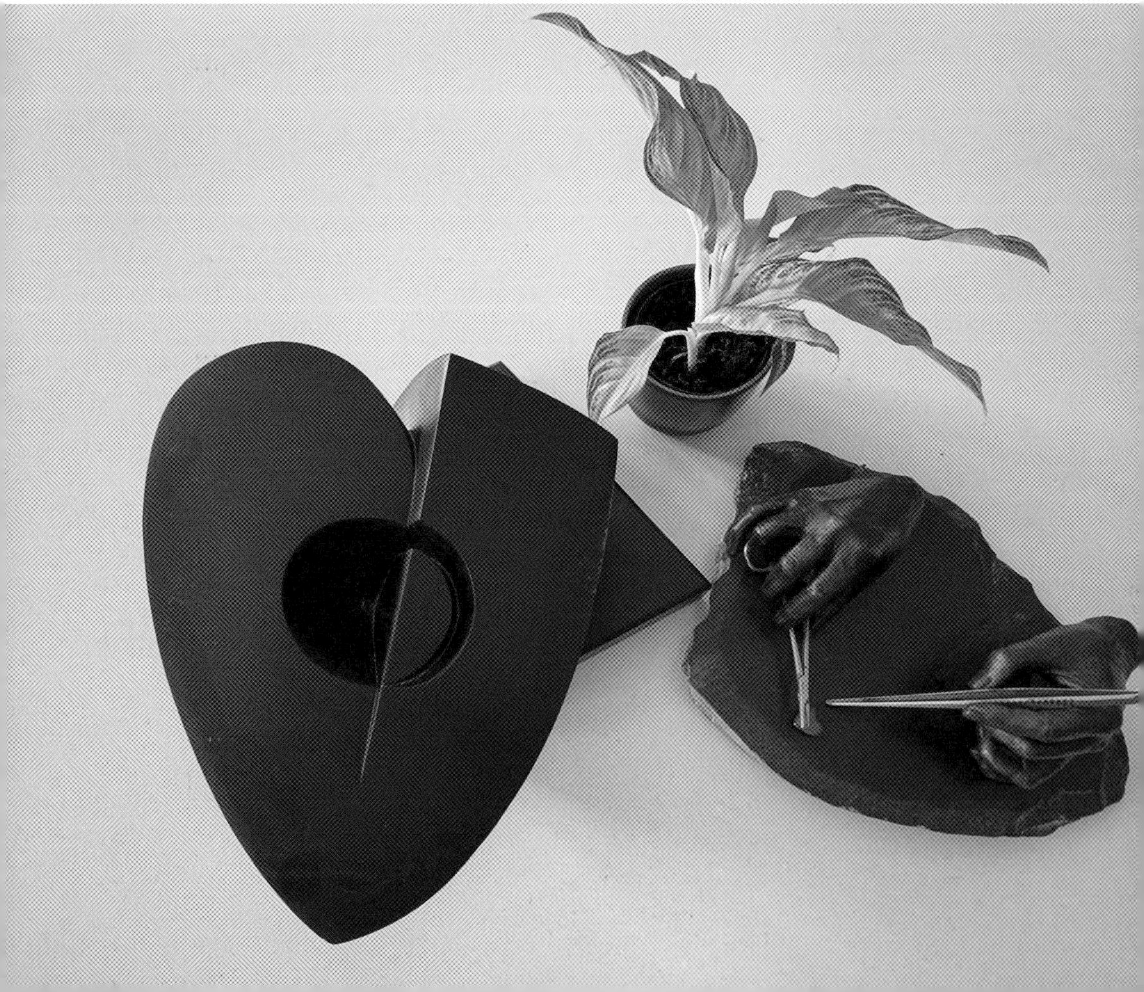

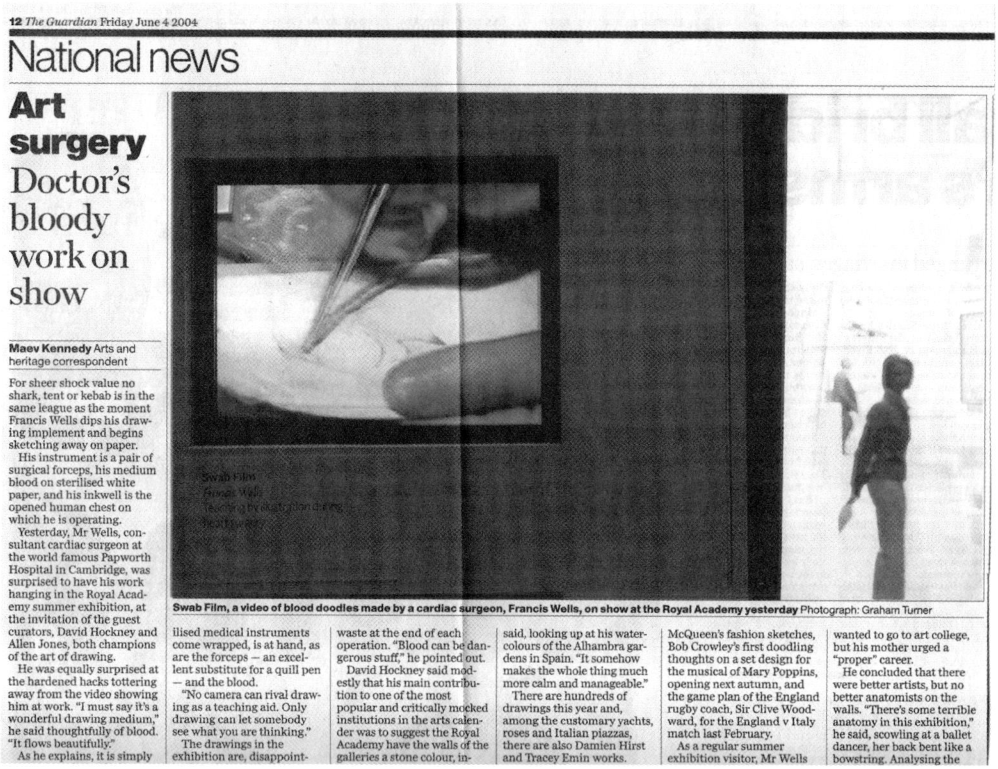

12 *The Guardian* Friday June 4 2004

National news

Art surgery
Doctor's bloody work on show

Maev Kennedy Arts and heritage correspondent

For sheer shock value no shark, tent or kebab is in the same league as the moment Francis Wells dips his drawing implement and begins sketching away on paper.

His instrument is a pair of surgical forceps, his medium blood on sterilised white paper, and his inkwell is the opened human chest on which he is operating.

Yesterday, Mr Wells, consultant cardiac surgeon at the world famous Papworth Hospital in Cambridge, was surprised to have his work hanging in the Royal Academy summer exhibition, at the invitation of the guest curators, David Hockney and Allen Jones, both champions of the art of drawing.

He was equally surprised at the hardened hacks tottering away from the video showing him at work. "I must say it's a wonderful drawing medium," he said thoughtfully of blood. "It flows beautifully."

As he explains, it is simply ilised medical instruments come wrapped, is at hand, as are the forceps — an excellent substitute for a quill pen — and the blood.

"No camera can rival drawing as a teaching aid. Only drawing can let somebody see what you are thinking."

The drawings in the exhibition are, disappoint- waste at the end of each operation. "Blood can be dangerous stuff," he pointed out.

David Hockney said modestly that his main contribution to one of the most popular and critically mocked institutions in the arts calender was to suggest the Royal Academy have the walls of the galleries a stone colour, in- said, looking up at his watercolours of the Alhambra gardens in Spain. "It somehow makes the whole thing much more calm and manageable."

There are hundreds of drawings this year and, among the customary yachts, roses and Italian piazzas, there are also Damien Hirst and Tracey Emin works. McQueen's fashion sketches, Bob Crowley's first doodling thoughts on a set design for the musical of Mary Poppins, opening next autumn, and the game plan of the England rugby coach, Sir Clive Woodward, for the England v Italy match last February.

As a regular summer exhibition visitor, Mr Wells wanted to go to art college, but his mother urged a "proper" career.

He concluded that there were better artists, but no better anatomists on the walls. "There's some terrible anatomy in this exhibition," he said, scowling at a ballet dancer, her back bent like a bowstring. Analysing the

Swab Film, a video of blood doodles made by a cardiac surgeon, Francis Wells, on show at the Royal Academy yesterday Photograph: Graham Turner

Above: Cutting from *The Guardian*, 4 June 2004, describing the installation video by the author in the Royal Academy Summer Exhibition 2004. (*Author's collection*)

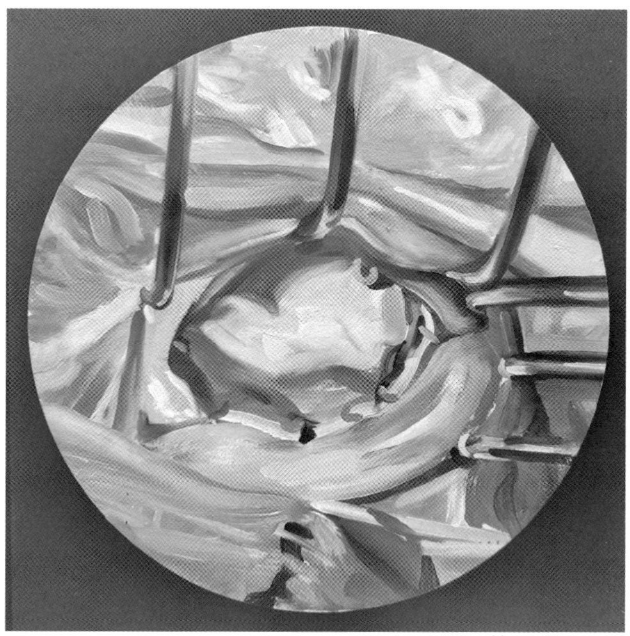

Right: Perhaps one of the strangest self-portraits ever. *Mitral Repair II*, part of a pair of before and after repair oil paintings on board. A gift of the patient. (*Author's collection*)

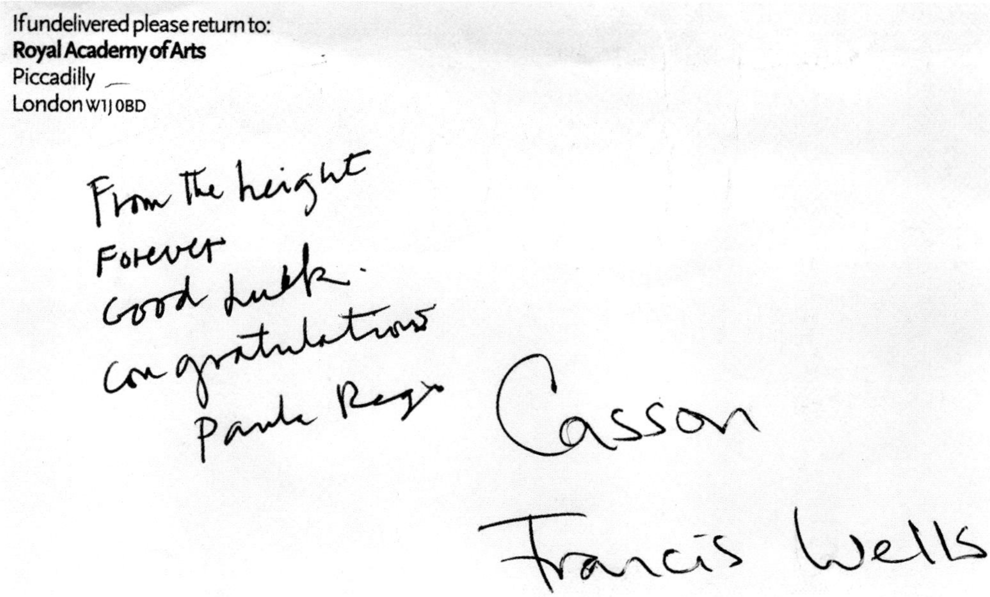

Above: Note of congratulations from Paula Rego scribbled on the envelope containing the prize cheque, on sharing the Hugh Casson Prize for Drawing with Rego and Frank Auerbach, Summer Exhibition 2004. (*Author's collection*)

Below: The author standing in front of his exhibits in the Royal Academy Summer Show 2004. (*Author's collection*)

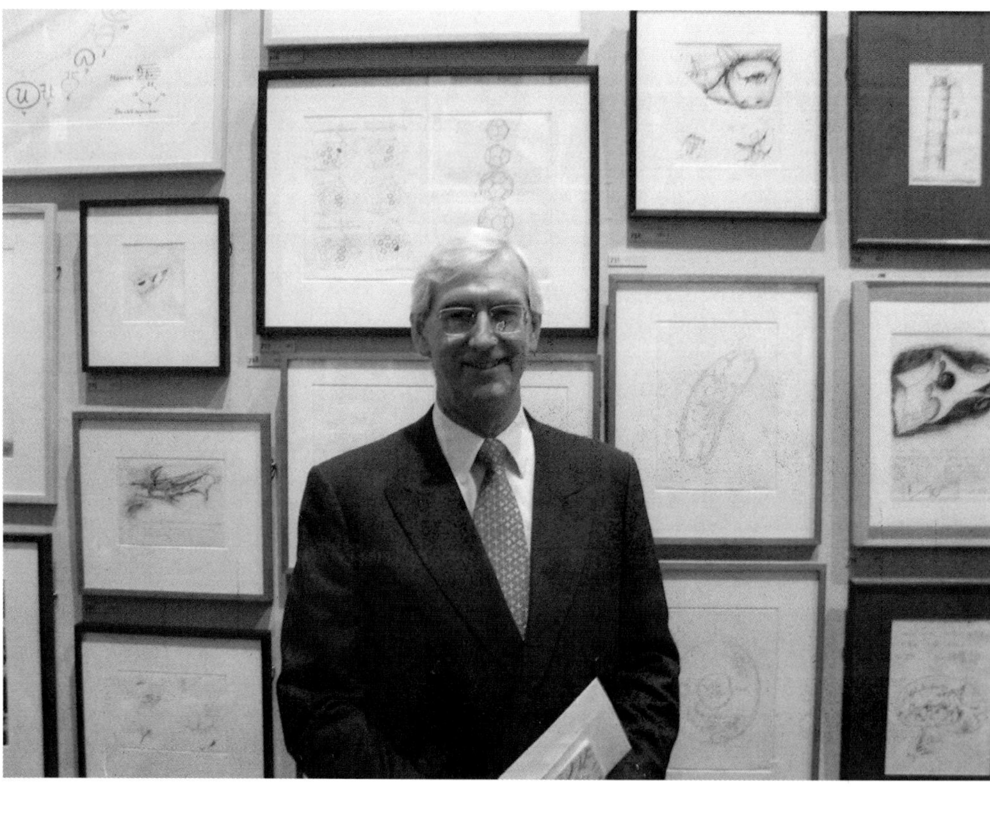

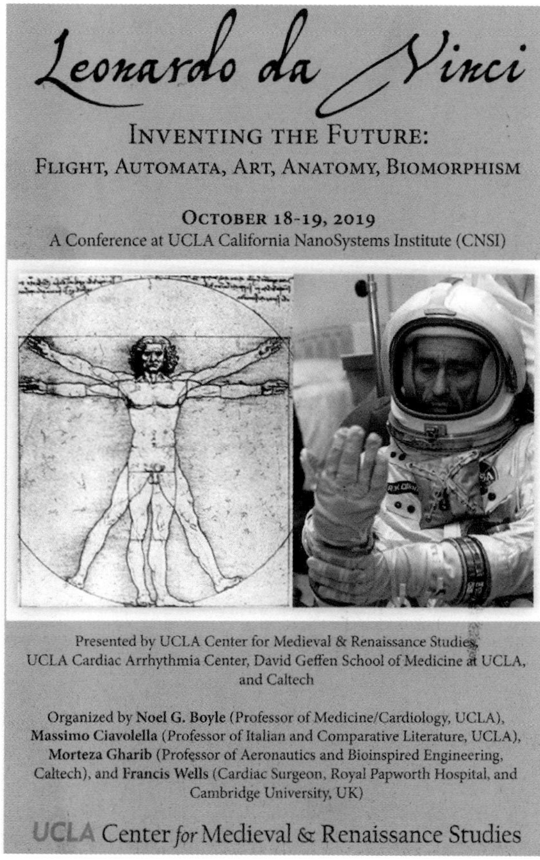

Right: Programme cover for the 500th anniversary meeting of the death of Leonardo da Vinci held in UCLA Nanoscience Building in 2019. (*Author's collection*)

Below: Newspaper cutting from *The Times*, No. 68504, 28 September 2005. (*Author's collection*)

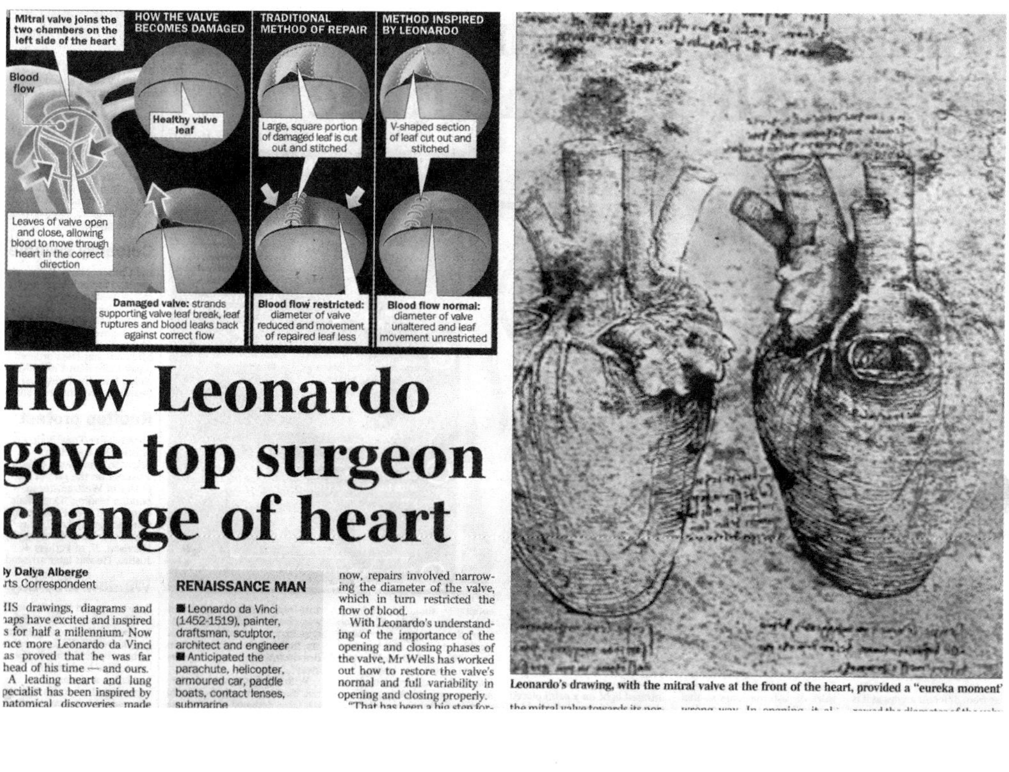

How Leonardo gave top surgeon change of heart

y Dalya Alberge
rts Correspondent

IIS drawings, diagrams and aaps have excited and inspired s for half a millennium. Now nce more Leonardo da Vinci as proved that he was far head of his time — and ours.
A leading heart and lung pecialist has been inspired by natomical discoveries made

RENAISSANCE MAN

■ Leonardo da Vinci (1452-1519), painter, draftsman, sculptor, architect and engineer
■ Anticipated the parachute, helicopter, armoured car, paddle boats, contact lenses, submarine

now, repairs involved narrowing the diameter of the valve, which in turn restricted the flow of blood.
With Leonardo's understanding of the importance of the opening and closing phases of the valve, Mr Wells has worked out how to restore the valve's normal and full variability in opening and closing properly.
"That has been a big step for-

Leonardo's drawing, with the mitral valve at the front of the heart, provided a "eureka moment"

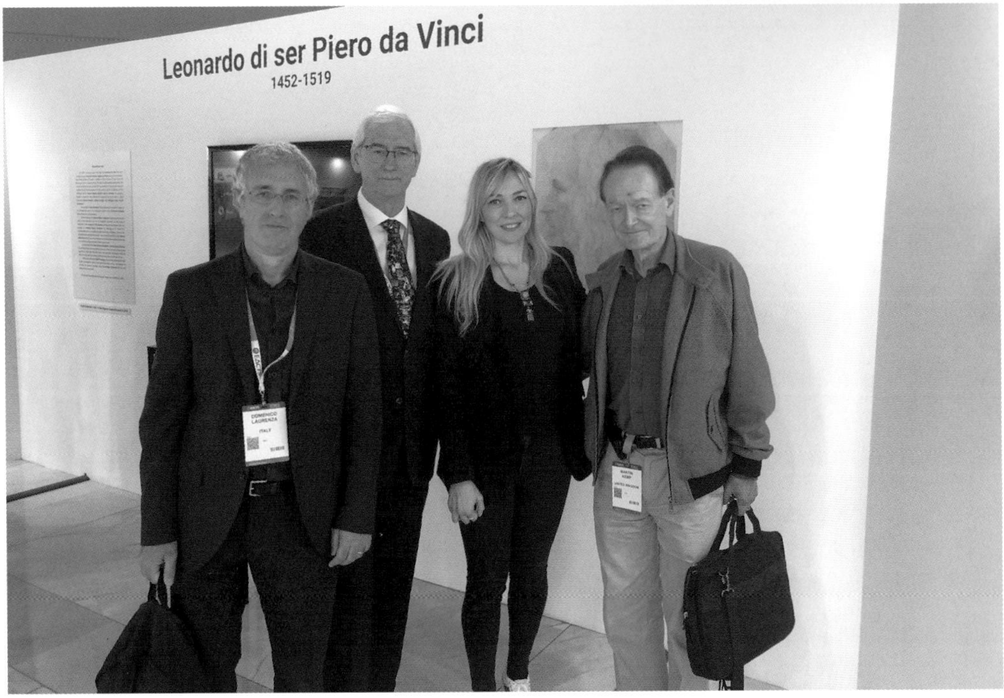

Above: At the opening of an exhibition of cardiac anatomy drawings by Leonardo da Vinci at the European Association for Cardiac and Thoracic Surgeons in Lisbon, October 2019. From left to right: Domenico Laurenza, the author, Sarah Taglialagamba and Professor Martin Kemp. (*Author's collection*)

Below: Sara Tagliagamba, the author and Roberta Ballestriero at the conclusion of the Leonardo exhibition in Los Angeles, 2019.

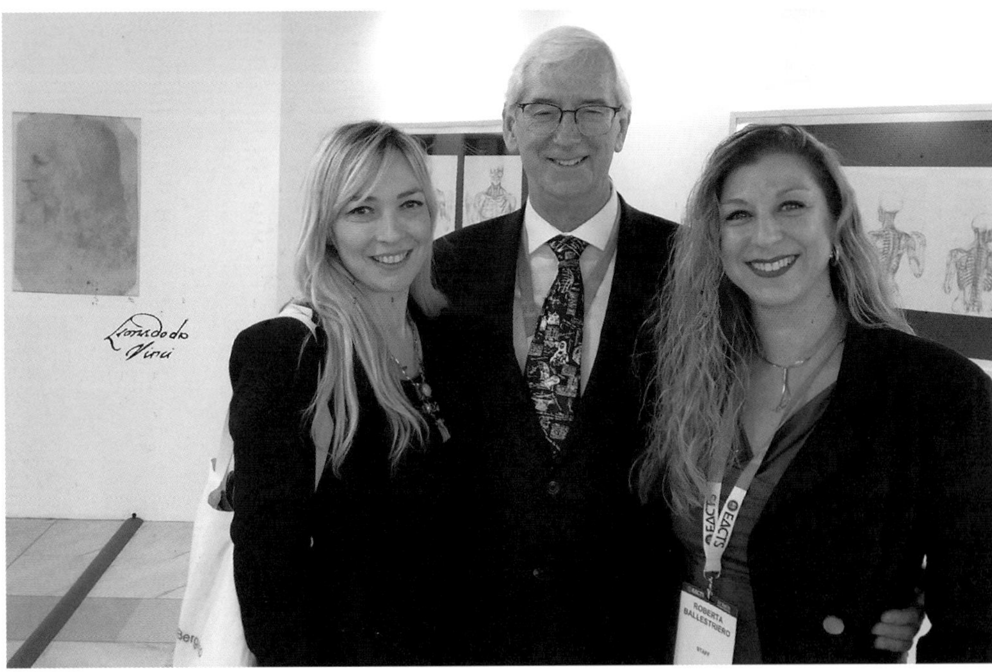

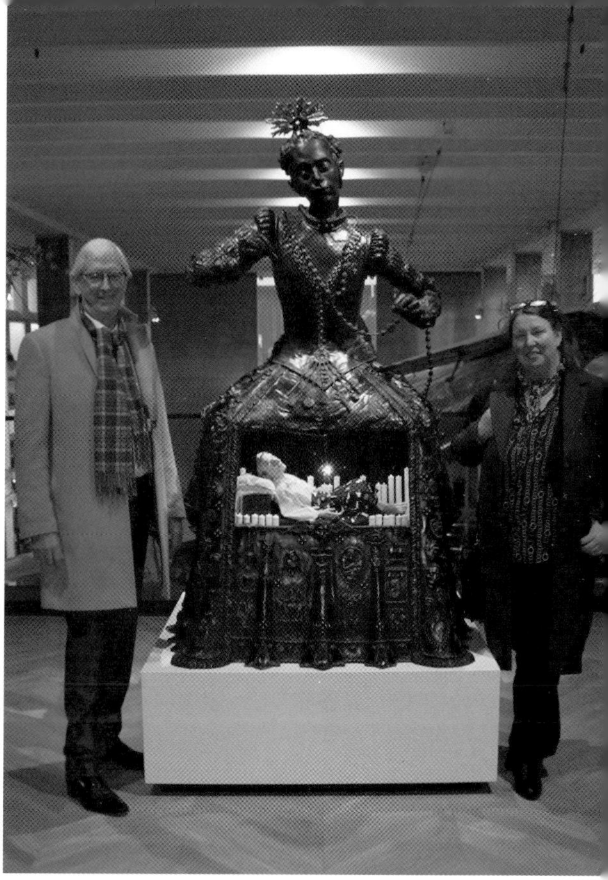

Right: With sculptor Eleanor Crook and her bronze statue made for The Science Museum, Medicine Section, London. (*Author's collection*)

Below: Wax sculpture of mitral valve surgery in the open chest by Eleanor Crook. My hands and those of my partner were used for the sculpture. Exhibited in the Royal College of Surgeons, London. (*Author's collection*)

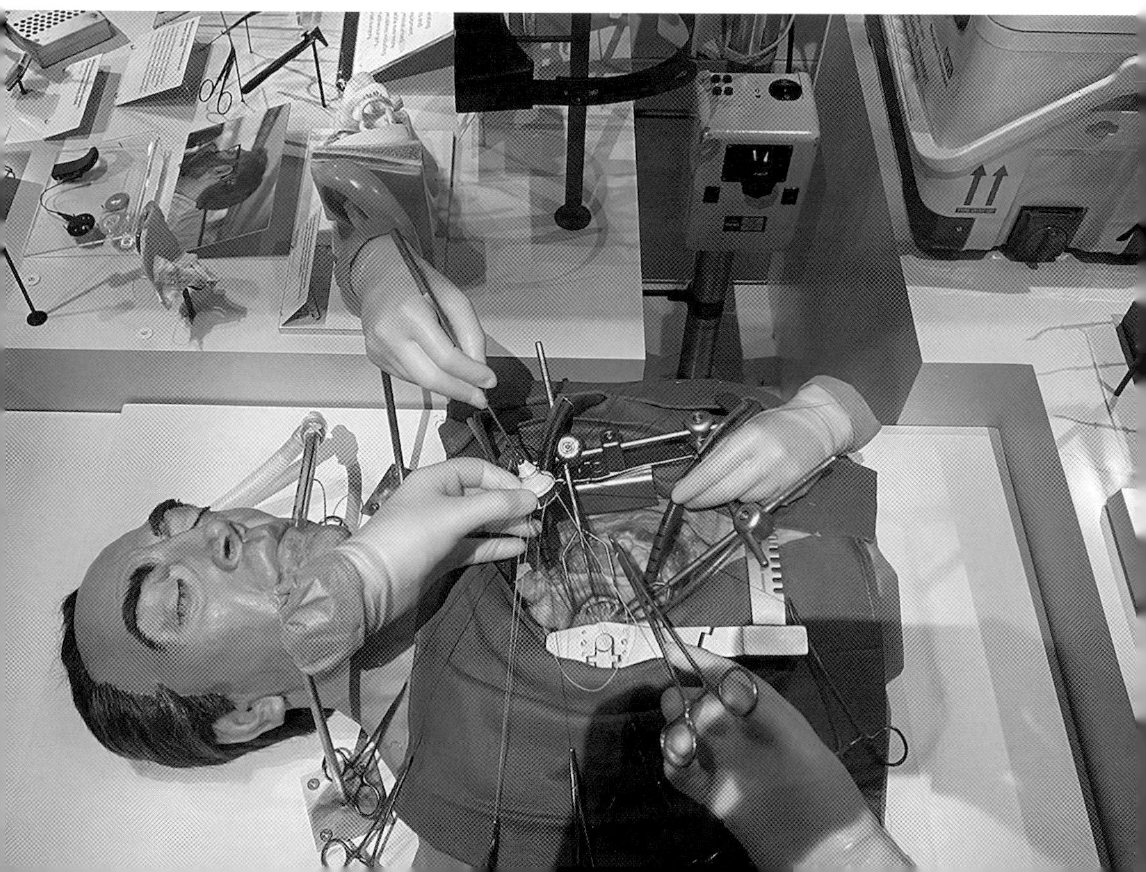

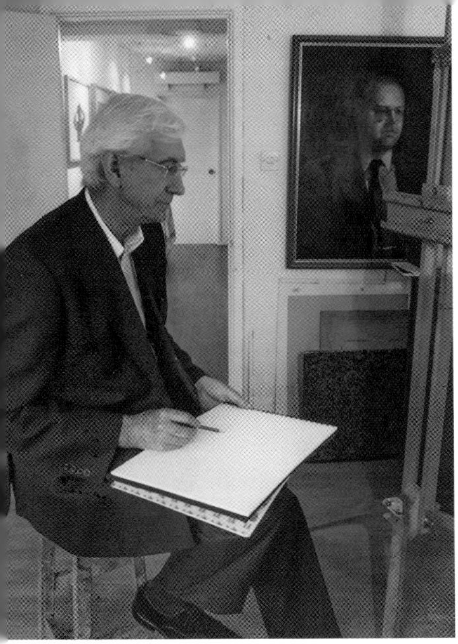

Drawing. Looking and seeing: the key to all surgery. (*Author's collection*)

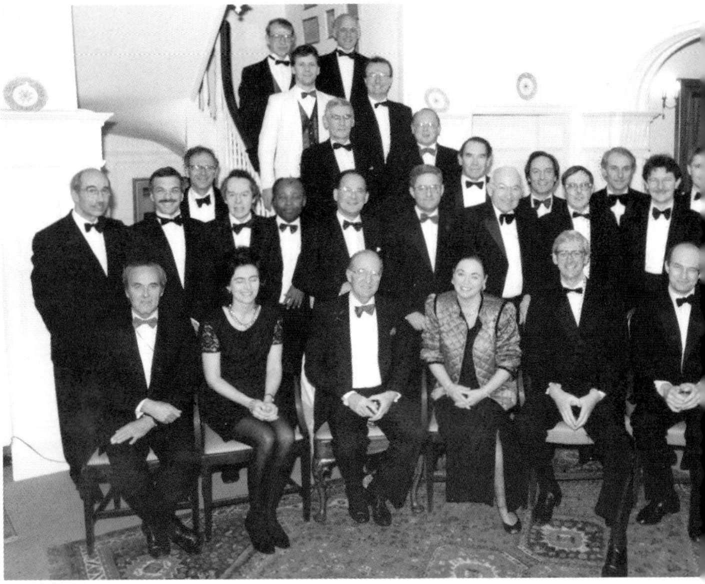

The consultant staff at the retirement party for the much loved Dr Bob Verney organised by the author. Left to right, front row: Hugh Flemming, Susan Stewart, Bob Verney, Dot Verney, the author, Steven Large. Middle row: Peter Stovin, Len Shapiro, Bill Newsom, Ray Lattimer, Amo Oduro, John Stark, David Stone, Ben Milstein, Ian Hardy and Nat Carey. On the stairs: John Kneeshaw, Peter Schofield, Mike Petch, Steve Bridge, John Wallwork, Terence English, Derek Appleton and John Shneerson. (*Author's collection*)

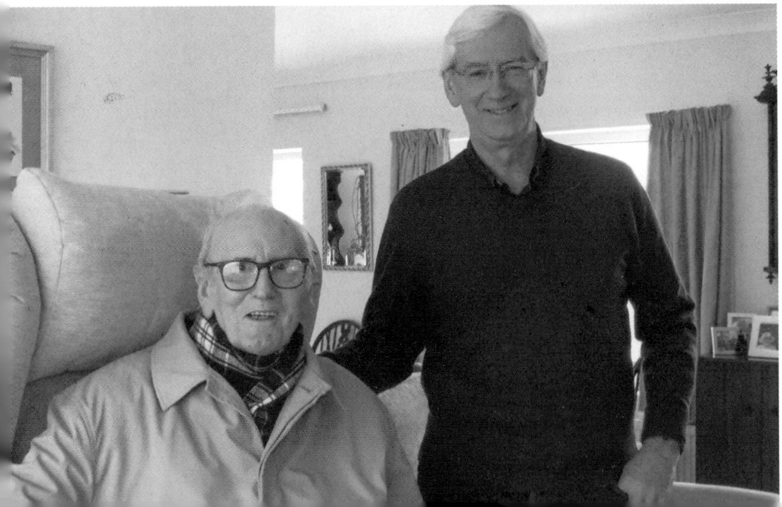

The author with his father Frank Wells senior in his home in Clun. (*Author's collection*)

An issue that we didn't know the solution to, was whether putting a slightly smaller lung into a significantly over distended chest in a patient with emphysema would result in a fixed space around the lung. Emphysema is a disease strongly associated with smoking and results in the coalescence of the air spaces, the alveoli, into giant bullae. These bullae cannot contribute to gas transfer and hence become enormous, wasted-space-occupying balloons preventing the normal mechanics of lung expansion on inhalation. In the normal situation the lung adheres to the chest wall through surface tension. That is the same force that sticks two plates together when wet after being washed. If the lung is not against the chest wall that cannot happen, and breathing would be impossible. In Emphysema the diseased lung is greatly over expanded pushing the chest wall upwards and outwards. The question was whether there was any elasticity remaining in the chest wall allowing it to collapse down onto the more normal sized lung. To our great relief we discovered from the first such patient that was what happened, and our concerns were dissipated. There were so many things that are now so obvious but then were completely unknown.

In addition to being on the rota for retrieval and implantation of the endo-thoracic organs, I was responsible for the assessment and acceptance of patients for lung transplantation. Patients with end-stage lung disease were referred from all over the United Kingdom. Assessments involved the immediate family, in light of the support that the patients would need after their transplant. Some of the most moving cases were teenagers and young adults with cystic fibrosis with their whole lives ahead of them. They had suffered hugely to that point with frequent hospital admissions and very limited meaningful therapy available. At first, we treated them with heart and lung transplantation, but the number of donors available for this was extremely limited. We were able to show latterly that double lung insertion alone would suffice in the absence of serious heart failure. Therefore, we moved on to isolated double lung transplantation quite quickly, as the donor organs were more accessible.

The manifestation of rejection was through the small vessels in the heart and the small airways in the lung. In the heart, rejection produced an inflammatory reaction within both the heart muscle and the coronary arteries. This form of coronary disease was diffuse and impossible to manage with coronary bypass grafting as it extended out to the periphery of the vessel in a graduated way. In the lungs, the attack was on the smaller airways producing a gradual obstruction called bronchiolitis obliterans. The introduction of cyclosporin-A began to ameliorate these problems, but they remain today as the enigmatic spectre of failure in transplanting those organs.

I continued to contribute fully to the transplant programme for more than thirty years. I will never forget the feeling of satisfaction of driving home after a successful operation with the first rays of sunlight in the early morning, with the foxes, pheasants and muntjac deer wandering around on empty roads. There was a huge sense of camaraderie amongst all of us on the team, from nurse specialist to consultant colleagues.

The response of the patients to their transplant varied a lot. A general sense of relief and gratitude was common. However, there were also some amusing asides. A few days following my first lung transplant, I was visiting the patient to check on their progress. After the usual clinical questions and pleasantries, I asked overall what observations the patient had as all of their responses were breaking new ground. With a very straight face the patient replied that, generally he was feeling very well and enjoying his new found ability to breathe easily and deeply, something that the fortunate rest of us take for granted. He added that there was only one disturbing feature and that was the thought of coughing up someone else's phlegm. The statement was met with stony silence until the patient himself broke the moment with a loud laugh. Relief was felt all around the room.

The ability to innovate was much simpler at that time. When John and I wanted to develop a solution to preserve lung function during removal and transport of the organ we sat down one Saturday evening with a glass of whiskey in hand and thought it out from first principles. We did not need ethical approval nor endless, often unproductive, laboratory work on animals which may not have responded in the same way as in a human. The result worked well at first use and continues in use today.

Soon after I arrived, Terence asked me to join him in a new adventure: the total artificial heart. Robert Jarvik, in his own words, a medical scientist, not a practical physician, had developed a dual chamber mechanical pump whilst working in the University of Utah. The Jarvik 7 was mechanically functional, but a large and clumsy device with inherent problems of thrombus formation giving rise to embolization. The pumping mechanism was driven by compressed air delivered through drive lines that had to breach the skin and enter the chest. As a result infection ascending along these compressed air externalised drive lines was an ever-present risk. However, it was the first truly functional device since the early stumbling efforts by Domingo Liotta and Denton Cooley in 1969. Dr. Cooley had famously fallen out with his mentor Michael DeBakey over the use of that total artificial heart [TAH].[1] Domingo had developed isolated ventricular assist devices with the support of DeBakey, who had at the same time opposed the development of a total artificial heart. Despite his many requests to develop and use such a device, DeBakey steadfastly refused to work with him on the project. However, Denton agreed to use the device that Domingo had developed in his programme in the same institution that DeBakey was then in charge of.

Whilst Dr. DeBakey was out of town, Dr. Cooley was faced with a patient who was slipping away but whom he thought would be suitable for support with the TAH. He decided to go ahead and implant the mechanical heart. Despite quite severe technical difficulties in implantation, it worked satisfactorily for a while. However, the patient died after a short time. DeBakey discovered what had happened by reading about it in a newspaper and was furious. The rift was so chasmic that Denton Cooley left and set up a rival heart institute just across the street from that of Dr. DeBakey. Their relationship was fractured until very close to the end of DeBakey's life when a reconciliation took place, which was cemented when Dr DeBakey was awarded the Congressional Gold Medal by President George W. Bush in 2008. DeBakey was then ninety-eight years old and had gone through a long recovery period from an aortic dissection repair. After a few abortive attempts by Denton to re-establish contact and a friendship, Dr DeBakey invited Denton to be a guest of honour at the award ceremony in the rotunda of the senate house. At that meeting he promised to send a replica of the medal to Denton in recognition of his contribution over the years. He wrote this accompanying note:

> Dear Denton, I am enclosing herewith a replica of the Congressional Gold medal given to me last week. I would like to share it with you since I think you deserve a part of this award. Our pioneering work in cardiovascular surgery was jointly done by us and the "first" successful clinical cases that were reported helped to usher in the specialty of cardiovascular surgery. We can take pride in that observation. With kind regards, Mike.

Denton wrote back to him and ended his letter with the following:

> Please know that I am comforted by the events of the past few months, which have restored our former relationship. Let me join so many others in congratulating you upon your life and accomplishments.[9]

Not long afterwards in 2008, Dr DeBakey died. This not before the two men had the chance to firmly cement their renewed relationship with reciprocal awards from their respective foundations. DeBakey had pioneered vascular surgery, but a lesser-known fact about him is that he was the one that came up with the idea of moving surgical personnel close to battlefield frontlines to save many severely injured soldiers in the Korean and later the Vietnam wars. They became known as the M.A.S.H. [mobile army surgical hospitals] units. Dr Cooley died in November 2016. Christian Barnard said of him:

> It was the most beautiful surgery I had ever seen in my life ... No one in the world, I knew, could equal it ... Dr Cooley's skill was matched by his grace and kindness.

These were my emotions after spending time with the great man both in the operating room and outside of it. Cardiovascular surgery had lost perhaps the two most important innovators of our specialty.

Willem Kolff had done much of the initial work on the total artificial heart whilst at the Cleveland Clinic in the 1950s. Robert Jarvik had designed the Jarvik 7 artificial heart working with Kolff. The programme at Papworth was enabled by Terence English's role in the Humana Corporation. Terence had begun to operate privately at the Wellington Hospital and had been promoted within the organisation, recognising his organisational skills. In 1982, William DeVries carried out the first implant of the Jarvik 7 in Salt Lake City. By that time calves with the device implanted were living up to seven months.

The first patient to receive the device was Barney Clark, a sixty-four year old dentist from Seattle with end-stage heart failure. The patient suffered multiple strokes but survived for 112 days. Terence had been approached by Bob Jarvik, who suggested that the device might find use in the Papworth transplant programme, at that time one of the largest and most successful in the world. They met over dinner in St John's Wood. Terence was cautious but thought that it might be useful as a bridge to finding a suitable heart for transplantation in patients that were close to death. A problem that he foresaw was one of funding. However, Jarvik had already thought of that and had approached the Humana Corporation, who had agreed to work with Terence and Papworth. By then Bill DeVries had left Utah to work within the Humana Corporation in Louisville Kentucky and had done two more implants with Alan Lansing in the Humana private hospital. Success was slow in coming. Humana had just bought the Wellington Hospital, where Terence had been appointed director of cardiac surgery. According to Terence it appeared that Humana and Jarvik were hoping for the implants to be in the Wellington, but Terence, quite sensibly would not agree to that because of inadequate back up. If it was to be done it would be at Papworth.[2]

Following a productive meeting between Terence and the Humana management a generous sponsorship was put together by the Humana

Corporation in return for public acknowledgement that they were funding the development. Local health authority approval was gained and Terence generously approached me to ask if I would like to help him with the project. Of course, I said yes. Four of us were on board with this. Don Esmore, a senior surgical fellow from Sydney, Dereck Wheeldon, our senior technician at Papworth, me and Terence. We needed to gain experience of the device by doing several implants into calves. The animal programme was based in Salt Lake City.

We visited Salt Lake on four occasions to carry out the necessary laboratory work. The laboratories were extremely well appointed and staffed with excellent professionals. All went well, and our calves survived with functioning devices. Salt Lake City has excellent skiing nearby in Snowbird and other resorts. A good friend of Terence from his mining days was Frank Joklik, president of the Kennecott Copper Company, who owned the largest open cast copper mine in the world, so big that it can be seen from space. We had dinner with him and his lovely wife Pam, an ex-British Airways stewardess. After a considerable amount of wine had been drunk the suggestion was made that we all go skiing the next day. Neither Terence nor I were accomplished skiers, and we had no gear with us, but Frank was able to help out and the skis etc were hired at the Snowbird Ski Resort. A wonderful morning of falling over and eventually some fast [well it felt fast to me] downhill skiing was achieved. Apparently, my headlong down-hill dash, mostly out of control, caused great hilarity to Terence, but concern to Frank and Pam as they thought that my death was imminent. However, we all survived without event, and I was hooked on the sport from that time. We went skiing again the next time that we were in Salt Lake. This time, however, Terence felt guilty as the acquired sun tan might give us away when we returned home and show that we had been having a bit too much of a good time.

I had cause to return on my own for further experience, but once the work was done, I took myself back up the slopes to enjoy them. I went by bus from downtown Salt Lake City. Whilst standing at the bus stop, I met three others on their way to Snowbird. We began to chat and the usual 'So, where'ya from?' came out. On answering, Cambridge, UK. One of them looked excited and asked: 'Do you know Len Shapiro?' The answer was: 'Yes, I know him very well. We work together and have done for several years.' The person asking the question was a cousin of Len's. I called Len and they chatted away, 7,000 kilometres apart. An extraordinary coincidence.

In principle, the surgical implantation of the Jarvik 7 mechanical heart was simple. Remove the old sick heart; sew the so-called rigid plastic quick connects to the atrial remnants; then the compressed air driven pumping chambers are snapped into place over the cuffs of the quick connects. The problem arose from the fact that the residual atrial tissue was very frail and the connects required a lot of effort to snap over the cuffs. It was very easy to poke a finger through the back of the left atrial tissue. Once the heart pumps had been connected, reaching the damaged and bleeding area was extremely difficult. The other potential difficulty was in closing the chest once in place because of its bulk.

There was quite a long wait until an appropriate recipient was identified. We needed a deep chested patient within which the device could be accommodated comfortably. Eventually an appropriate patient was found and we set about the first implant on 4 November 1986. Terence, John and I operated together.

The procedure went smoothly, and it was fascinating to see a human being kept alive with a mechanical artificial heart. The device driver was a large machine on wheels. It took up much of the available space at the bedside. Derek Wheeldon and Roy Gill, our two senior pump technicians, had learnt how to match the output of the device to the needs of the patient and all looked satisfactory. I sat with the patient until late in the evening before driving home. Finally, I parked the car in our garage, and as I was about to get out of the car, our success was announced on the midnight news. My first experience of hearing my name headline the BBC news.

The patient woke the following morning and was stable and able to communicate. A small stroke then ensued, encouraging us to speedily find a replacement heart for him. Within a few days, a suitable human heart donor became available, and sensibly, rather than wait we took the decision to remove the device and implant a human heart. Interestingly I do remember some gentle pressure from our industrial partners to let it run longer to see how the device performed but we ignored that and followed clinical judgement. The removal was quite a difficult procedure, but all went well, and the patient lived for a further two years.

As it transpired, that was the first and only experience with that device outside of a clinical trial, more of which later. The device was clumsy, time-consuming and vastly expensive for practical use. Also the complications of thrombus formation and embolization causing strokes etcetera, were too prevalent. Ascending infections along the compressed air drive lines was a real problem and though several iterations of the fixing device to the skin were developed, it remained a problem. For the patient it was extremely noisy, and it dominated the room in which it sat. It was like being fixed to a very large, old style washing machine. This remained the case for many years and as yet, despite advances, the many potential problems with mechanical devices have not been completely resolved.

A colleague at the London Hospital Terry Lewis was also working on the possible role of mechanical assist devices and we began to co-operate in this, but the resistance at Papworth prevented meaningful progression of this project.

At that time I became interested in other devices and tried such things as an intravenous oxygenation device, [the I.V.O.X.] for patients with advanced lung failure. The idea was to pass a bulky catheter with multiple hollow fibres, into the inferior vena cava, (the largest vein in the body) through which oxygen was flowed. The oxygen would then pass out of the fibres along a pressure gradient, entering the blood and then combine with the haemoglobin in the red cells. The first problem was inserting the hollow fibres through an introducer into the femoral or iliac vein. This was difficult because of its bulk, and blood loss could be substantial. It also suffered from the problem of clot formation and venous embolization. We abandoned it after trying it in a number of patients with end stage lung disease, mostly adult respiratory distress syndrome. This is a condition in which the terminal airway sacs of the lung become excessively leaky as a result of an abnormal inflammatory assault, and the patients drown in their own blood. At that time the condition had a mortality in excess of fifty percent irrespective of any treatment that was tried. It was an area that I had explored in my research project in Alabama, more of which later.

We also looked at the Jarvik isolated left ventricular assist devices, but the mood was not to support these devices. At that time, Terence English was moving on to become president of the Royal College of Surgeons and John Wallwork had taken over as director of the transplant programme. I was very heavily tied up running the general thoracic surgery and was not in a position to drive these devices forward. John had set his heart against using mechanical devices acting as a bridge to transplantation for terminally failing patients. As a result he had been asked to take part in a debate at a meeting of the International Heart and Lung Transplant Association in North America. The debate was on the merits or otherwise of mechanical heart assistance as a bridge to transplantation. He, of course was opposing the motion. We travelled to the meeting together.

When the time for the debate arose, John went first. He had no data and simply paraded around the stage with his double-breasted jacket open and his one hand in pocket and the other gesticulating. His case was somewhat rambling and an attempt at philosophising. He made a somewhat inadequate case against the motion. The opposition presenter was Dr Robert Bartlett.

He was both an accomplished speaker and vastly experienced in the use of mechanical devices in heart and lung problems, being one of the earliest exponents of extra corporeal membrane oxygenation in babies. Dr Bartlett was speaking for the motion, supporting the use of mechanical support to bridge a patient to transplant. His presentation was accompanied by slides packed with data and he made an overwhelmingly compelling case. When it came to the vote, sadly John lost massively with me, out of loyalty, as one of his supporting voters. Whilst this was somewhat humiliating for us, the Papworth team, there was also logic behind John's arguments. The devices available were inadequate to the task and consumed enormous amounts of time. The results were poor at best. There was and still is an argument for focussing funds on ameliorating advanced heart failure, both by prevention and better medical management. Therefore the subject was not closed, however, as the costs involved were huge and a full cost-benefit analysis did not exist. On the aeroplane home it was agreed that we would organise a study comparing best heart failure medical therapy to mechanical assistance. Over the next few months, we drew up a protocol, arranged funding, which was considerable, and obtained ethical approval. There was such an interest in the subject world-wide that we seemed to be pushing against an open door.

An important part of the deal that John and I agreed was that we would not go public with the story until we had completed the study, and we had the results to present to professional colleagues.

The first case was done on a Thursday morning. The following day I went to a prearranged educational meeting for trainees at Attingham Park Hotel. On leaving my hotel room on the Sunday morning, rather as in the DeBakey Cooley story, I was confronted with a *Sunday Times* newspaper outside the door with the headline 'First Artificial Heart in Man' and a full band width photograph of John at the top of the front page. It was not true on several counts. Artificial hearts had been used before, not least by Terence and me in 1988, and it was not a total replacement but an assist device. Moreover, it had broken our agreement of silence until the study was completed. He had clearly sought a journalist to announce the procedure.

When back at Papworth on the following Monday morning, I confronted John in his office with a copy of the newspaper. At first, he thought it all rather amusing, but when the medical director and the chief executive joined us, the mood changed. It became very unpleasant and not surprisingly we lost the support of both Medical Director Michael Petch and the C.E.O. Stephen Bridge. It was the beginning of a sad rift between the two of us. Although the case went satisfactorily, no more were done and the study closed very prematurely.

Horses' Hearts

In the mid-1990s, I received a call from the offices of Peter Rossdale, the leading horse veterinary surgeon in Newmarket. Peter Rossdale had been the vet who had been involved in looking after the famous racehorse Shergar that disappeared and has never been found. He had heard of my experience in reconstructing valves within the heart and wondered if I would go and look at a very expensive foal in heart failure at the Godolphin stables, the home of many famous horses and breeders. I agreed to meet him there.

On arrival, I was taken into the yard where a beautiful foal of about three months was lying down and breathing very heavily. I was invited to examine the poor animal and given a veterinary stethoscope. Feeling my way along the horse's chest, in an obviously amateurish manner, it rapidly became apparent that no stethoscope was necessary. There was a massive thrill, a palpable murmur (a murmur is an abnormal heart sound generated by turbulent flow) arising from an abnormal communication within the heart. Echocardiography revealed both a narrowed aortic valve, producing aortic stenosis and a large shunt between the aorta and the pulmonary artery, a persistent ductus arteriosus. This is a normal connection when the animal (and human) are within the womb, to bypass the lungs, as they are not working at that stage. Immediately after birth, on drawing the first breaths, the haemodynamics change and with the help of locally produced prostaglandins the duct closes, and the normal postnatal circulation is established. The persistence of the duct is one of the most common congenital problems and is easily fixed. Many will close with the appropriate administration of prostaglandins, but those that don't can be closed with simple clipping through a small opening in the chest wall. In a large animal such as the horse, however, this would be a more challenging proposition and had never been done before. The equipment didn't exist for such an exercise.

The first thing to do was to reverse the heart failure that was causing such distress for the horse. A diuretic was indicated. This is a drug that encourages the kidneys to secrete much more urine, thereby reducing the circulating volume and the fluid load on the lungs. We considered how much to give. In a normal adult male the dose would be between twenty and forty milligrams of the drug Lasix©. In a horse of this size though I was out of my depth. We considered the mass of the horse compared to a seventy-kilogram man and scaled up the dose accordingly. With some trepidation we administered 200 milligrams. As we watched the horse began to flood the yard with a river of urine. After a while its breathing steadied and slowly, with help it became possible for the horse to stand. So far so good. I felt confident that we could deal with the duct, but the aortic stenosis was going to be a much bigger challenge, as replacement with a tissue valve would not last long because the valve would calcify and fall apart within the first three to six months. A mechanical valve would present the need for the animal to be given the anticoagulant warfarin for life. With that comes the constant risk of bleeding in the brain and other organs. Any trauma to limbs or body whilst taking anticoagulants could be catastrophic, and so that option was out. The only option was if we could open up the valve enough to relieve the obstruction but not so much as to cause severe regurgitation through it.

A date was set for the procedure. I assembled our perfusionists to run the heart lung machine and recruited John Kneeshaw to the team, John is an excellent cardiac anaesthetist. The perfusionists calculated that we would need double the capacity of oxygenator and reservoir to cope with the volume of blood. These would need to be connected in series.

The day arrived and we set off in convoy for the Royal Veterinary School at Potters Bar where they had the necessary facilities. The anaesthetic and operating room was unsurprisingly voluminous. Whilst the perfusionists set up their equipment in the theatre, John and I prepared to receive the horse. A young 'equestrian lad' led the foal in and it was stood next to a large air bed with projections for its legs. The first step was to put the animal to sleep. The drug used is aptly called immobilon. It is a combination of etorphine and acepromazine maleate. It has a massively greater potency than morphine. It was given into the jugular vein of the horse who then rapidly subsided, 'immobilised' and with the help of the lads and a sling under its belly, lifted onto the table. Step forwards the anaesthetist to put the breathing tube into the airway. John, with his nice clean white coat stepped forwards, only to be shocked to see another lad enter with a tube so large that he was carrying it across his shoulders. In slight shock, John stepped backwards into a fresh pile of horse manure and skidded onto his back. Amongst raucous laughter, he regained his feet and his composure but triggered another bout of laughter when the brown excrement was seen on the back of his, now not so clean, very soiled white coat. We were then told that the procedure would have to be interrupted every ten minutes or so whilst the air bag was partly deflated and shaken vigorously to reduce the local pressure on the muscles of the horse, as they become ischaemic relatively quickly.

We moved through to the operating suite and after preparing the chest with sterilising fluid and placing the sterile gowns around the area, the senior vet made the incision in the thorax. As surgeons for humans, we are deemed not to be of sufficient quality to operate upon animals. Because of the extent of the ribs, it was necessary to remove a significant portion of the fourth rib. We were then able to deflate the lung and to gain a view of the heart within the pericardial sac. The roar of the abnormal flow of blood and the accompanying palpable thrill was very prominent, and also quite startling.

Carefully I opened the pericardial sac and exposed the heart. Its movements were dramatic because of the severe haemodynamic situation. We placed pipes in the ascending aorta and the great veins to establish cardiopulmonary bypass. We were then able to manipulate the circulation giving us access to the duct, which was huge. Although very short it measured a good three to four centimetres across and was cramped between the aorta and the pulmonary artery. Although access was not easy, I was able to get clamps on it and then to divide it ready to be closed at both ends. The tissues in that area are very friable and easily torn, and so every move had to be made with the utmost care. With this accomplished we turned our attention to the aortic valve. We stopped the heart with large doses of cardioplegia (heart stopper) and exposed the valve. The problem was clear. The three leaflets had not separated properly. I gingerly incised between the cusps just enough to enlarge the orifice but hopefully not enough to produce massive regurgitation, which would cause the horse more harm than good. There was nothing further that we could do. We restored the blood flow to the heart which started promptly and with considerably less dynamic motion since the duct had been closed. The pipes were removed, and the vet took over to put the chest back together again. I must admit that I had found it every bit as stressful as a human operation and to a degree more so because of the unfamiliar nature of the job. The horse recovered, and although it could never race, I was told that it could still be part of the breeding programme as it came from a very famous mother.

Following on from this, I was invited to visit the horse physiology laboratories where I saw perhaps the most impressive sight I will ever see in a laboratory. A thoroughbred horse was exercised on a treadmill at full gallop whilst connected to a cardiac output monitor and a modified Douglas bag to measure oxygen consumption and carbon dioxide production. Standing close to this magnificent specimen in a small room was humbling indeed. The sheer power that the horse developed whilst travelling at close to 40 mph on a treadmill was truly breath taking. An output of three to 400 litres per minute can be achieved.

Following this I was asked to consult on a horse with a fungal abdominal aortic aneurysm. An aneurysm is an abnormal dilatation of an artery, in this case, the aorta as a result of a fungal infection. To assess the aneurysm an ultrasound probe was passed into the horse's rectum and on up into the colon. The aneurysm was large and risked rupture if the horse was exercised.

There were no adequate treatments for this condition. In a human it would be excised with full antifungal therapy. This had not been achieved in a horse before. Having seen the size of the problem we needed to plan for a procedure that we might consider. In a quadruped, much of the abdominal contents extend under the lower margins of the rib cage, which extends almost to the pelvic rim, making access very difficult. Also the abdomen is very deep and there were no retractors available to hold the bowel out of the way to allow access to the aorta. I was invited to attend a post-mortem to assess the feasibility of any attempt to replace the horse's aorta. With the help of the vets, I set out to assess the accessibility of the aorta. I suggested trying a large plastic bucket with the bottom cut out and cut down the side to allow it to be rolled up. Then with the vets holding the bowel out of the way the rolled plastic bucket was introduced down to the level of the aorta and allowed to unfurl. We then used some large roller towels to hold the bowel back with friction. This jerry-rigged system seemed to work. The next problem we encountered was that the instruments were not long enough to reach the surgical field. Sadly no longer ones were available. At that point we realised that without new, specially designed kit it was not going to be possible.

Later, as a result of these endeavours, Walter Swinburne became a friend. His father, also Walter Swinburne, had been Irish flat champion in 1976 and 1977. Walter Junior, aged nineteen, rode Shergar to victory in the Derby in 1981, winning by ten lengths, the greatest achievement until that time. Michael Stoute was the trainer. He went on to win the Derby twice more and the Prix de l'Arc de Triomphe in 1983. During this time, I was invited to his father's beautiful home for dinner and he regaled me with fascinating stories from the racing world. In 1996, Walter Junior had a bad fall and was in a protracted coma with multiple fractured ribs. I am not sure that he ever recovered from this and he sadly died prematurely following a fall from a low window only 12 feet above the ground, aged only fifty-five. It was defined as an accident by the coroner.

At that time I discovered that mitral regurgitation was a common lesion in thoroughbred racehorses. I wondered whether the intense breeding programme to enhance speed and durability had outstripped the ability of the heart to develop at the same rate and the huge cardiac output overwhelmed the valve function, but I didn't have the time to pursue this with the vets.

Through this association and others that developed clinically, I was honoured to be invited to the race meeting in Newmarket when Lester Piggott's daughter had her first winner, having taken over from her father and mother. The great trainer Henry Cecil was with her on that day, and

I was privileged to be taken into the Winners Enclosure with them. It was a fascinating period for me.

With growing experience and ever more significant international awareness of the mitral valve programme at Papworth, the invitations to travel and lecture on the subject grew rapidly. I was quietly very pleased to be developing something of a reputation in the sub-specialty around the world despite the obduracy I encountered at Papworth. It seemed to me at that time that anything that was not to do with the transplant programme, was not really appreciated. Transplantation had come to dominate the raison d'être for Papworth in the eyes of management.

One of the many opportunities that presented itself to me at that time came at very short notice. I was called by colleagues in Edwards, a valve technology company based in Irvine California and asked to travel to New York to lecture at an important valve conference. The session that I was being asked to contribute to was on the Friday of the same week. However, I had promised my son Nicholas that I would be present to support him at his school's sports day on the Saturday of that week, where he was competing in a number of events. I politely declined as it would not allow me to be back in the country in time to keep my promise. In those days getting to family events was extremely difficult through the sheer volume of work at Papworth. A few hours later the organiser rang back to say that if she could guarantee that I would be back in time for the event on Saturday would I reconsider? I stressed again that my condition was non-negotiable. Sometime later they rang back to say it was all arranged. Would I please be at Heathrow in the first-class lounge for an early morning flight to JFK in New York. I had never flown first class before and found it extremely comfortable. On arrival in New York I was met at the airport by a driver in a suave black limousine that swept me through the early evening rush hour to the Plaza Hotel on the corner of south-central park and fifth avenue. Dinner was a glitzy affair and after a relatively early night, (the Americans do like to eat much earlier than Europeans), I was met by the organisers in the lobby where I was waiting with my overnight bag packed and ready to go back to the airport following the lecture. On leaving the hotel Hillary Clinton swept past me with her entourage entering the hotel. Dressed in a light blue suit, she looked immaculate and even managed a smile as she passed by.

My lecture on mitral valve reconstruction appeared to go down well and as soon as my session was over, I was again wafted away in a very handsome black air-conditioned limousine to the airport. It was then that the trip became really interesting. Rather than going back to the routine check-in area for British Airways, I was led into the Concorde entrance. The excitement built rapidly as the realisation dawned that this was to be my rapid transfer back to the UK. The organisers had kept their promise in fine style. Following the most courteous and rapid check-in I had ever experienced, I was escorted by not one but two elegant and polite female hostesses to the lounge. Once plied with champagne and caviar, I settled in for the short wait until departure. I noticed that there were very few fellow travellers. Amongst them was an entourage of four adults and one child, clearly in a party together. One of the party was an extremely tall and fit-looking youngish man who was engaged in light conversation with a woman dressed in a shell-suit and large sunglasses, so popular for travellers at that time. I didn't recognise either of them, but I have never been one for following the glitterati. The other two in the party were quietly sitting with the child who was playing quietly with a doll.

The time came to board and I found myself sitting in an aisle seat close to the bulkhead with the woman in the shell suit next to me. Across the aisle from me was the very tall man who was having great difficulty fitting into the small seats of Concorde. The other woman, clearly identifiable as the nanny for the child sat in front of us.

Preparation for take-off, and the take-off itself, were as exciting as it only can be on the Concorde. The pilot had great fun telling us what we could expect that was so different from a normal passenger flight. Rapid acceleration, a very steep angle of climb and a kick in the back as the afterburners were turned on. Then once at a good height the afterburners would turn off and it would feel as though we had just suddenly stopped as our speed and the thrust dramatically fell away. That once we had cleared Cape Cod, we would be going supersonic and there would be another kick in the back as the afterburners were switched on once again as we climbed to 60,000 feet when we would begin to see the blackness of space above us. Also to notice the speed on a display on the bulkhead. We would reach Mach 2 or faster than a speeding bullet at over 1,500 mph. As if that wasn't exciting enough, I then discovered that the tall gentleman that I had recognised across the aisle from me was Michael Jordan, the world-renowned basketball player.

The lady next to me began to chat to him across me and I asked her if she would like to change seats so that she could talk more easily but she declined and began to chat with me. She gleaned the information that I was travelling back for my son's sports day and she immediately leant over to Michael Jordan and asked him to sign a Concorde card dedicated to Nicholas, which he very kindly did.

As the flight progressed, we settled into a very interesting and polite conversation about many things. As final approach began over Bristol, my flight companion asked me what I did as it hadn't come up before in our conversation and I told her I was a heart surgeon. I then asked her the same question and she said that she was a singer. She asked my name and I told her, following which I did the same. The reply stopped me in my tracks: Madonna. It was all so matter of fact and pleasant that it seemed almost natural. Friends who hear me recount this story are more impressed or amused that I didn't recognise her than the actuality of sitting next to her.

The following day, she had been seen at the Bluebird Club in London, which had been reported in *The Times*. In the article, they stated that she had not been recognised there either on account of changing the colour of her hair and dressing down. I suspect that she had quite enjoyed a conversation that wasn't in any way in adoration of her but just a normal chat. Sadly, I was never to fly Concorde again, but I was home in time for my son's sports day.

Thoracic Surgery

I had been interested in embryology and congenital heart disease since my medical school days. Naturally, from that interest, I had a feeling that I would enjoy paediatric cardiac surgery. My jobs with Christopher Lincoln at Brompton and John Kirklin and Al Pacifico in Alabama, had begun to prepare me for this. However, as I progressed through the latter part of my training, it became clear that there would be few if any consultant jobs at the right time for me. I therefore abandoned that idea and focussed on the more general specialty of thoracic surgery.

I had gained a lot of gastro-intestinal tract surgery experience, as well as managing thyroid problems during my general surgical training and had been taught thymic surgery by Joel Cooper. Ben Milstein had already developed the first oesophageal and the earliest vascular surgical practices in East Anglia and had brought me up in those specialties. The breadth of work in thoracic surgery meant that it would be a very interesting life. The wide variety of diseases that needed to be managed appealed to me as a good alternative to paediatric cardiac surgery. I was therefore quite excited to take over all aspects of Ben's practice. I found myself immersed in all aspects of surgery of the oesophagus, lung, chest wall, thymus, retro-sternal thyroids.

The Oesophagus

Cancer of the oesophagus can be very depressing to treat and few surgeons wanted to be involved as the surgery was perceived as being taxing, often demanding access to three body areas, the neck, chest and abdomen, and in the wrong hands, general results were poor. However, the things that I had been taught by Bill Everitt in anastomotic techniques, the handling of tissues, and the post-operative management by Ben Milstein, gave me confidence to develop the specialty. During the next twenty plus years I carried out over 350 oesophagectomies with a mortality of under five percent and an anastomotic leak rate of less than two percent.[3] The average operative mortality in the UK at that time was twenty-five percent.

A large part of our success came from the excellent nursing care that the patients were afforded. This was despite the fact that we did not have a high dependency unit at Papworth and the intensive care was always occupied by cardiac patients. Visiting surgeons could not believe that the patients were extubated on the operating table and then recovered in the corridor of the theatre suite, before moving directly to the ward. Our results were all the more remarkable when those conditions are considered. Despite many requests for the development of a properly staffed and equipped high dependency recovery unit, no funding was forthcoming. It was one area where I lacked support from my consultant colleagues. Also at that time we didn't have a computerised axial tomographic [CAT] scanner. Pre-operative assessment and any surgical staging had to be done with more basic investigations. Despite this, with thorough and careful pre-operative evaluation, the number of truly inoperable patients that found their way onto the operating table was low.

There were many memorable patients, but one that stands out in my mind was a lady who had an oesophageal cancer but was ninety-two years old. Whilst an inpatient at Addenbrooke's hospital she had been turned down for any treatment because of her age. At that time she was in the final stages of writing the biography of her great uncle twice removed John Couch Adams, who had discovered Neptune. He was born in 1819 in a family of tenant farmers in Cornwall. Adams was considered by many of the time to be truly the natural successor to Isaac Newton. Indeed he was the one who was asked to edit Newton's papers when they were bequeathed to St John's College in Cambridge. By watching the perturbations of Uranus, he had proposed the presence of a new planet Neptune. He had submitted his mathematical calculations to the astronomical society, but they neglected the ratification for almost a year.

Meanwhile, just afterwards in France, Urbain le Varrier submitted his workings to the French society, who ratified them almost immediately, taking the prize. Adams had never received the recognition that he deserved, and my patient was in the process of completing her work to attempt to restore Adams to his rightful position of the discoverer of the planet. She was desperate to finish her book describing his life and achievements, and by some means or other discovered my name and whereabouts. I was summoned by the family for a consultation. Despite her advanced age, I was immediately impressed by the great strength of her character and otherwise good condition. I agreed to help her and transferred her from Addenbrooke's to Papworth hospital.

Two days later and with some trepidation, the operation went ahead. It went extremely well. True to form she was up and about quite quickly, threatening her own imminent discharge to get on with her work. The book was completed, and she lived another three years.[4] Afterwards, she wrote in a letter to me:

> With the author's compliments, thank you for your skilful rescue from Addenbrooke's on Saturday 25th September 1993 for which I most grateful.

Sadly, in the absence of advanced scanning techniques, some patients were found to have advanced metastatic disease on opening and only supportive care was possible. To amend this situation, I began to push hard for a CT scanner to be installed at Papworth.

In addition to the malignant conditions, we provided a full practice for benign oesophageal problems. Before my arrival as a consultant an oesophageal physiology laboratory had been begun under the direction of Ben Milstein. It was one of the first in the country. Calling it a laboratory is something of an exaggeration. All that we had was a mobile trolley with the equipment laden on top of it. At least it was mobile. As a result, we were able to assess and treat patients with acid reflux as a result of a hiatal hernia, offering full range of anti-reflux procedures and all of the dysmotility problems. These facilities were not available at Addenbrooke's at that time, and so we were taking patients from a wide area. I worked closely with Dr John Hunter, the senior gastroenterologist at Addenbrooke's. Between us we dealt with some highly complex cases, many turned down or who had failed treatments at other places.

In the latter years of the 2000s, as general surgery was contracting with ever more super-specialisation, some general surgeons were vying for oesophageal cases and calling themselves upper G.I. tract surgeons, often with little real experience. The anomaly here was that few if any were trained in thoracic surgical techniques and the anatomical truth is that eighty percent of the oesophagus lies within the thorax. At that time, as director of thoracic services I had petitioned for a gastro-enterologist joint appointment between either Addenbrooke's or Huntingdon hospitals and ourselves. I was in the process of trying to reinvigorate the thoracic services at Papworth. I had managed to get several developments that I had sought, in reorganising the thoracic services (more of which later) through the management executive, but sadly they were not far-sighted enough to back this development. The result was inevitable. The physicians are the source of referrals in the NHS and as such control the flow of work.

Once surgeons claiming to be upper gastroenterological surgeons had been appointed to their institutions, the referrals flowed to them and away from us. This was a shame for our thoracic surgical trainees and indeed perhaps for the patients. As the general surgeons became more involved the oesophagectomy rate decreased in the region, and more tumours were simply held open with stents, in my view depriving some patients from a potentially curative procedure. Additionally, we slowly lost the benign service as well. Little or no regard was given by outside management to our excellent results. It was a significant lost opportunity for the unit.

A Sleepy Project and Other Developments

One of my thoracic physician colleagues John Shneerson was an international expert in respiratory support dealing with sleep apnoea and other conditions causing respiratory failure. In 1987 he had become interested in phrenic nerve palsy, which impaired diaphragmatic function in tetraplegic patients and some other conditions. Gerhard Baer, an anaesthetist, and Pasi Talonen, a physiologist and engineer working in the University of Tampere in Finland, had been developing a device for diaphragm pacing. John had established a working relationship with them and asked me to join him in the project.[5] My role as surgeon was to implant the electrodes around the phrenic nerves to stimulate the diaphragm rhythmically. The concept had first been developed by Professor William Glenn of Yale University. Glenn had also worked on an artificial heart and was a very respected cardiac surgeon.

Developing the project required several trips to Tampere. The laboratory work was interesting, but the fun ensued in the evenings when I was taken out into the woods for Finnish Sauna. I had no idea what I was letting myself in for. We drove for more than an hour into the forests around Tampere and stopped on the banks of one of the more than 1,000 lakes that Finland is famous for. During my first visit there was deep snow on the ground. We parked in the woods and entered a non-descript wooden building: the sauna. The scented wood was beautiful and the warmth very inviting after the biting cold outside. Once inside, I was surprised to find everyone stripping all their clothes with great excitement and loud chattering voices. With British reserve suppressed, I joined in. We entered the sauna, something of which I had had no previous experience. I was told that the real men sat on the top bench, in the greatest heat.

In attempt to keep the British sangfroid, I joined the hardy Finns. It was hot, very hot. Sweat began pouring from every surface of my skin, dripping from my forehead as though in a shower. After what seemed like an age, and with a loud whoop, they sprang up and headed for the exit. Just outside were small spirit glasses, which contained a colourless liquid. As each one passed, he grabbed a glass and swiftly drank it in one move. I followed their lead. Raw spirit hit the back of my throat like a flamethrower. Reeling from the shock I ran after them. They continued to head, naked, down a wooden path to the lake where they all jumped in. I followed. It was freezing. After a great deal of shouting and laughter and with testicles now firmly re-imbedded on my posterior abdominal wall, we climbed out and headed back into the sauna. This was repeated over and over, the number of times I lost count of. Each time singing of Finnish folk songs broke out. As my blood 'spirit' level rose and any remaining inhibitions disappeared, I couldn't resist contributing a few British songs – Auld Lang Syne, the national anthem and Rule Britania. To their great credit they all joined in with me at the top of their voices. On the way back to the hotel, a journey that I remember little of, I do recall them telling me that on one occasion with the lake frozen over, they had lost a colleague under the ice. It was his last sauna. I was glad to learn of it on the way home.

Back at Papworth, we began the programme and patients were selected for the procedure. It was simple in principle, but fiddly in practice. Pasi and Gerhardt travelled to Cambridge for each implant and became good friends. The programme came to an end when we discovered resistance building up around the electrodes on the phrenic nerve, causing early failure of the device.

We went on to develop a programme of intra-tracheal oxygen [ITOC] catheters to help patients with chronic respiratory failure. This was an alternative to the use of nasal cannulae or facemasks giving the patients more comfort. We developed a method of tunnelling the catheter to overcome problems of catheter displacement and fracture.[6] It was an interesting time of new ideas.

It was an exciting period with new adventures popping up constantly. The surgical technique of first rib resection for patients (almost always very young) with compression of important nerves in the neck was practiced by few surgeons in the UK. The condition is called thoracic outlet [or inlet] syndrome. Ben had developed this to a fine art, removing the rib through the armpit with a small incision. At first sight, this is quite a scary procedure as you found yourself operating through a small dark hole shaped like a cone, with very important structures deep within it at the cone's apex. The instruments needed to free up the rib and to remove it were large and long. Behind the rib were the artery, vein and nerves that supplied the arm. One slip could cause the functional loss of this limb. In this condition, the artery and nerves to the arm are compressed in a scissors-like manner between the clavicle [collar bone] and the first rib. There are two principle types: neurogenic and vascular. Occasionally in very severe cases, both obtend in the same patient.

In the neurogenic type, the symptoms are radiating pain and electric shock-type sensations along the arm and into the hands. In the vascular type, there is restriction to blood flow in and out of the arm. Both can be quite debilitating and are still underdiagnosed. By excising the first rib, the previously compressed nerves from the cervical spine, the brachial plexus and its cords and branches, the artery and vein to the arm can drop down into the space that is created, thereby removing the compressive force on them and relieving the symptoms. Despite being able to give sufferers enormous relief. It was offered by no other surgeons that I knew of in the country. Therefore the potential referral base was huge. It was quite a scary operation in the hands of the untrained and required a good knowledge of anatomy and a steady hand. This axillary incision gave a very acceptable, almost invisible, cosmetic result. To achieve the best exposure an assistant was needed to stand on a step, 2–3 feet high, to wrap their arms in a convoluted way around the flexed elbow of the patient who was positioned on their side. If the height difference was correct the arm could be elevated simply by the assistant standing up straight. This eliminated the likelihood of the arm being lowered as the case progressed, thus obstructing the view. Meanwhile the surgeon had to burrow up to the first rib, strip off the attached muscles to the very front and back of the rib without damaging the major artery, vein and nerves that ran over it. Then to introduce a long pair of shears right up to the cervical origin of the rib and sheer it off, repeating the exercise at the front. Needless to say, the sight of such a procedure frightened many surgeons. For a while I travelled around various thoracic surgery departments demonstrating the procedure.

The results, however, were excellent. One young lady stands out in my mind. She was a second-year medical student who was getting such terrible pain in both of her arms and hands that she was on the verge of giving up her studies. She had visited several other physicians and thoracic or vascular surgeons but had been told that there was nothing wrong with her and that there was nothing that could be done. She sobbed uncontrollably when I informed her that I thought I could help her, but to be safe we would do the side of her non-dominant hand first. The result was excellent and after completing the other side, the young woman was transformed. She graduated as a doctor, fulfilling her ambition.

Thoracic Surgeon to the RAF

Shortly after my appointment to the Papworth staff, I was asked to be the consultant thoracic surgeon to the RAF in Ely. This was the hospital for air force personnel and their families. Papworth was the most local thoracic unit. It had been one of two RAF hospitals from 1940. As leader of thoracic surgical services at Papworth, it was a natural appointment. Soon after accepting the (unpaid) post I was summoned to RAF Coningsby for an induction course. Coningsby is a quick reaction alert base with squadrons of fighter jets on site, ready to respond at a moment's notice. It had been the home of 617 squadron, also known as the Dambusters, and later a 'V' bomber base, and more recently the home of the RAF Battle of Britain memorial flight. It was the base that I had visited as a teenager in the combined cadet force.

After a morning of lectures on various scenarios and an excellent lunch I was taken out for some 'field work'. A fighter jet (a Tornado) had supposedly crash-landed at the base and the pilot was trapped in the aircraft with the jet engine still running. I had to approach the aircraft with the rescue crew and to assist in the extraction and first aid for the injured pilot. With no instructions of how to approach the aircraft, I suddenly heard the officer in charge shout out 'You're dead'. Apparently, I was in just the right position to be sucked into the jet engine and shredded like confetti, not a comfortable thought. After having been told of the correct approach and how to open the canopy, we set about extracting the pilot and applying first aid. Practical instruction aside, a good time was had by all and after further education of how to behave around a 'live' jet we adjourned for well-earned drinks and dinner in the mess. Thankfully, I was never summoned to such an emergency. My most frequent duties were treating airmen and women with spontaneous pneumothorax and a few other minor surgical conditions. Eventually, in 1992 the medical base moved from Ely to Peterborough and my tenure of the post in Ely ended, but I was invited to continue to back up the Peterborough section. This resulted in the referral of a lot of American personnel, a whole other challenge, not least for reimbursement.

Since my appointment in 1985, I had developed a large mitral valve reconstruction practice, more of which later, and could repair almost all patients' valves with, what is conveniently referred to as, degenerative valve disease. This name implies an actual degenerative disease state within the valve tissues, but realistically it is the result of poor distribution of forces upon a congenitally malformed valve which closes under high pressure. I was able to apply this experience to young RAF pilots with this condition. This allowed them to continue with their life-long ambition and keep flying, the source of their very strong self-identity. Replacing the mitral valve with prosthetic valves in younger adults, raises the spectrum of relatively early failure of the prosthetic valve, particularly if it is a tissue valve. The alternative of mechanical valves commits the recipient to a life of drugs to reduce the rate at which the blood clots, thereby raising another range of potential complications and grounding the pilot. The tissue valves are derived from pigs. The valve that is used is the aortic valve, which is then mounted in a circular metal stent with a Dacron and foam coating to allow the placement of retaining stitches. An alternative is ox pericardium fashioned into valve leaflets which are then similarly mounted to enable sewing into the heart aperture between atrium and ventricle. They are individually hand made by highly skilled workers sitting in long rows in large high grade sterile rooms in California. The level of skill that these technicians (usually female) exhibit is higher than that which most surgeons can reproduce. They are high quality seamstresses producing life giving devices.

The implantation of either type of these prosthetic devices will prevent pilots from flying military or civilian aircraft because of the risk of catastrophic failure. As a result I had a steady stream of pilots both military and commercial referred to me for reconstructive surgery. With their mitral valves repaired, and after a relatively short period of rehabilitation, they all returned to active duty. Each of them gave me some wonderful images of either their aircraft or themselves in flying gear. They seemed to be competing with each other to present the most impressive gifts. I have some wonderful pictures as a result.

After several years of treating them, many of the pilots came together to arrange a special treat for me to say thank you. Shortly after an initial contact I received an invitation to visit RAF Yeovil. I was asked to be there by 8.00 a.m. Not knowing quite what to expect I set off in the early hours. The day began with a welcome breakfast, forces style, accompanied by several flight officers that I recognised. They were all back on full flying duties after their surgery. After breakfast I was taken to a briefing room where I was informed that I would be spending the morning on a flight simulator for an Apache helicopter. The chief instructor for the RAF with the flight controller for the simulator guided me through it. It was very exciting, learning to take off, hover and to try landing on the deck of an aircraft carrier. There is the usual joystick for left and right turns, a rudder bar to correct yaw and a massive lever like a handbrake to the left of the pilot's seat, which increased or decreased the rotor speed. The rate of ascent felt incredible. I didn't try the opposite direction for obvious reasons. Succeeding, initially, in an imitated flat calm, they dialled up the weather to a mild gale, and things became very much more difficult. It was a morning of high concentration, some drama and a lot of fun. My spectacular crash into the ocean in a high gale was mercilessly painless.

We then adjourned for lunch in the officers' mess. This was a very grand affair as there were a group of pilots about to be deployed to Afghanistan in attendance, along with the camp commander and some of my ex-patients. The conversation was lively with the excitement of the moment, and I felt very lucky to witness that group, and had a real feeling of pride that these young men and one young woman were my compatriots. Excellent wine was on offer, but disappointingly none was given to me. I was soon to discover why. After drinking, the health and good fortune of the pilots leaving for their tour of Afghanistan, I was taken over to the first-floor window. The camp commander pointed down to the tarmac outside. There was an ominously black Apache helicopter sitting there. The commander turned to me and said, 'That is your aircraft for the afternoon, sir.' I was stunned into silence and filled with excitement and not a little apprehension.

I was then taken to a changing room, where I was fitted out with a flying suite and helmet. I was introduced to the chief instructors for both the Marines and the RAF. I was going to be in very good hands. We walked over to the helicopter and climbed on board. I was settled into the right-hand front seat with the chief instructor on my left in the number one seat. The rotors were fired up and I was invited to place my hands gently on the controls, with actual control in the hands of the instructor. We rose slowly to about 50 feet, the helicopter was turned to face the officers' mess and there were the pilots now watching on the balcony as we dipped the nose in salute, whereupon they raised their arms to return the salute before we turned away and rose steadily to about 1,000 feet. It was extremely emotional and I had to fight back a tear in my eye, with a big lump in my throat we flew off towards Glastonbury Tor. As we were approaching, I was being encouraged to familiarise myself again with the controls. To my left-hand side was the large arm controlling the rotor speed; pull it upwards and the helicopter began to rise more quickly, lower it and the reverse happened. The other controls, the rudder bar and the joystick had the same effect as found on an aeroplane, something that I was fairly familiar with from my experience in Chipmunks in the RAF CCF.in the sixth form at school.

Once I had found my feet so to speak, the instructor said, 'OK, you have control. Now fly around the Tor maintaining a steady height.' Quite gingerly, I took over control and around we went in a large arc. After a full revolution, he said, 'Now, I'll show you how we do it in action.' Suddenly, the helicopter lurched to the left and accelerated in a very tight turn, such that you could feel the increasing G-force on the whole of the body. The aircraft shuddered violently, and we had turned 360 degrees in a very short time. We then set off along the M4 corridor and again I had control. Nearing Bristol we made a turn back towards Yeovil. When nearly there, we came to a disused airfield. We flew towards an old hangar and the instructor said, 'OK, let's see how you can do holding it at the hover.' There was quite a side wind with rain falling steadily. I gingerly took over the controls again and was able to hold it at about 100 feet facing in the right direction against the wind for about a minute. My instructor was pleased and then we set off on our final leg back to base. When almost there we rose to about 5,000 feet and came to a hover. I was instructed to look to my left for one final surprise. There, through the murk appeared two Harrier GR 4s closing at about 500 knots with the pilots at full salute. As they passed, the jet wash blew us backwards some yards and then they were gone. We returned to base. What a trip it had been.

We landed and had tea. In my imagination I could feel a little like my father's cousin Cyril Babbage in his Battle of Britain flight log, 'Scrambled at 3.00 p.m. found Jerries at 15,000 feet, engaged 2 ME 109s and back for tea!'

That evening was the Taranto night dinner. This important event in the life of the Royal Fleet Air Arm celebrated the attack by twenty-one fragile Fairy Swordfish on the bulk of the Italian fleet, moored off the port of Taranto. The 'Stringbags' as the Swordfish were otherwise known, were remarkably sturdy aircraft, which could 'hang around' for a considerable time in the air. On the evening of 11 November 1940, flying from the aircraft carrier Illustrious, the Swordfish in two strike wings one hour apart made their daring attack. The harbour was seriously damaged, and significant damage was inflicted on several Italian warships. Only one Swordfish was lost. There is credible evidence that the Japanese took a great interest in this first strike against the Italian navy and may have designed their actions against Pearl Harbor around it.

The evening was a black tie event and was unforgettable. Much fine wine was drunk and fun and games began early with a few thunder flash blank grenades rolled under the table accompanied by loud explosions. The evening continued into the early hours. The following morning was also memorable for the size of the headache, resolved with buckets of very black coffee and an excellent forces English breakfast. We said our goodbyes and I set off back to Cambridge with some very special memories. The men and women in our armed forces are special folk. I feel privileged to have been able to help them to keep their wings.

Some Skullduggery in the Chest Department

In late 1992 whilst serving on the Thoracic Services management group, word reached me that there were advanced discussions between our chest physicians and senior Addenbrooke's management, to move chest medicine from Papworth to the university teaching/district general hospital Addenbrooke's. The quoted reasons were firstly, that asthma, principally encountered in the young, was moving into the hands of the general practitioners. Secondly, that advanced inflammatory lung disease was seen in the older patients and was frequently accompanied by multiple other morbid conditions and therefore would be better managed in the general hospital setting and thirdly, lung cancer patients would be better managed in closer proximity to the oncology department. Also, patients needing respiratory sleep and other support (R.S.S.C. service) were being managed in Newmarket Hospital, where the service had been set up. The plan was to move those services to Addenbrooke's as well. This move would have eviscerated the thoracic services and effectively isolated thoracic surgery, which would have to follow. Thus threatened the continued coherence of Papworth. What to do?

After discrete enquiries, it became clear to me that this was likely to happen if there was no intervention. In addition, a letter had come into my possession, passed on by a loyal clinician at Addenbrooke's describing the plans for the move. The situation was even more fraught for me, as the chairman of the thoracic group at that time was a highly respected Papworth chest physician who was a great support to me and a friend. However, my loyalty to the unit overrode those emotions and with great trepidation, I reported these occult plans to Mr Bridge, the chief executive at that time. He agreed that we could not allow this to happen. The outcome was that the physicians implicated in this 'house coup' were called to account by the hospital management, and after initial denial, the letter was produced and the lie was revealed. Sadly, this resulted in the call for the chairman of the thoracic services group's resignation and a severe reprimand for the others. The coup had been defeated. I was asked to take over as chairman of the group.

A Major Reorganisation

Coincidentally, I had been referred a patient with the diagnosis of lung cancer, for whom only palliative care was appropriate. Looking back through the patient's notes it was clear that the patient had been so long in the system that any chance of meaningful treatment had been lost. The time from initial visit to his GP was over eighteen months. It had taken several months to get past the putative diagnosis of pneumonia, with multiple courses of inappropriate antibiotics and return visits to the surgery with cough, loss of weight and coughing blood. Eventual referral was to the Accident and Emergency department, and only then onward referral to a general physician and hospital admission. The patient was very belatedly passed on to a physician whose specialty was for the care of the elderly. (The patient was in his early seventies.) Only after a further period in their hands was he referred to me for a thoracic surgical opinion. There had been no attempt to diagnose the clearly visible tumour with tissue biopsy, nor to gauge the extent of the disease. This was clearly quite unacceptable, but on wider discussion with colleagues it became clear that this sequence of events was more common than should be the case in a modern medical society. Also, it brought home to me just how far behind we were in the management of lung cancer when compared with the rest of Europe and the USA.

I began to think about what I would want for me or a member of my family in such circumstances. It was pretty obvious that the speed of diagnosis was paramount, and then for the tumour to be accurately staged before being passed onto the hands of the appropriate specialist with the minimum of delay. Following presentation to the GP, full history and examination, an early chest radiograph with an expert's report should be followed by referral into a specialist unit if the patient had possible signs of a malignancy. I had the notion that a suspicious GP should be able to make an urgent referral which would allow the patient to be seen at the start of the following week, where full and detailed investigation would be done, and a biopsy of any lesion could be completed. In addition, appropriate counselling and a detailed explanation of what was likely to follow, would all be fitted into that first appointment. All results were to be collated and ready to be imparted to the patient by the Thursday of the same week. In other words, a 'two-stop shop'. At that second appointment the treatment plan would be put in place. For this to be brought into operation, we needed to completely rearrange the working week of several of the physicians and radiologists, and to appoint cancer specialists and specialist radiologists.

Also, to overcome the claims of our wayward physicians I wanted to introduce up to date specialist areas to cope with the changing world of chest medicine. One of these, was to service patients who had cystic fibrosis moving on from childhood into teenage and adult life; an adult cystic fibrosis unit so that the 'grown-ups' would not have to sit with the children and their differing needs. On the back of this development, it seemed sensible to have a specialist unit for inflammatory and infectious lung diseases.

Thirdly, it seemed another obvious development was to move the respiratory support unit (the RSSC) from Newmarket into Papworth, rather than the proposed move to Addenbrooke's. Finally, I wanted to develop the oesophageal services further as mentioned earlier.

I prepared a lengthy paper to these ends and presented the ideas to the board of the hospital. They listened intently and to my surprise supported all of these developments other than the appointment of the gastroenterologist which seemed to be one step too far for them.

Having got these ideas past the hospital board, there was then a huge amount of work to do to make all of it happen. Much of it was surprisingly easy and we seemed to be pushing at an open door. The main initial obstacle came in the form of the Public Health Director at that time. Generally, the outcome for patients with lung cancer was awful in Britain for the reasons outlined, namely complete lack of focus.

We have always lagged behind several countries in Europe where the disease was being diagnosed much earlier, making effective treatment much more available. Also, there was a nihilistic attitude towards the disease held by many physicians. This was revealed to me in a very surprising way. At the first meeting with the Director of Public Health for the Cambridge area, I laid out the case for the development, and was horrified to hear him say that the health authority was going to remove funding from the management of lung cancer because the results were so bad. This was diametrically opposed to my ideas for the modern development of a programme of treatment for this disease and the direction of travel in the USA and on the continent of Europe. I was deflated by this seemingly ignorant proposal but hoped that it was said partly with his tongue in his cheek and that he was goading me to make the case for development. Fortunately, I had taken my computer with me, and at that point I was able to show him the results of properly staged patients who were operated on in early-stage cancer from European and North American studies. I was able to convince him that the proposed plan was utterly wrong and what we needed was appropriately targeted funding for the modern management of the disease. He listened intently, following my arguments carefully and, being an academic himself, he rapidly reversed his initial position and agreed that we could develop the plan and represent it to him when in its final form. A sign of intellectual strength is the ability to reverse an opinion in the face of good evidence, and I will always be grateful to him for that change of heart.

We were up and running, but we needed the support of the GPs to ensure early referral. In addition, we needed the facilities for a service that could respond appropriately to the increased volume of referrals that would inevitably occur, and in a timely fashion. Therefore my next plan was to organise a meeting with as many of the local GP leads in our region as possible. Mr Bridge, our chief executive, was very supportive. The trick was to make it look as though the demand for improved service came from them, the frontline of medicine.

With Mr Bridge's approval we hired the conference room at Madingley Hall, near to Cambridge, and I asked several of the GPs to present the problems from their perspective. The public health team were in attendance and with up to date oncological and surgical data, the case was forcefully made. Support began to come from all quarters. The one remaining temporary obstruction was from Addenbrooke's. We needed the support of the Regius Professor's office. That ancient position was founded by Henry VIII in 1540. It is a powerful position in Cambridge medicine and clearly we weren't going to move forwards without their support. Perhaps I was too strident in my views, and the initial response was once again depressingly negative. I was not going to take no for an answer as I felt passionate about the need for that development. Further meetings pressing the case were arranged and with the support of my chest physician colleagues, and Papworth management, we received the final go ahead to develop the service.

Oncologists and chest physicians with a special interest in lung malignancy were appointed, along with specialist nurses. It was clear to me that we needed the support of the wonderful MacMillan palliative care nurses who were so expert in managing patients with advanced disease, and who could bring end-of-life support when needed. In conjunction with this, I felt that a 24-hour hotline for worried patients and their relatives was an extremely important facility. This would enable them to call for help and support whenever they were significantly concerned. All of this was put in place. None of it could have been accomplished without the willing support of everyone involved, which included the management team.

I have previously mentioned the need for a CT scanner. That expensive but vital piece of equipment was needed to enable the proper staging process of the disease. Whilst in Alabama, my good friend Dr. Eamon Braetnach had been one of the pioneers in the development of the radiological staging of the disease, enabling appropriate treatment. The scanner was central to this. Indeed perhaps the most important development in the management of cancer has been the introduction of accurate disease staging. Here was a problem. How to find the very large sum of money, over one million pounds, for the initial outlay for a state-of-the-art scanner. Dr Richard Coulden was one of our best radiologists who had a deep interest in this area. Working closely together we came up with the idea of hiring out the use of the scanner in the evenings and weekends to support the orthopaedic surgeons at Hinchingbrooke, the closest district general hospital. They were keen to gain access to the scanner and the combined income allowed us to make the purchase. All that was left then was to organise the rotas of consultants and nursing staff to cover the service. Senior consultants, reputationally difficult to organise, all willingly changed their weekly programmes to make the service work. This included those not directly involved in the lung cancer programme, who also obligingly moved their schedule, allowing the flexibility that was required. The esprit de corps was excellent, creating an environment that greatly enhanced the general patient care.

We were then able to offer a very streamlined service. Once a patient had seen his or her GP with symptoms and signs suspicious of malignancy, an appointment was made for the patient to be seen on the Monday of the following week. Thus no patient would wait for longer than one week to be seen by a specialist. All tests would be completed on that day and reported by the Thursday of the same week. Our oncology multi-disciplinary team met on Thursday morning of the same week to discuss the patient and to arrange the next steps in the management of each patient to be planned. That same afternoon, the patients with their families were seen in the outpatient clinic and informed of the results and the plans for them. Specialist nurses were on hand to offer emotional support and to answer any further questions.

This new service reduced the mean waiting times from first suspicion to treatment for patients with lung cancer from 6.5 months to 3.5 weeks. A huge improvement. Its impact on patients was recognised with an NHS award from Frank Dobson, the then secretary for state for health. Furthermore, it was complimented on the floor of the House of Commons, and as such is recorded in Hansard as the gold standard for treatment. My first major success in policy change. It was more exhilarating than a successfully completed operation and to this day is one of my proudest achievements. It has grown enormously from that early start and remains one of the foremost cancer services in the United Kingdom.

Cystic Fibrosis

As discussed, the old guard of chest physicians had attempted to desert Papworth and move to Addenbrooke's, citing the increasing reducing relevance of chest medicine at Papworth. In my attempt to counter these criticisms, I had begun to think of ways to make Papworth more relevant in the modern thoracic medicine world. I knew a lovely family who had two out of three children with Cystic Fibrosis, a terribly debilitating disease that manifests with thick obstructing mucous production in the lungs and the bowel. Their lives could be a miserable round of repeated chest infections and hospital admissions with a significantly reduced life span. I searched the literature on the current state of the management of the disease for these unfortunate children. It soon became clear to me that, happily, survivorship was improving dramatically, and more were surviving into young adulthood and later. As far as I could see, other than in Manchester, all patients with the disease were seen in the same clinics, children and adults together. It seemed to me to be likely that their needs would be different and that we had an opportunity to develop an adolescent and adult service at Papworth.

I presented the idea to the board, and it was accepted as a welcome new development. We then set about finding and appointing the necessary staff. Most importantly was the physician to lead the specialty. There were two excellent candidates in the running. One heavily orientated to research, and the other a very warm physician, also with a good clinical research portfolio, whom I thought would be the right person to build and bond a team. The day of the interview arrived.

The interviewing committee was large, with thirteen members. It included representatives from the teaching hospital, chief among them the Regius Professor of Physic and our own chairman and chief executive. As the interviews progressed it became clear that the Addenbrooke's contingent were heavily biased by the CV of the researcher. Other than me, our side seemed complacent and willing to follow their lead. Finally with the interviewing over, it came to the discussion and the vote. The first round of voting went twelve to one against my preferred candidate. I was not happy. I felt that we were heading down the wrong path and I began my challenge. After over an hour of discussion, the vote swung in favour of my candidate. Triumph! As we rose to leave the Regius was grunting about the lack of appreciation for research at Papworth and the chairwoman, whom I was sitting next to, wrote in her notes, in Latin, 'This is a black day for Papworth,' [hoc est niger dies in Papworth], thinking that I wouldn't understand. Suddenly, those years of school Latin, 'bonus bona bonum, etc.,' became of use. I whispered in her ear, 'We shall see.' Following the meeting Stephen Bridge, the chief executive, wrote to me:

5.10.1993
Dear Frank.

Now that we have successfully appointed Dr. Bilton may I say how grateful I am to you for your tremendous efforts in bringing about this achievement.

Not only have you put in a tremendous amount of time with your shuttle diplomacy between the various partners concerned, but right through to the end, i.e. in the actual interview room you demonstrated your commitment to making this post work and ensuring that we got the best candidate.

I know that Audrey Stenner is also appreciative of your efforts and admires your articulate and persuasive manner in arguing your case.

Obviously, as you made this one look so easy, I will have to find you a more difficult one in the future!

Kind regards

Steve

I continued to build the programme for development of the service and was invited to present to the board my ideas. This went well and sometime later, the chairwoman Audrey Stenner wrote the following:

25.05.1995

Dear Frank

I want to thank you for the talk you gave to the board this morning, which was exactly what I wanted in that it was both a review of previous objectives and a look to the future. Excellent.

The whole board joins me in thanking you for this morning's impressive presentation.

Audrey

Dianna Bilton was a wonderful success and came to command the respect and affection of all, patients, relatives and staff alike. Her retirement many years later was met with real sadness.

I continued as clinical director of the thoracic unit for another six years until 2001, during which time we were able to develop all of the modernised sub-specialties other than the gastro-enterologist post. As a result, the oesophageal service evaporated and with it a significant body of expertise.

From the outset of my consultant career, I had a full practice of thoracic and cardiac surgery with a sprinkling of vascular surgery. Within the sub-specialty of cardiac surgery, I always found valve surgery interesting. There had been a steady evolution of alternatives for valve replacements. From the very early ball-in-cage type devices to what we affectionately called the toilet seat valve, the Bjork-Shiley single tilting disc valve. That valve was very successful and had excellent flow characteristics. The housing for the single tilting disc was made of titanium, with the supporting struts welded to it. Then one day, in an attempt to improve haemodynamic function, the design was changed in a way that increased the forces on the struts that then began to fracture. This was against the advice of the engineers who predicted that metal fatigue would be a real risk. Disaster. In a very short time, the welds began to break, releasing the carbon occluding disc to escape into the aorta of exposed patients. The result was a massive and sudden regurgitation of blood into the left ventricle of the heart, causing the patients to collapse in heart failure. There were deaths and as the news spread, patients and their relatives began to panic.[7]

Their spouses were buying stethoscopes to listen to the replacement valve of their loved one, even going so far as to stay awake for most of the night listening and waiting for disaster to strike. I had chosen not to use that valve, so none of my patients were vulnerable. This was payback for following the excellent advice of Dr Kirklin in Alabama, 'Pick a valve that has been around for a long time and use it for a long time.' Colleagues received many phone calls from worried patients at all times of the day and night. Multiple lawsuits followed and the valve was withdrawn from the marketplace. The company made things worse for themselves by being slow to admit the problem and indeed tried to blame a fictitious engineer for faulty welding. This was followed by an iteration with a single strut cast in one piece of metal which was an excellent valve, but sadly the name of the company had been tarnished so badly by the experience and the massive lawsuits that followed that this valve too was withdrawn.

A different solution to the problem was the double tilting disc valve, which had butterfly-like wings, produced by a company in Minnesota. It was designed with the help of Dr Walt Lillehei, and it completely changed the game. Marketed, somewhat tongue in cheek, with the name of St Jude, 'the patron saint of lost causes and hopeless causes', it rapidly became the market leader and has remained a successful valve ever since, with other companies copying the basic principles. The valve leaflets are made from pyrolite carbon. A material pure in carbon atoms and cast at very high temperatures in a strong magnetic field. This causes the atoms to align perfectly, producing an ultra-smooth surface, which is resistant to clot formation in the blood stream. It is the same material from which the heat-resistant tiles on the underside of the space shuttle are made. They can resist atmospheric re-entry temperatures of 17,500 degrees centigrade. It amused the patients to think that should they find themselves entering the earth's atmosphere unprotected, at that speed their valve would survive, but sadly they would not.

Over the last forty years, the valve market has been beset with many new valve types, a lot of which have fallen by the wayside through underperformance. Staying with established well-functioning technology and not chasing the limelight with newer developments remains my gold standard. Let others deal with early valve failure. It is astonishing to me how easily so many colleagues are tempted into that trap.

The Mitral Valve

The mitral valve was so named by the sixteenth century anatomist Andreas Vesalius, because in his eyes there was great similarity between the up-turned mitral valve and a bishop's mitre. He wrote the following in his magnum opus *De Humani Corporis Fabrica*, published in Basel in1543:

> Because of the membranous circle of the venous artery, the left atrium, is split into only two membranes you would not be wrong in comparing them to a Bishop's Mitre if you compare the part encircling the head to the membranous circle and its processes to the front and the back points of the Mitre.

His description defined the characteristics of the valve, being of two principal leaflets and the sub-valve apparatus of the cords and papillary muscles.

The first person to describe the role of the atrioventricular valves in supporting the function of the ventricles and not just as a flow control was Leonardo da Vinci. He did not publish his work, and his revelations lay dormant for the next 300 years. My interest in that Renaissance genius has fuelled a cross fertilisation of ideas that continues to stimulate and invigorate specialists across the world in many fields of endeavour, even today.

Thoracic and cardiac surgery are very different entities. Thoracic surgery is more akin to general surgery, with a wide variety of potential problems involving the lungs, the chest wall, diaphragm, the other intra-thoracic contents such as the oesophagus, the thymus, thyroid gland, the parasympathetic and sympathetic nerve chains and the chest wall itself. Practised comprehensively, it demands the knowledge and ability to work not only within the chest but also below the diaphragm and in the neck. It encompasses a sound knowledge of oncology to deal with the many malignancies that the thoracic surgeon will be confronted with, and he or she must have the ability to discuss knowledgeably with the oncologists. Multi-disciplinary teams are, quite rightly, here to stay. At one extreme the thoracic surgeon is important in gaining tissue for diagnosis and the staging of a tumour, and at the other he, and more frequently these days, she, are the only ones that can offer the highest likelihood of cure of an early-stage malignancy, with its complete and timely removal.

Cardiac surgery on the other hand is more akin to fine modelling to correct morbid anatomical changes within the heart. One of my earliest mentors Christopher Lincoln, a fine paediatric heart surgeon, was wont to say, in a loud voice,

> Wells, all you need, to be a good heart surgeon, is the ability to place a stitch accurately, in any position and at any time, and the mentality of someone who enjoys making model aeroplanes.

There is a lot of truth in this. Patience and accuracy, with the ability to persist and focus with intense concentration in potentially stressful situations, often for many hours, is essential. An obsessive/compulsive personality is helpful. Also the ability to question yourself, and to undo, and to do again something that doesn't look just right is essential. In the modern world it is common to work through more than one shift of nurses and indeed, these days, trainee doctors, all of whom work to set shift patterns. Sadly for modern trainees, this does dilute their training experience in an already shortened training programme. It was common to work a full day in the operating theatre, then to find yourself dealing with complex and stressful emergencies through the night with a patient's life on the line, only to carry on into the next day with another full list. None of us complained about that as we had been brought up to see it as the job. Today, that has been largely stopped for all but the consultant staff.

Something that the general public and the hospital managers have not grasped nor really tried to understand is the performance status of a surgical operation. We speak of 'performing' an operation and indeed there is an element of performance in it. Performance stress is a real thing, and not really accounted for by surgeons in general, nor dealt with in the training and preparation of young surgeons for the task ahead of them. Musicians, high performing athletes and other groups working at a high stress levels spend time preparing themselves for their performance or event. There is none of that in surgery. Indeed it is still regarded as not having the 'right stuff' to speak of such soft ideas. Talking of these things is commonly regarded as a weakness in this high ego environment and thus not discussed. Yet the toll on the surgeon can be huge and carry through to personal lives, destroying relationships and rendering the surgeon open to challenge over what is externally seen as bad behaviour, when it is actually a human being under great stress. Preparation for any cerebral-manual task is essential in so many other walks of life and yet that doesn't occur in surgery.

Performance anxiety needs to be addressed. Professor Roger Kneebone, professor of surgical education at Imperial College London has formed a centre for 'performing in science' and has demonstrated how being able to deal with performance anxiety is crucial in the specialty. When an operation has been particularly stressful and complex it is really essential for the surgeon to have time to sort their thoughts out afterwards. Practically every surgeon is left on their own with no time to reflect on performance. Focus is on completing the paperwork and then pushing on with the next case, driven by the demands of management who have a poor understanding of what is involved in our profession.

This can be a very lonely experience, especially with the amount of litigation that hangs as a sword of Damocles over some unfortunate surgeons. The situation is amplified in many surgical departments nowadays with the advent of the hot desk area, where the surgeon has no private space in which to reflect on the procedure just completed, or as is often the case, to take a short break to rest a little and recoup for the completion of a long and demanding case.

The lack of appreciation by management of these issues and to try to understand the reality of the life of a surgeon is thoughtless, and sometimes cruel. Their attention is too focussed on bottom line finances and patient turnover, and less on caring for the staff and thence the care of the patients. To ask for help is one step away from suspension for inability to perform appropriately. Hence it is not surprising that no one wants to talk about it.

In an attempt to address some of these issues, several years ago I arranged weekend retreats for trainees at a hotel in the middle of the country. The time to think through a procedure or general management of a patient, followed by a much longer period of discussion between trainees and consultants revealed a lot of hidden anxieties. Learning to deal with these stresses is very important. The situation in the modern health service is compounded by the frequent lack of adequately skilled and knowledgeable supportive staff. Elite performance, which dissecting another human being demands, requires the appropriate level of support from the other staff in the operating theatre. Too often that is not available. Everyone in the theatre environment has to realise that everything that goes on in that room is for the patient, the most important person present. Too often discipline is lax and the pressure on the surgeon can mount exponentially in that situation.

The development of health care as a business model carries a huge responsibility in worsening the situation. In our old hospital, our chief executive Stephen Bridge had a great sense of corporate care and at the end of every week could be found going round his consultants (mainly surgical as the physicians had largely gone home by 6.00 p.m.) to enquire how we were and how he could help us. The current management are rarely, if ever, seen and yet are very quick to criticise, causing them to lose the respect of their surgical consultant staff, whilst piling the pressure onto them. In a broken health service as is the case in Britain today, the pressure to perform in inadequate facilities is huge and good for neither patients nor staff.

Cynical non-cardiac surgeons have fun suggesting that there are only four or five operations in the specialty: coronary artery bypass, valve replacement and valve repair for some, with the occasional myxoma thrown in. Of course, this is not true, in addition to which, the variation in the presentations of these conditions and the demands on the surgeon vary enormously. Then there are all of the congenital abnormalities that the paediatric heart surgeon has to deal with. In every case, the life of the patient is on the line and mortality in the specialty has been an issue over the years, highlighted in the Bristol Babies affair. We were the first specialty to report in the public domain, each surgeon's mortality for public scrutiny. There was a suggestion that this caused some surgeons to turn down the more at-risk cases, but with excellent risk stratification of patients now available that is less of a problem. Our colleague at Papworth, Samer Nashef has done a fine job in producing one of the most useful risk scoring systems, used internationally, the Euroscore. This allows sensible analysis of the pre-operative risk for most patients treated in significant volumes, and for a sensible discussion of outcomes, including death, with the patient and relatives.

It is true, that as a seventeen year old, the idea of being able to successfully transplant the human heart triggered my nascent interest in cardiac surgery, but it never became my first love. However, working at Papworth meant that I needed to be involved in the transplant programme. Of course, a good outcome is wonderful for the person involved and I have never felt negative about the complete change in life that a new working heart and/or lung(s) can offer someone at the edge of life and their families, and I am a wholehearted supporter of the practice. It's just that for me, there are more interesting and challenging procedures that demand more surgical expertise. There are truly wonderful outcomes from transplantation, beautifully illustrated by a patient into whom I transplanted a new heart over thirty years ago, He has recently passed his ninety-third year and is still playing golf three times a week and shooting regularly in season. He wrote the following to me, inviting me to a most important birthday,

> Dear Mr Wells, I am planning to celebrate my 90th birthday together with the 31st anniversary post-transplant. I would be delighted if you and your partner can join me and my family on that day, kind regards, Ted Warner.

Once the surgery is completed, the ongoing management of the patient is largely the responsibility of the transplant physicians, making sure that the patient stays on the tight rope, balancing between infection and rejection. In recent years the advances in post-operative management have been enormous and the results are quite startling compared to the early days, with five-year survival of over ninety percent now the norm.

Much of the media hype surrounding the procedure of heart transplantation stems from the medieval idea that the soul, and through that spirituality, is intimately linked to the heart. For much of history, touching the heart was seen as something reserved for the gods and their representatives on Earth. Think of the rituals of the Inca people and many others. This attitude permeated into the practice of medicine until well into the late nineteenth and early twentieth centuries. The famous German general surgeon Theodor Bilroth is often quoted as saying that he who operates on the human heart deserves the scorn of his colleagues. His remarks were limited to early and fumbling attempts to repair injury to the heart, usually in the form of a stab wound or draining fluid from the pericardial space around the organ. The means to differentiate between a big heart and a heart surrounded by fluid did not exist, other than by informed clinical examination.

Many patients were killed by large bore needles injuring the heart, resulting in severe haemorrhage and death by tamponade of the heart. A similar claim was said to have been made against Sir Henry Souttar, a British surgeon who performed the first mitral valve operation in 1924 when he opened what he assumed was a valve narrowed by rheumatic disease. It has been a popular claim that Souttar was not referred any further patients because the physicians that he worked with accused him of operating on the seat of the soul. In fact, research by Professor Tom Treasure has demonstrated that the predominate lesion of the valve was of regurgitation and stretching it made the situation worse.[8] Despite this, she lived on for another seven years with some improvement of symptoms.

I have always enjoyed the challenge of reconstructing structures and the artistic qualities that it demands. As mentioned earlier, paediatric surgery had been my first love but when I would have been ready for a consultant's job, it was likely that there would be no vacancies in what is a very small specialty.

Thus, the reconstruction of heart valves beckoned. I had been very impressed by the Carpentier approach to the mitral valve presented in his honoured guest lecture to the American Association for Thoracic Surgery. From the start of my consultant post, I began to develop the skills that this practice demands. Alain Carpentier, worked in L'Hôpital Brussais in Paris with his wife Sophie, a biochemist with an interest in tissue preservation. They were so dedicated to their work that they lived in a relatively small flat on the top floor of the hospital for several years. Sophie Carpentier developed the biochemical concepts that led to the possibility of preserving the function of bioprosthetic valves. Her contribution cannot be underestimated.

Alain was working on a better understanding of the regurgitant (leaking) mitral valve and had devised a classification system of mitral valve dysfunction that he called the functional classification. The concept was simple but ingenious. He had grouped the observable valve lesions into three types with subclassifications that spoke directly to the lesions that the surgeon would encounter. To each he mapped a surgical solution. Type I is annular, or orifice dilatation or leaflet perforation. The treatment for which is the reduction in orifice size with a band sewn around the atrio-ventricular junction or patch repair of the hole in the leaflet. Type II is elongation of the supporting leaflet cords or papillary muscles or rupture of those structures. For each there was another set of solutions. Type III is leaflet restriction with rheumatic disease or ischaemic restriction, for which further solutions are described. This allowed the surgeon who infrequently dealt with such problems to have a logical approach to finding a solution but also allowed for comparison of results between surgeons and units.

This approach he disseminated to surgeons from around the world through a regular series of meetings called 'Le Club Mitrale'. These were organised by Judie Vivian, valve product manager for Edwards Laboratories, whose headquarters were in Irvine California. Judie was, and still is, a rare dynamo of energy, delightful and intelligent, who effortlessly moved between internationally renowned cardiac surgeons, charming all as she went, from the most polite to the most aggressive. The meetings were organised with great efficiency so that the attending surgeons had travel, accommodation and meals all organised in fine style.

Everyone could focus on studying Professor Carpentier's teaching. For the operations a special boom camera had been designed for the meetings and the resulting images were like none seen before. The observers in the gallery could see the valve very clearly. Normally measuring on average 3.5 to 4.0 cms, it was projected 6 feet in diameter. There was always a moderator in the audience interacting with Alain, who was wearing a headset and could speak directly to the audience describing every step of the procedure.

Patrick Perrier and Gilles Dreyfus were frequent local moderators and did a splendid job in keeping things lively and the questions focussed. After each case, Alain came to the lecture theatre and explained in great detail the procedure he had just completed and took endless questions, never losing patience and spending as long as it took to satisfy everyone's desire to learn. Each night there was a delicious meal in excellent restaurants in the centre of Paris hosted by Judie and her colleagues. Discussion on what we had witnessed went on well into the night. They usually lasted three days so that by the end of it we had seen a wide range of cases. Not all went smoothly, and we probably learnt more from the difficulties that we witnessed than the straight-forward cases. Occasionally, Alain joined the dinner festivities late, as he had to take the patient back to theatre and replace the valve. Further learning for all of us. Don't push too hard to repair, the long-term outcome for the patient is what matters most.

I had attended two of these meetings before being asked by Alain to be a moderator for future ones. These were very exciting times, hosting the questions and the interaction between Alain and the audience. Remembering that I was still very early in my career I found it a little humbling as I was expected to educate more senior surgeons from many different countries. My growing experience and desire for more knowledge, however, stood me in good stead to do that. Many enduring friendships were made through our fascination with the complexities of the mitral valve.

Back at Papworth, I had completed 100 repairs without complication and with a sound result. I chose to present the work to my local colleagues; a home audience is usually the most hostile that one can encounter, and this proved to be no different. Having presented my series with what external colleagues considered excellent results, two of the three consultants rose and accused me of experimenting on their patients and left the room. Only Michael Petch, the most junior consultant cardiologist there at the time rose to support me and the work that I was doing. I was delighted that the detractors were proved wrong with the passage of time. The paper was published in the *Heart* journal and the word began to spread. At that time in the late 1980s I was almost alone in the country repairing these valves with any regularity. However, to me it seemed the correct approach and I steadfastly continued, and my experience grew. The patients were not coming back for repeat surgery. At the same time, I was able to teach several of the trainees many of whom have gone on to be successful mitral surgeons around the country.

Soon I felt that the word needed to be spread further afield within the UK and other European countries and decided to organise a course along the lines of Club Mitrale at Papworth. Enter once again Judie Vivian who, with her employers Edwards, wholeheartedly supported me. We were given access to the same film crew as the one that helped with Alain's Club Mitrale.

My natural inclination was to ask Alain if he would be kind enough to help me and to moderate the course, reciprocating my role for him. We met at a European meeting, and I approached him to ask the question. His response was brisk and in the affirmative, asking how many he cases he wanted me to do. That was not the idea at all and when I said that I would be doing the surgery his response became negative, stating that he didn't work that way. I replied that what I wanted to achieve was a masterclass, with him being the master and me the pupil. He would guide me through the operation from the lecture room. It would be a different way to bring out the finer points of the surgery and also a chance to discuss options for surgical resolution of the lesions encountered. He thought for a moment and with a very broad smile, said, 'Ok, but on one condition'. I tentatively asked what that would be, having no idea what was coming next. 'I will do it provided that you find Napoleon's stomach for me.' I gulped with surprise but replied that we had a deal. With that he turned and joined another conversation. I found Judie and told her what had happened. I think that she was somewhat surprised that he had agreed to do it, as he had not worked with anyone outside Broussais in this area. I was left wondering just what I had let myself in for. As far as finding Napoleon's stomach was concerned, all that she could say was, 'Well, good luck with that,' with the thought in her mind that it was never going to happen.

The story behind Napoleon's stomach revolves around the fact that he died in British captivity. Following his defeat at the battle of Waterloo he was exiled as prisoner on the remote island of St Helena. The French complained that his British captors had poisoned him as all of the symptoms that he was complaining of could be confused with arsenic poisoning. Arsenic had been detected on analysis of his hair suggesting that was the case. However, in the nineteenth century, arsenic dyes were used in the preparation of flock wallpaper. The rooms in the house in which he was imprisoned were of this type. The arsenic detected in samples of his hair probably arose from that source and not a mendacious British jailer. Prior to his death he was reported as complaining of severe abdominal pain and weight loss with frequent vomiting. He had been given a mercurial drink the night before he died to try to help with his abdominal pain and this too raised suspicion of poisoning.

The post-mortem was carried out by a Corsican doctor Dr. Francesco Antommarchi, in the presence of sixteen people, which included seven British doctors. Severe ulceration of the stomach was found. The cause, gastric cancer, but myth clouded the truth for 200 years. On the bicentenary of his death, a review of the available data was carried out and the conclusion drawn that Napoleon had died of an ulcerating cancer of the stomach.

I did not have the benefit of this review and set out to find out for myself. I began by calling the museum curator of the Royal College of Surgeons in London but drew a blank. I was surprised to discover the lack of knowledge about the stomach, as I did know that the material from the post-mortem which included the stomach had been sent to the college. I continued my search through all of the other royal colleges in Scotland and Ireland but still drew a blank.

The planned date for the meeting was approaching and I was no nearer to having an answer. In desperation I called back to the London college and asked again, if they had any information on the death of Napoleon, and in particular did they have his stomach? The same curator that I had spoken to before, answered in the negative, but then paused and said, 'wait a minute the curator that was here before me and who has been in the curator's post for several decades is visiting today'. The phone was quiet for a while whilst I waited, and then I could hear voices in the background and the previous curator lifted the phone and spoke the magical words, 'I think I can help you.' Huge relief flooded over me. She went on to tell me that they had had Napoleon's stomach up until the Second World War. It had been kept as a part of the museum collection, which had been started in the eighteenth century, by the famous scientific surgeon John Hunter.

As the Nazi blitz of London began, most of Hunter's museum specimens had been moved for safety to Down House, Darwin's old home, then in the possession of the college. However, before everything could be moved, the college had been struck by a bomb and much had been destroyed, including the pot with Napoleon's stomach. Once again, I was deflated but she went on to tell me that they still had the written report from the post-mortem and photographs of the specimen. Would that do? 'You bet it will!' was my excited reply. She offered to send the information to me. Sure enough, two days later it all arrived by special delivery.

Triumphantly, I was able to call Alain and tell him of my success, and he agreed to keep his side of the bargain. The meeting was on. I named the meeting 'The French Correction' in his honour and mimicking the title of the film *The French Connection*. Thus, a series of Cambridge meetings was born; a Portuguese correction, a Canadian and two American corrections followed. The format of the meeting was in the style of Le Club Mitrale with the exception that I didn't pre-select the cases but took them in turn from my waiting list so that the reality of a surgeon's practice would be followed, and the master Alain Carpentier was in the audience and not operating. That task fell to me.

The day before the meeting began Professor Carpentier was awarded an honorary fellowship at the Royal College of Surgeons. It was the perfect occasion to present him with the evidence that Napoleon had died of advanced stomach cancer and not poisoning. We gathered together with Professor Sir Magdi Yacoub, in front of the statue of John Hunter in the entrance hall of the college for a small presentation ceremony. The information now resides in the Pompidou Museum in Paris.

The meeting was to start on the Thursday morning with a welcome reception in a Cambridge college the night before. During the day on the Wednesday I set up two trial cases so that the systems and connections to the lecture theatre could be tested. Alain was present and all went well. The meeting lasted for two and a half days. I had commandeered two parallel theatre sessions for each day. The day began with a lecture from Alain on his strategic approach to the valve. As my colleague Dr Len Shapiro presented the case, I readied myself in the operating theatre. We then went live with the surgery. An excellent senior trainee had opened the chest for me and prepared the patient for cardio-pulmonary bypass. As I scrubbed in, I must admit some feelings of trepidation. I began to expose the valve and go through assessment and demonstrated the findings to the audience. Alain was extremely supportive, and his comments were all very valuable both to the audience and to me. The first case was relatively straight forwards, and all went well with a perfect repair at the end of the procedure. Once done I went down to the lecture room to join the audience for more detailed discussion.

Whilst that was happening another senior trainee was setting up the second case, and I returned to the operating theatre to start again. The same format was followed and the surgery proceeded under the watchful eye of Alain. The second case was similarly straightforward but in each one Alain was able to bring out important learning points for us all. It was truly working out as a masterclass for me. I was learning at a faster rate than anyone else in the audience. After lunch I did two more cases, which seemed to be getting more difficult each time, but all yielded good results with perfectly functioning valves. At the end of the day we adjourned to King's College for a reception and dinner.

Day two began similarly to the first. However, as the day progressed the cases became more and more complex. This was simply the serendipity of taking patients from the waiting list without prior selection. It was real life surgical practice. By the end of the second day, with ten successful cases behind me, I was quite exhausted. Buoyed up by the clear excitement and enjoyment of the attendees I was ready for the last morning, which comprised a series of lectures from Alain, me and Len Shapiro, my cardiology friend, with an extended question time. Following lunch, it was time to take Alain to the airport for his flight home. Once he had left, I collapsed in complete exhaustion and slept for twenty-four hours. Attendees had come from all over the UK and mainland Europe and the accolades flowed in over the coming days and weeks. It had been a triumph, but most importantly Alain had been delighted at the outcome. The information on Napoleon is back in French hands. In keeping with the fake news movement of today, there are those who still choose to believe that Napoleon was poisoned by his British captors. All in all it had been very satisfying.

After a few months of reflection and a good report conveyed to me by Judie Vivian from Edwards Laboratories who had funded the meeting, we decided that we should make this a regular event. I was in the fortunate position of being able to invite many of my surgical heroes: Tirone David from Toronto was our guest for the Canadian Correction; Craig Miller from Stanford, California for the first American Correction; Manuel Antunes from Coimbra, Portugal for the Portuguese Correction; and Randy Chitwood for the second American Correction. Each surgeon brought their own distinctive style and character to the event. All were generous in their support and excellent guests, spending as much time as the delegates demanded from them. As every meeting progressed, my experience and knowledge grew. There were no clinical problems, and all patients recovered well. It is important to state that every patient willingly gave their consent to be included and also entered the spirit of the programme, showing great interest in who the special guest was. I will always be grateful to them.

At the time of Craig Miller's attendance, I had an exciting car – a TVR Cerbera 4.5 litre, which was immensely powerful, if somewhat unreliable. During his visit to Papworth, Dr Miller wanted to be taken for a ride in it. With his Stetson hat, from which he was rarely separated, firmly on his head he 'mounted up' and we made a speedy run around the quiet back roads of Papworth. That had him clutching his Stetson on his lap with white knuckled hands. Every time we have met since, he has relived the moment with a big smile.

Randy Chitwood was the guest for the last meeting of the series. During the evening of the first day, I received a call from my father telling me that my mother had become unwell and had been admitted to hospital. There had been a significant progression in the multiple sclerosis from which she had suffered for over thirty years. She had developed pneumonia following influenza. Her respiratory muscles had become very weak and there was a concern that she might not survive the weekend. I had a conversation with Randy telling him of the situation. We agreed that I should leave the meeting and drive to Shropshire to be with her. As soon as I had finished the last operation of the day, Randy generously took on the responsibility of hosting the dinner that night. It is 150 miles from Cambridge to the hospital in Shrewsbury.

When I arrived, my father was with her. She was clearly very unwell. The multiple sclerosis from which she had suffered and fought against so courageously for more than three decades had savagely weakened her muscles for breathing. Despite being in her early eighties and having lived with the disease for so long, she really wanted to live but was having great difficulty in breathing. I could see that she needed help to clear her secretions. I knew that a small tube placed in the trachea through a little incision in the neck could bring her great relief. I discussed it with the chest physician responsible for my mother's care. He would not agree to do it, saying that they didn't have the necessary equipment. I offered to bring what was needed from Papworth, but he still would not agree. My father who had always conformed with authority asked me to desist. It was very hard watching my mother suffer so greatly when I had the knowledge and skill to help her but was prevented from doing so.

After staying all night at her bedside, I drove back to Cambridge in the early hours getting back in time for the second day's surgery. After a short rest and a large black coffee, the day went well. On completion, I returned to Shropshire to spend the night with my family again. Things were deteriorating quickly for my mother, but she insisted that I return to Cambridge to see the meeting through. Her determination to support her children so obviously dominant right to the end. With great trepidation and not knowing if I would see my mother again, I set off back to Cambridge to complete the meeting. On the way back, again in the early hours, I was stopped by the police for speeding along the A14. The policemen were very understanding and became more interested in the car than my misdemeanour. One of them checked on my story of being a surgeon at Papworth whilst the other asked to see the engine under the hood. After informing me that they could have charged me, they let me go. I drove carefully the rest of the way.

On the Sunday of that weekend, I took Randy and his wife to Ely Cathedral for a pre-arranged guided tour, and then for a good lunch before they left for the airport. He had shown himself to be a good friend in difficult times. Afterwards, I drove back to Shrewsbury and sat with my mother until she died in the early hours of Monday morning. That was the last of the Papworth Mitral Meetings.

Foreign Travel

As my reputation in surgery of the mitral valve grew, invitations began to arrive from interesting places to lecture and to operate. In 1996, Iran, which had been closed to most visitors after the change of regime, was beginning to open. I was contacted by Mrs Jaleh Hearne, a woman working for St Jude Medical in the UK, to ask if I would consider a visit to her country to begin to spread the word about mitral valve reconstruction. I was very interested in the idea and quite excited at the thought of spending time in that beautiful country. As is so often the case, putting the politics and warring factions to one side, there is so much history and beauty to experience there. I find the history the Middle East, and Persia in particular, very interesting and the art from those countries beautiful and intriguing.

The plan was to visit the Tehran Heart Institute to lecture on the subject, to see cases and to mentor interested surgeons in the operating theatre. I jumped at the chance. Jaleh was closely related to one of the five generals who left the country with the Shah of Iran when he was overthrown in 1979. She had not been allowed to return until that time. Over the intervening years she had been acquiring medical equipment and teaching material to send to her Iranian medical friends to help them provide the necessary care.

The first trip of two that I made was to Tehran. On 27 April 1995 we flew out, first class, on Iranian airlines. Grand though that sounds, it was tempered by the fact that sitting at the front of the cabin I was confronted with a large screen on which was played in an almost constant loop a propaganda film showing the victorious hordes of Iranian cavalry driving the infidel Americans out into a glorious sunrise, all accompanied by booming Iranian music. This was relieved by buckets of the finest caviar washed down with fresh orange juice. No alcohol allowed. We landed at Tehran airport at 4.00 a.m.. As I stepped out into the perfumed, warm night air I was struck by the silence. There were no other aircraft arriving. The arrivals hall was a massive military hangar-like building, completely stark and without any adornments other than two huge images on the wall facing us, one of Ayatollah Khomeini and the other of President Hashemi Rafsanjani. They were at least 20 feet high.

We were guided into a queue by revolutionary guards bearing Kalashnikov rifles with grenades hitched to their belts. Jaleh was wearing a burqa and a hijab. However, her ankles were just showing the bottom of seamed stockings. Immediately the dress police, with switches in hand, descended upon her, tapping her ankles and shouting at her to cover up. We were then confronted with a series of border post checks. First, we had to pass through the revolutionary guards who carefully checked our passports.

Following that was another desk manned by what seemed to be a group of religious clerics. They again checked our passports and asked the purpose of our visit. Next were the female revolutionary guards who were much more aggressive towards us. Finally came the customs check. Jaleh had a large briefcase filled with teaching videos for the surgeons we were about to visit. She was challenged to open it. As soon as they saw the videos she was taken by both arms and marched off to a room away from the arrivals hall. As she was being taken, she turned to me telling me not to worry as her nephew was waiting for me outside and would take me to the hotel.

At this point I was surrounded by crowds of people all bustling to get out. Amongst them were a lot of young men in orange suits all clutching at my bags and my arms shouting at me in Iranian. I became quite anxious as I had no idea what was going on. They turned out to be taxi drivers. Being tall, I could see over their heads and to my relief, saw Jaleh's nephew waving frantically at me and shouting at me to get through the crowd. I managed to do this, and was whisked off in his large SUV just as the sun was rising, leaving Jaleh behind. It transpired that the authorities were suspicious of the content of the videos, suspecting that they were full of propaganda. They made her show each one from beginning to end before they allowed her to pass out from the airport.

As we approached the outskirts of the city, with the sun rising, we arrived at the Azadi Tower, a large arch on Azadi square marking the western entrance to the city. I asked if we could stop for some photos. My guide said that he would only slow down but not stop, as the square was surrounded by shadowy groups who were drug and arms dealers and that it was a very dangerous place to stop. As my eyes acclimatised to the light, I could see these silent crowds standing in the shadows. We quickly moved on to the hotel where I was staying. It was the old American Hilton that had been abandoned when the Shah left the country. The hotel was completed to the fourth floor only, with the exposed girders of the higher floors reaching up into the sky. I was greeted warmly by the hotel receptionists. As we separated for me to freshen up, my host told me that I was being picked up at 6.00 a.m., just an hour hence. As soon as I got into the room, I called home to let my wife know that I had arrived safely. As soon as I picked up the phone, I heard some strange clicks and other noises on the phone. It was being tapped. I just had time to unpack and go through my slides (no power point at that time), before being picked up.

We were driven to a large conference centre on the outskirts of Tehran that looked a little like the National Exhibition Centre in Birmingham. All along the outside walls were large banners draped like giant sashes with Farsi script writ large across them. At first sight to my untutored eye, they seemed somewhat intimidating. However, they probably carried simple messages of support for the religious leaders, or even advertising slogans. I was greeted by a large entourage of medics who were utterly charming and warmly welcoming. I discovered then that it was a meeting of the Asian Cardiac Society with cardiologists and surgeons from all over southeast Asia as well as the middle eastern countries. I was taken first to the slide ready room and my presentation was loaded onto their projection system. Then we lined up ready to process into the hall. At the head of the procession were several Mullahs, followed by a guard sporting an assault rifle and in full battle fatigues. Then came the president of the society followed by me with other guards behind me and then several others, probably the committee, bringing up the rear. The corridor to the hall was narrow and lined with what appeared to be corrugated metal sheets, not a little claustrophobic. Then a door opened and in we went to a vast hall with several thousand attendees who all leapt to their feet.

Revolutionary music was being played very loudly as we processed to the front of the hall. I was seated on the left-hand side, at the aisle end of the front row. When everyone was in place, and the religious leaders had taken their places along with the president and council of the society on the large stage, the proceedings began. First, there were readings from the Quran, followed by a welcome introduction from the president and then a short movie, again showing the exodus of the villainous Americans chased by the gleaming Persian knights on spectacular horses.

Then there was a long speech in Farsi. I was there with Asghar Khaghani, a delightful cardiac surgeon from Harefield, who had arrived a day before me. Asghar speaks Farsi and initially he looked very comfortable in the environment. However, as a native Iranian they found fault in the way he was dressed and quietly reprimanded him for it. Although I couldn't really make out what was going on with any certainty it appeared to be about the open collar on his shirt.

Asghar was the opening guest speaker, and I followed him. Following an introduction in Farsi, I could hear my name being clearly enunciated. I took it as my cue to get up and to mount the stage for my presentation. I spoke for the invited forty-five minutes, and all went very smoothly. When I had finished there was a steady stream of excellent questions, all addressed in excellent English, some with a heavy American accent but many more European sounding. There were two more presentations before we were escorted ceremoniously out of the room and taken up into a gloriously large chamber adorned with beautifully woven rugs and huge cushions. We sat on the giant cushions and jasmine tea was brought to everyone. The whole of one wall was a glass window that looked out onto the snow-capped Caspian Mountains. The room was filled with the scent of lavender and jasmine. Shortly after we had settled the main door opened and two guards entered, once again heavily armed, followed by a small entourage which headed towards me and the president of the society. He swiftly jumped to his feet and I followed suit. I was amazed to be introduced to President Akbar Rafsanjani, one of the founding fathers of the Islamic Republic. He generously thanked me for coming and supporting the doctors of Iran. As swiftly as he had arrived, he left after speaking to few others. My experience of personal relationships throughout that visit and the next one were uniformly courteous.

I spent the next two days in the Tehran Heart Institute doing ward-rounds of the patients and time in theatre with the surgeons. The standard of surgery was very high and all of them were extremely well educated and very experienced.

On the last day, I was taken on a tour of Tehran and was enthralled by the culture, so different from our own. I made several new friends there and wanted to return.

Two years later in April 1997, Jaleh took me on a trip to Isfahan. It is said of Isfahan, that of all the beauty in the world, half of the beauty is there. It really is a very beautiful place. We flew with British Airways to Tehran on 2 April and changed aircraft for the flight to Isfahan. There was a drive of about forty minutes through desert country to reach the city. We were staying at an old camel motel. It was a stopping off point on the old silk road. On the ground floor were rooms with entries that were the outline of a camel's profile seen from the front. On the floor above were the rooms for guests. It was shaped as a square. In the centre was a beautiful garden with fountains and lovely flowers. The air was filled with the scent of jasmine. For me the meeting and surgery were somewhat incidental to the exposure to the culture. I felt close to the old Persia. I travelled with cardiologist Rodney Foal and his lovely artist wife. We visited the old polo ground in the centre of the city. It is the Naqsh-e Jahan square. At one end of the square is the beautiful great Nizam al-Mulk mosque.

The giant wooden entrance gates to the mosque are covered in uncut precious stones. They had stood there for almost a millennium. On asking if there were problems with theft, I was reminded of the extreme punishments that were meted out to any aspiring criminals. Once inside, the scale of the beauty is difficult to give justice in simple words. Just inside the entrance is a large granite urn dwarfing me, with the words of the Holy Quran carved on its surface. The skill to achieve it with such precision is breath-taking. The main dome has a dual skin separated by about 20 feet. The acoustic result allows the Mullah to speak with an ordinary voice and be heard throughout the courtyard. All the surfaces are covered with the most beautiful carvings and paintings in classical Persian style.

Walking around the square with London cardiologist Rodney Foale and his wife we attracted a lot of attention. Lady Foal had been shopping in a fashionable store in London and was wearing a beautiful turquoise blue burqa. All the local women were dressed head to toe in black. I discovered that if the woman is covered from head to feet, the colour of the burqa didn't seem to matter.

Around the edge of the very large square was an extensive market with an enormous number of souks. Looking into them, they disappeared into a dust laden gloom and darkness, summoning images of stories from the Arabian nights. Everyone we met was very friendly and welcoming.

We were told a story from an early kingdom when Isfahan was under threat from a foreign army much larger than the resident army. In an attempt to deter a war, the head of the army in Isfahan invited the invading generals to a show of arms within the square. The local army had just enough soldiers to form a continuous file of men several soldiers abreast all the way around the square. As they left the square, it is said that they quickly changed into different dress before parading back into the square and this continued for many hours giving the impression of a vast army. The threat of invasion was removed.

During the second evening of our visit, following the day's lectures, a group of us were sitting with some local surgeons in the gardens enjoying a cup of jasmine tea and good conversation. Towards the end of the evening, one of the Iranian surgeons suggested we reconvene in his room where he had some alcohol. Knowing the consequences if we were caught, I demurred and left for bed. The next morning, I heard that he and a colleague had been removed during the small hours of the night and we didn't see them again. At that time, if the rules of the country were respected, a trouble-free visit could be anticipated. Whether that still holds I am not sure. It is a huge indictment on world politics that such beautiful countries become off-limits. Travelling to meet the wonderful people of the country would do so much to defuse international tensions.

On the last day, I had expressed an interest in buying a silk rug. I was taken to a wonderful old souk just off the polo square where the long-suffering owner pulled out rug after rug. I offered to help but was gently told that I should sit and enjoy the revelation of so many beautiful things. After a significant time, I finally settled on a beautiful blue and silver silk rug and Jaleh began to negotiate terms on my behalf. At that point, police cars, with sirens wailing, pulled up outside and police rushed in calling my name. My first reaction was of concern that my time had come, and I was about to be arrested. In fact, a minister in the government had developed pre-infarction angina and they wanted me to go with them for advice. I was escorted into the coronary care unit and asked to review his data. It was clear that he was settling with the appropriate medication and would need an angiogram, following which he could be operated on if it was deemed necessary. They thanked me profusely and then it was time to leave for the airport. I had hoped that I might find the rug wrapped and ready to take with me as a thank you, but to no avail.

There was one last episode of excitement for me. As we reached the end of the drive through the desert back to the airport, I reached into my jacket for my passport, but it wasn't there. In a panic I searched through my pockets and my bags. No passport. Not the best country to get caught trying to leave without a valid passport, I thought to myself. As soon as we had dropped Rodney and his wife at the terminal, we raced back through the early dawn to the hotel. As we approached, I could see the organiser of the meeting standing on the front porch of the hotel, calmly smoking a cigarette, probably reflecting on a job well done. He was jolted back to reality when we raced up to the hotel, the apron to which was tiled with marble flagstones. As the driver braked the car skidded with a loud screech up to the bottom of the steps causing him to leap out of the way. As I jumped out of the taxi, I quickly described the problem. We raced to reception who calmly handed over the missing passport. They had taken it on arrival as it had to be inspected in the local police station. I had forgotten to ask for it and they had forgotten to return it as I checked out. As I was getting back into the taxi, I could see steam rising from the radiator grill and wondered if we could make it back across the desert to the airport safely and in time. The long-suffering taxi driver courteously summoned another taxi for me whilst he sorted out his overheating vehicle. We managed to get back to the airport in record time. I ran from the taxi to check-in, leaving the second driver raising the hood of his car to inspect the engine as his car and developed similar problems. I just made it to the flight in time.

Once on board I was sat next to a young Iranian engineer. We began to chat. It transpired that he had been sent to buy the last giant tunnel boring machine that had been used to core out the English/French channel tunnel. I enquired why. He calmly informed me that there was a strong feeling that the next world war would be fought over water, and they were in the process of connecting the massive aquifers beneath the Caspian mountains to capture the melt water to ensure their long-term water supply.

My journeys to Iran were over. I had had a wonderful time in an exciting culture and met some delightful people. It is so sad that returning is fraught with difficulty and perhaps a little danger, but I do hope that one day that will be possible.

Between these two visits, I had been asked to go to Cairo to supervise the examination for a Ph.D. student. He had been initially attached to the cardiac surgical unit in Leeds but had not received the support he needed. He sought my help and had transferred to be under my wing, to complete the work and prepare the manuscript for his thesis. With the work complete and the thesis submitted he was called to defend it in the old-fashioned way, in front of the faculty and his whole family and friends. His work was sound, and the results commendable, however, there seemed to be an issue with one of his professors who was asking him silly questions to which he, the professor, didn't know the proper answers. This left me in quite a conundrum. How to defend the candidate without offending his professor in front of the assembled audience. With some careful turn of phrase, I managed to extricate the candidate from a poor situation. When it was all over and he had been awarded his degree, I was introduced to his family who were charming and grateful as they could see what had been going on. His uncle happened to be the director of the Cairo Museum. As a thank you, I was given a marvellous tour of the museum, which at that time was still chaotic. However, I was able to see many of the Tutankhamun artefacts that were not available for public viewing. I was then taken on a wonderful tour of the Valley of the Kings at Luxor. I was taken into several of the tombs that were still being explored. They had put me up at the Nile Hilton in splendid style. On my return to Cairo, I had a grand tour of the Pyramids and the Sphinx before leaving for home.

We are very fortunate in our specialty of cardiothoracic surgery. The number of surgeons in academic university posts around the world is relatively small. International communication is high in the cutting-edge sub-specialties. Also, my time in Alabama generated a lot of lifelong friends. I was elected a member of the American Association of Thoracic Surgeons and the European Society very early on and I have attended most of their meetings over the decades. This has taken me to most major cities in North America, Canada and Europe. Academic international meetings aside, I have been invited to many centres to do demonstration operations and to mentor others.

Ethiopia

Other outstanding memories for me, are the missions that I made with the charity the Chain of Hope to Ethiopia. This is an organisation that has at its 'heart' the provision of heart surgery for children in under-developed countries that have no ready access to treatment for cardiac pathology. It is under the directorship of Professor Sir Magdi Yacoub. Chain of Hope, La Chaîne de l'Espoir, had been originally set up by Professor Alain Deloche, a French surgeon who had also been instrumental in the founding of Médecins Sans Frontières and Médecins du Monde. Following a meeting at Brompton and a leisurely dinner, Professor Deloche asked Professor Yacoub if he would set up a branch in the UK and support the project. Instantly he agreed and enlisted his daughter Lisa to help to run and champion the charity. He found a staunch ally in Diana, Princess of Wales who became the patron. Professor Yacoub is a humanitarian and in addition to Chain of Hope he has set up centres in multiple sites around Africa, Jamaica, and Aswan in Egypt.

The small children's heart hospital in Addis Ababa, is a not-for-profit non-governmental institution. They have excellent nurses that staff the wards, the intensive care and the theatres. However, they have only one cardiologist, and no resident surgeons. Teams travel from some developed countries, which include anaesthetists, surgeons, nurses and perfusionists to run the heart and lung machine. The team takes all the equipment that is needed to operate safely on the children with them, the money for all of which is raised charitably through magnanimous donors.

Whilst the aims of this charity are wholly laudable, it has had its critics. Aldo Castaneda, head of paediatric heart surgery at the Boston Children's Hospital criticised surgeons who were travelling the world on behalf of charities, doing several operations and leaving carnage behind them. This has happened and is to be severely criticised and prevented. However, that is not tolerated by the Chain of Hope. Central to the charity's mission is the training of local surgeons to carry on the work and to progress the specialty within the country. Indeed as a result of Professor Yacoub's efforts there are now fully functioning units in Kingston, Jamaica and Aswan.

I made five trips for the charity, between March 2010 and September 2014, with a further trip in 2019. Each one has been both exhilarating and exhausting. We arrive at Addis at about 5.00 a.m.. The first hurdle is passing through customs with all of our medical equipment. On occasions we pass through unhindered but on others the customs men on duty seem to enjoy making it difficult for us and on one occasion there was no one present and a phone call to the minister of health was necessary to free everything up.

Then it's off in the van with our wonderful driver, always cheerful and very long-suffering. He often found himself hanging around for hours waiting to transfer us from hospital to hotel but always greeted us with a warm smile and firm handshake.

A hotel that we use quite frequently is ineptly called the Dreamliner. It is small and cramped and the beds are almost impossible to sleep on with a generous supply of bed bugs. On my first visit, the morning quiet was shattered with loud traffic noise and shouting. As I looked out of the window, I saw several trucks with gangs of young men armed with Kalashnikov rifles driving by. This was unusual but one was aware that interesting situations could arise out of the blue. On another trip a government minister was shot dead in his car just down the street from our hotel. The morning drive through the centre of Addis took us past the only museum that I know that is dedicated to terrorism the Red Terror Martyr's memorial museum.

The cardiac centre had been built in 2009 with money from an Arabian donor. It was next to, but unrelated to the main Addis hospital the Black Lion Teaching Hospital, or simply the Black Hospital as it was known. All of the staff have a joyous attitude towards life, and nothing is too much trouble for them. Their focus and attention to detail is something that I wish was found throughout our NHS. It is a joy to work with them. Their hours of work seemed irrelevant as they all stayed as long as it was necessary to complete the tasks in hand.

As soon as we arrive at the hospital, we begin an outpatient clinic to select the cases for surgery. This is one of the hardest things to do because as soon as the word is out that a team will be coming, parents stream in from many miles away with their children, often walking great distances over several days.

Whilst I was working through the children in the clinic, colleagues were setting up the intensive care and the theatres ready for use. At the end of a long day, we have to decide who we will operate on and then in which order. There are only six beds in the intensive care and therefore the first children we operate upon need to be moved through the intensive care in one day. Then we face the most difficult task of informing the parents of the children who cannot be operated on during that mission. It is truly heart-breaking for all of us. We know that several of them may not survive for much longer.

After a late night and an early morning rise, we started the surgery. We managed two or three cases a day, working late into the evening. Problems with equipment were common and on more than one occasion we had to send out to the market for bits of basic kit, such as a pair of scissors that had broken.

There are no porters, and so the brave little children walk into the operating room. They arrive with a parent and climb onto the operating theatre table. Two wonderful anaesthetists have accompanied me on these trips. The first, Gavin Wright has been a stalwart of the charity and been on many missions in all of the countries in which The Chain of Hope operates. We first worked together in Papworth hospital many years ago. After a relatively short period he moved to work at Harefield with Magdi. Gavin is an exceptional character and a real joy to work with. His care and compassion towards the children and the staff around him is exceptional. The other was Barbora Paraskova. Barbora is another exceptional character and outstanding anaesthetist who cares very deeply about her work. Her preparation for the missions was wonderful, taking toys and other small gifts for the children. She had several children's movies loaded onto her mobile phone which the children would watch as the central venous and arterial lines were placed under local anaesthetic. Both are what I would call surgeon's anaesthetists, not in the sense that they will follow our every demand, but that they understand the process of surgery and the surgical mentality and support us in the most professional way. Their guidance and opinions on management are always invaluable. Success in these situations is very much a shared responsibility and no surgeon could be in better hands than those of Barbora and Gavin.

Once fully anaesthetised the operation would begin. In all of the children we found massively enlarged hearts in tiny, frequently malnourished little chests. The heart valves were ravaged by the rheumatic process that underlay the problem. I felt that it was imperative that I repaired every valve that I could, as valve replacement was fraught with potential problems. If we used a mechanical valve then the child would have to take anticoagulant medicine to prevent the valve from being blocked by clots of blood that would form on the valve, obstructing its orifice. If we chose a tissue replacement valve, then they would degenerate within a very few years in these young children. Thankfully, with the experience that I had gained over the years I was able to reconstruct all of the valves bar one that a previous surgeon had tried to repair but had failed. The surgery was taxing and delicate but immensely rewarding. Long term follow up of these children has revealed that these reconstructed valves continue to function well many years later.

After the operation is completed, the child was woken up on the operating table and transferred to the intensive care unit, where a parent, was there to greet them and sit with them. Surprising to me was the fact that the child's relative more often than not was the father. The children were so very resilient. They never complained and endured any discomfort and pain with huge fortitude.

One of the most moving incidents that I experienced was the actions of a child that I had operated on in the morning. After completing a second operation and entering the intensive care to check on the progress of the first child, I was beckoned over to the bedside by the nurse, as the little boy had something to say to me. With no prior knowledge of the English language, he had learnt a few words that he wanted to say. As I leaned in towards him, he punched me lightly on my arm and whispered with a lovely smile spreading across his fragile little face, 'Well done doc'. It was perhaps the most moving experience of my entire career in surgery.

Whilst our surgical team is occupied in the operating theatre, my friend and colleague Sir Shak Qureshi, a wonderful paediatric cardiologist working at the Evelina Children's Hospital in St Thomas' Hospital London, is working through many catheter-based procedures in the small next door catheter laboratory. His work is phenomenal, and he is able to rectify significant congenital lesions of the heart under radiographic control. However, our relationship seems to be tarnished by some mysterious curse that comes into being when we are working together.

On one trip, I agreed to take on a very complicated redo operation after a previously protracted case on the day that we were flying home. Shak and his team finished their cases early and in their tired and demob happy states managed to eat all of the food that the hospital cooks had prepared for all of us. When my team came out of the theatre at 10.00 p.m. there was none left. A lovely kitchen worker offered to heat some food up for us. A big mistake. Just one hour after consuming it, and on the way to the airport, my intestines began to writhe like a coiled snake. Once on the aeroplane, an old Ethiopian Airlines Boeing 737, the nausea began, followed rapidly by severe vomiting and profuse diarrhoea. I had clearly consumed a large dose of bacteria. The door on the toilet cabin would not close properly and I sat miserably holding it whilst losing control of everything. When I did not reappear, Shak came to look for me and saw the terrible state that I was in. With the help of the anaesthetist, I was half carried to the back of the plane where there was an empty row of seats and laid out. By then, severely dehydrated, they set up an intravenous infusion on me. We had to land in Jordan to refuel and the pilot was keen to off-load me there. Shak and colleagues stepped in and reassured him that they would look after me until we reached London. Clearly, I had ingested a large dose of freshly agitated bacteria, probably staphylococcus.

The remaining journey was a blur to me. On arrival at Heathrow, I was medivacked from the plane to Hounslow Hospital. After a two-litre transfusion of fluid and heavy doses of antibiotics I began to improve. I tried to use the toilet to evacuate some of the fluid that was now streaming through my kidneys. I was told that I couldn't move, however, I knew that if I didn't very soon I would need a commode which was not forthcoming, the nurses being more interested in discussing their escapades of the night before or going outside for a 'smoke'. I asked for a cap for the intravenous cannula to allow me to disconnect the drip and to walk to the toilet. The nurse insisted that it did not need one and just disconnected the cannula from the drip. I stood up to walk to the toilet and on looking around saw a trail of blood that had flowed from my vein onto the floor. At that point I knew that I had to take my self-discharge and called a taxi, demanded my clothes and left.

Later that same year whilst attending a conference in San Francisco where Shak also happened to be, we met for a cup of coffee in Union Square before he set off to return to the UK. I jokingly said that as we had spent time together that I would probably be caught up in an earthquake or some other such disaster. We both laughed and went our separate ways. The conference over, I hired a car for a few days' break in the Napa Valley with a friend. Sure enough that first night after settling into a basement room, we were woken at about 3.00 a.m. to loud rumbling noises and a violent shaking of the house. There were shouts of, 'Earthquake, get out now.' We tried to open the door from the room, but it was frozen in its frame as a result of the movement of the house. There was a window that the upper half opened to the lawn outside, the other half below ground level. Luckily, we had left it open and were able to crawl through and escape. My first call was to Shak, who laughingly said he knew something would happen.

Each mission to Ethiopia yielded more moving stories and wonderful new friends. It was a period of my life that I will never forget and hold very dear to my heart. The very first person I operated upon was a teenage girl Abinet, who had severe heart failure. I needed to reconstruct both her mitral and tricuspid valves. She made an excellent recovery and now is married with a child of her own. She has set up a local charity building mud and thatch houses for homeless families and collecting food for them. A wonderful legacy for this important charity, bearing witness to the huge compassion and drive of Sir Magdi Yacoub and Professor Alain Deloche.

Sadly we have struggled to be able to train local surgeons as a result of some obduracy of the Ethiopian government. Apparently, they express concern that if they train their doctors too well, they leave for South

Africa or other countries where pay and conditions are better. Progress has therefore not been at the pace of Jamaica or Egypt. I hope to be able to accompany the team on more missions.

Highlights of the last decade have included invitations to lecture and to operate in China, South Korea, Thailand and Japan. Each culture so different and so interesting. My first trip to China was to Beijing and Shanghai. I was asked to lecture and run wet laboratory sessions in both cities. The trainees were so keen to learn and the sessions went on long after their allotted times. The reception everywhere I went was so courteous. Excellent meals and fascinating company. My lectures were delivered with simultaneous translation. Unfortunately, on the second day in the Beijing Heart Institute, the translation system broke down and so I was afforded a lovely lady surgeon who translated in paragraph-sized chunks of speech. In the middle of one of them I had placed an attempt at a light-hearted comment and illustration. At that point the translator stopped me and said, 'This a joke ha ha?' I said yes, and she said, 'Don't worry I make 'em laugh.' In the lecture when we reached this point, she transmitted the joke, there was a pause and then, as though brought in by a conductor, there was a thirty-second sound of loud forced laughter from 300 Chinese surgeons, which ended as abruptly as it began. Their faces returned to sombre looks until the end of the lecture. I never knew if it was boredom or tiredness that they felt.

Further trips to Shanghai, Shaoxing in Zhejiang province, Taizhou and Lishui have followed. Everywhere the staff and students have been exceptionally polite and welcoming. Each new visit was accompanied by excessive gifts of paintings, books and calligraphy. Quite out with any experience in our own country was the welcome given to me by the senior management of each hospital. The quality of equipment and instruments available for the surgical procedures is of a high order. The vast size of many of these institutions is also quite extraordinary in comparison to what we are used to in England. Each centre had twenty to thirty operating theatres working around the clock, treating many thousands of patients in a highly efficient manner. Several of the operating theatres have CT and MRI scanners attached to them. The training centres for young surgeons are extraordinary, with multiple robot machines to practice on. In contrast to our hospital, they have excellent institutional memory of the pioneers who have gone before. Shaoxing People's Hospital has a wonderful museum revealing their history, all housed in the most modern of settings that would do more than justice to any small museum or gallery at home.

An example of the generosity of spirit of the Chinese physicians towards their fellow carers and patients was their desire to help during the Covid crisis. From the beginning through to the height of the pandemic, the doctors in Wuhan linked with us at Papworth every Wednesday morning to pass on their knowledge and experience to help us.

In South Korea I was taken to Tegu by high-speed train at over 300 kph. Similar to Japan, the train is exactly on time, with neatly uniformed carriage chaperones seeing you to your seat and providing food, drinks and newspapers if required, all with a warm smile and a deep bow. In Tegu, the reputation of the South Koreans and alcohol consumption was in evidence at a dinner I was hosted on the night before I was operating. They were drinking 'boilermakers' in quick succession. These were pint mugs of beer with shots of whiskey, bourbon or Rye in a shot glass dropped in. Despite the copious amounts of alcohol consumed by the local surgeons, they were all up very early and fresh the next morning for the surgery.

For an experience I was taken to the Number 1 tunnel which was at the end of the demilitarised zone and passed through to North Korea, dug by the North Koreans for quick access to thousands of troops should a land invasion be started. There are hundreds of them, with more being discovered every year. Entering the tunnel I was bent double and we walked about half a mile underground until we reached a heavy metal grill preventing any further progression. This marked the border between the two countries. On both sides there were heavily armed guards, with each standing rigidly to attention, looking very aggressively at the other. Leading up to that point it was heartbreaking to see many South Korean citizens of all ages, sitting on the ground, many weeping, for the loss of their families trapped in North Korea. A tragic sight.

In Japan, trips to Osaka and Kyoto were enchanting with wonderful experiences of the polite and gentle Japanese culture. Chado, or as we know it, the Japanese tea ceremony, was everything that I expected it to be: polite, ritualistic and calming. Everywhere I went, including in Thailand, the local health professionals were charming, erudite and keen to learn whatever they could from us. I felt that on each trip I was learning more from them than ever I was able to pass on to them. In Bangkok, there is a very special surgeon, Dr Taweesak Chotivatanapong. We have known each other over many years, both of us being interested in surgery of the Mitral valve. Taweesak's particular expertise is in the surgical correction of Rheumatic Mitral valve disease, with perhaps the largest experience of this in the world. His warmth and charm is always at the fore in everything that he does.

It has been an absolute privilege and pleasure to experience so many different cultures and ideas. These are things that I will forever be grateful to the wonderful world of Surgery and its cross-boundary collegiate nature. All working to one end, to help our fellow human beings at their times of stress and discomfort. There can be few other occupations in the world comparably satisfying and generous of spirit.

A Journey into Politics

At the end of the twentieth century the waiting times for heart surgery in Britain were unacceptable with many patients waiting up to and over one year. The mortality of patients on the waiting lists was higher than following the surgery. The risks of a poor outcome were also higher as people who had waited for a long time were in a worse state at the time of surgery. The government wasn't listening to the reports from clinicians and as usual hospital managements seemed deaf to the problem. One Friday evening, I was listening to the BBC Radio 4 programme *Any Questions*. There was a discussion on the NHS in the usual politician's platitudes. I was so angry about what I was hearing I decided to call the sister programme *Any Answers* the following day. Surprisingly, I was called to speak first and David Dimbleby, the chairman of the programme gave me almost the first twenty minutes of the programme. I tried my best to explain the devastating effects of the wholly inadequate service that patients were having to endure. As soon as the programme finished my telephone was hot with calls from colleagues all over the British Isles congratulating me on my contribution. Finally, the phone quietened and after about an hour there was another call. I immediately recognised the voice. It was that of Mr Dimbleby, thanking me for my contribution and asking me if I would like to take part in a future programme soon. With some trepidation I agreed.

A week or so later, I was invited to travel to the Robert Jones and Agnes Hunt Hospital near Oswestry, North Shropshire to be a part of the team. The other members of the team were to be Michael Meacher MP, Minister of State for the Environment, John Bercow, Conservative MP and future Speaker of the House of Commons, and Sir Simon Hughes of the Liberal Democrats, with David Dimbleby in the Chair. I was invited to a pub supper before the programme with the team, which was when I met the others for the first time, and was also informed that we would not know the questions that would be asked until we were live in the programme. Michael Meacher was late, arriving in a government car armed with a pile of briefing papers. Bercow was garrulous and quite superficial in his conversation. Simon

Hughes was more serious and very pleasant but with statements on the health service demonstrating a serious lack of frontline knowledge.

After refreshments we walked over to the hall where the programme was being recorded. Oswestry is not far from my home in south Shropshire, and I thought that I would play the home boy card. David asked me how I would like to be introduced. I replied, 'the butcher's boy from Clun'. He looked rather askance at me asking me if I was sure, I replied in the affirmative, but that he could add anything that he wanted to about my subsequent career as corollary evidence of my knowledge of the NHS.

We were sat on a stage behind a table with Bercow on my right and Meacher on my left with Hughes beyond him. Dimbleby sat on a separate small table. There were several minutes of warm up by a comedian and then just before going live on air we were introduced to the capacity audience. As I requested, David introduced me as the butcher's boy from Clun and a huge applause followed. Clearly my affiliation had connected with the assembled crowd, largely local farmers. Immediately I felt a little more relaxed.

The questions from the floor began, most of which I cannot remember. There was a question on Clause 4 relating to the LGBT community for which I offered my support, but then came the big one, the one that I had been asked to be present for; the National Health Service.

I launched into my everyday experiences of it and what it was doing to the people who needed our help but could not get ready access. At one point I remember comparing the organisation of a Trabant factory in Russia to the current state of the health service. Remarkably, Michael Meacher leaned over and whispered in my ear that he wished I was in government with him. Quite what that meant I have never been sure. Considerable applause followed my comments. It was clear that many in the audience, or their relatives were suffering long waits for attention from the NHS. There is a real risk of having your views amplified by the echo chamber effect but I spoke from the heart and ever worsening experience of the service that we were able to offer.

It was after this programme that everything became very interesting. I was invited to take part in several other programmes including a programme titled *Doctors on Trial*. Jon Snow chaired a courtroom-style debate at the London Weekend Television studios on the South Bank. This was part of the backwash from the awful Bristol Babies furore. Doctors, in particular heart surgeons, were vilified and accused of causing huge harm and unacceptable mortality in children with congenital heart disease. It had received huge publicity and engendered rage against the profession. This was the environment that we were stepping into. There were two teams lined up against each other: the doctors, in other words us versus the media influencers. Both teams had been provided with professional barrister support. Dame Helena Kennedy QC and Andrew Neil, past editor of the *Sunday Times* newspaper were the prosecutors. Before the programme went live we had an hour or so briefing with our barrister for the defence. Alongside me I had the President of the Royal College of Surgeons. Against us was Claire Rayner, a retired nurse and television journalist accompanied by other early media influencers whose names I cannot remember.

As we walked into the studio, we were confronted with an audience seated in a semi-circle around a central podium. We had to sit immediately in front of them. They were supposedly selected by an independent company to represent many different points of view. As we approached our seats to sit down, we could hear very hostile remarks against us, the doctors. The word, 'Killers', could be heard amongst the hubbub. Clearly not a particularly unbiased audience.

I was the first to be called and as I took the stand Helena Kennedy rose to ask the first question. I knew from some earlier courtroom experience when acting as an expert witness in medical malpractice trials that the jury were the ones who had to be convinced of the argument and so I aimed all my comments to the audience. As soon as Dame Helena had asked her question, I framed my answer so that she couldn't get a second one in and spoke as coherently as I could. I could sense her frustration burning into my back as I had turned away from her. The tactic worked and she didn't get a second question. The rest of my team followed suit.

Perhaps the most disappointing person was Claire Rayner, who was hypercritical of doctors in general and surgeons in particular; however, when it came to the vote, we, the doctors won comfortably. As we left the studio, I met Andrew Neil coming the other way. He bashed past me without acknowledging my greeting and stormed off. Clearly a very bad loser. Once back in the green room, I approached Claire Rayner to try to find out the reason for her aggressive stance towards us surgeons. Smilingly, she said that her comments were all just an act and that she loved the surgical mind and would never go to a surgeon who was not outspoken and to a degree, arrogant and sure of his/her abilities. She then turned to my daughter Joanna who had accompanied me and made a lovely fuss of her. The politics of television. It was a healthy lesson for me.

Later, I was invited to appear on the politics show with the health minister to discuss the waiting time problems for patients with heart disease. David Frost was to be the interviewer. On the Thursday before the Sunday morning programme, I was operating and the phone rang in the operating theatre. It was the Chief Executive Stephen Bridge. He had received a call from the health minister threatening to remove the funding for our new intensive care if I went ahead with the programme. Stephen said, of course, in the interest of freedom of speech he wouldn't stop me, but the message had been clear. As soon as I finished the operation, I called David Dimbleby informing of what had happened. He was horrified and contacted Number 10 Downing Street. Either he or David Frost visited prime minister Tony Blair to raise the issue. The next day, the Prime Minister announced to the press a very significant increase in the funding of heart surgery; he had made the decision without discussing it at cabinet, which raised a moderate furore, but the decision stuck. His decision was lauded in the medical profession and other changes that he and his government made dramatically improved the health service, a change that has not been matched since. Whether or not my intervention had any influence I will never know but two things make me think that it did. First, the timing of everything and the second came from a chance meeting ten years later between Stephen Bridge and Lord Hunt a then health minister. Stephen was asked how his 'Rottweiler Wells' was. A rather uncouth question from a minister of the crown suggesting a considerable degree of ire.

My own experience of politicians has been one of duplicity and, although they often offer warm words, it rapidly becomes clear that their responses to any kind of challenge are carefully worded to avoid direct answers to questions that they find hostile to their cause. Words are used like shields to protect themselves from any form of deep questioning. Whatever their reassurances, other than the significant developments brought about by Tony Blair, they are almost all guilty of massive neglect. They have ridden on the back of the idea that 'we are all so fortunate to have the NHS, which is free at the point of delivery', and thus trumpeted as the best health care system in the world across the ages since its inception. True it is free for most at delivery, but, oh dear, how woeful that delivery often is. Difficulty in getting to see a general practitioner, is common place, often being confronted by a nurse or paramedic in place of a properly trained and qualified doctor.

It goes without saying that there are still many very good GPs who work hard and deliver an outstanding service, but excellence is patchy. Once through the GP blockade, the average patient faces huge waiting lists, and access to ever more dilapidated hospitals. With poor cancer survival and perinatal statistics, what is there to be proud of? This decay and neglect have forced the current secretary of state for health Wes Streeting to declare the whole system broken. Well, whose fault is that? I believe that the fault lies not just with the politicians but also with the public who continue to accept the mantra that the NHS is a world leader. For decades now they should have been demanding more. Those who are fortunate enough to travel widely in the world know that this is just not the case. It is clear for all to see when eyes are wide open that the UK has been left behind by many countries. Whilst recent government initiatives are beginning to have an impact, there are still over 90,000 patients who have been waiting for more than a year for treatment with close to 6 million waiting to start consultant-led treatment.

Across the decades, several politically led reorganisations have empowered NHS management to seize all control of the day-to-day management from the medical professionals and to place it in their hands, some of whom are business school trained but whose eyes are more firmly fixed on the financial bottom line whilst paying lip-service only to the real care for the patients. At this point in time the management structures, both within the hospital setting and in the community, are so top heavy with functionaries who cannot see the clinical wood for the structural trees and who have distanced themselves so far from their consultant and senior nursing staff, that they really have little concept of what the true needs of an efficient, caring and holistic care system should be. Morale amongst the professions is low in many parts of the country.

Whatever the politicians and the managers like to tell us, healthcare, as dispensed by the state, should not be a business led by profit in the usual sense. It is a service that needs the efficient administration of the taxpayers' money to fund the necessary resources on the frontline of doctor patient interaction. They should not be talking about profits and financial excess at the end of the financial year, but what services have they improved or put in place to enhance the care of the patients. If the money has not been spent on auditable improved clinical outcomes, then the hospital management should be penalised, not lauded. In the case of the NHS, the shareholders are the patients but unlike in business they don't have the opportunity for an annual review and the ability to evict the board if they are failing. Only at a general election can their voices be heard.

There are rafts of unnecessary staff in the management offices, many on salaries that exceed the doctors and certainly the nurses. Every manager often has an assistant manager; they all have other functionaries and secretaries and many of the secretaries have their own assistants. There is so much unnecessary paperwork and a plethora of meetings that produce little to nothing.

This change has infected the nursing profession as well. Having quietly praised Tony Blair, he holds a significant responsibility for the inception of the modern matrons. These posts are so far removed from the original concept of the hospital matron as to make the name stupid. Hospitals are now swarming with dark blue clothed nurses on quite huge salaries telling others what to do, but rarely lifting a finger in direct patient care. This change followed the College of Nursing's character change for nurses emblazoned as 'Nursing 2000'. This successfully took many nurses away from patients, enforced degrees upon them such that much of the day-to-day care of the ward patient is conducted by assistants supported by physicians' assistants. All of this makes the fully trained nurses and doctors ever more remote from their patients. This in turn engenders laziness and slopy attention to detail.

In the medical schools, the change of teaching methods and the downgrading of detailed anatomical and physiological knowledge means that some doctors approach patients with inadequate knowledge of the functioning body. This too often leads to massive overuse of investigations as a blunderbuss approach to a problem. What has happened to the good history and full clinical examination supported by sound anatomical and physiological knowledge, leading to a differential diagnosis and then appropriately targeted investigations to hone the diagnosis?

So much time is now taken up with wokist-style education, focussing more on social mores than scientifically informed knowledge, backed up by a sound work ethic and discipline. The teaching methods of the 1960s, 1970s and 1980s are scorned these days, but those decades turned out better doctors. Much of the teaching of the basic sciences is done by non-medics and people without biological science in their backgrounds. The whole of medical education needs shaking up and the restoration of sound teaching of the core subjects with rigorous examinations to ensure adequate levels of knowledge. The educationalists need to be removed from the process.

Will that happen? I doubt it until the really poor levels to which the system has sunk are exposed. So many young doctors are voting with their feet and moving abroad. It remains to be seen how well they do in the face of perhaps better trained local professionals.

At a recent reunion of the forty-four students in our year marking the fifty years since our graduation, everyone was of the same opinion. The shrinkage of expected standards and the move towards paramedical care and away from 'proper doctors' has significantly diminished the quality of the service and added significantly to its costs. This has become so marked that it is commonplace to find elderly physicians forming loose alliances to look after each other as old age creeps upon them in response to the falling standards.

Although our training and the hours we worked as junior doctors were in need of reform, the exposure that we had then gave us great depth in experience and thus in our ability to work fluently in the care of our patients. A well-trained surgeon could deal with a multitude of problems aside from his/her final specialty. Now, if for example a patient has a retrosternal goitre (enlarged thyroid gland within the chest), instead of being managed by one well rounded surgeon, it invokes the need for at least two consultants, halving their time to do other things and doubling the costs. In several areas, multiple surgeons are required nowadays to achieve what would have been done by one person.

The reduced training time has been forced upon us by a lack of planning by politicians to meet the growing need. Now they are playing catch up with no thought of the real loss of quality and the increase in costs.

Following an operation I carried out on a prominent politician, he asked me for my thoughts on the health service. Somewhat reluctantly, as I do not like to mix politics with the care of my patients, but at his insistence, I suggested that what was really needed was a ten year rolling all party commission, heavily informed and advised by senior and experienced clinicians, to come up with a real sustainable plan for the service instead of the kneejerk reorganisations every few years headed by people far removed from the frontline. His response was that perhaps I would like the same thing for education, transport and the like. I suggested that it would be a good idea. His response was very telling. He said, 'So what would we all do then?' This fixed in my mind that so many of the political classes are in the job for themselves, power and aggrandisement and not really for the people that they are supposed to serve. A very sad reality.

As Winston Churchill amongst others said,

> Many forms of government have been tried and will be tried in this world of sin and woe. No one pretends that democracy is perfect or all-wise. Indeed it has been said that democracy is the worst form of Government except for all those other forms that have been tried from time to time.[9]

13

Life as a Consultant Surgeon

> The best portion of a good man's life are his little, nameless, unremembered acts of kindness and love.
>
> William Wordsworth

Amongst many in the public there is often a perception of glamour and a sense of awe around the idea of being a heart surgeon, perhaps only matched by the aura of being a brain surgeon.

Perceived by many over the centuries, and by some to this day, as the seat of the soul and emotions, the ability to interrupt its action and to correct pathology within it has been seen to need almost God-like qualities. Of course, the truth is far from these imaginings. Quoting Woody Allen in his comedy *Hannah and Her Sisters*, a 1986 Rollins and Joffe production, 'The heart is a very, very resilient little muscle. It really is.' The Renaissance genius, Leonardo da Vinci pointed out five centuries ago that, whatever properties we wish to bestow upon it, the heart is at its simplest, a pump made of muscle that requires its own blood supply, just like any other muscle. He reluctantly conceded a form of divine intervention, in one passage stating that it was designed by the 'great Master', recognising its natural exquisite structure.

We now acknowledge it as such but refined by millions of years of evolution. This exquisite piece of biological engineering has been created by functional needs and has not been satisfactorily or sustainably reproduced by any man-made attempts. Beating at least 34 million times a year throughout an average life time it is a wonder of nature. The complex interstices of muscular chambers, valves and supporting cords are beautiful to behold. The syncytium of muscle fibres that contract incessantly, and which can vary their power and rate and volume in response to changing physiological demands is truly remarkable. It is indeed a great wonder of the natural world. To be in a position to be able to spend one's working life manipulating and repairing it is truly a privilege granted to but few people following extensive training and experience.

Surgical correction of lesions on this organ requires great skill, dexterity and mental agility to deal with all that may befall the surgeon during the procedure. As with all operations there are those that are quite straightforward but then there are those that present situations that one may not have encountered before and tissues that demand the greatest care. Often times, the surgeon will find that a balletic like stance and manual agility is needed to place a stitch in just the right place and depth. Valve reconstruction and the correction of congenital lesions demands a high degree of imagination and the ability to see in three dimensions Every operation has the possibility of ending in disaster and the death of the patient. Each heart has its own unique characteristics, modified by the onset and progression of disease. In the most advanced cases of heart failure there is a grey area of the unknown as to how it will respond to the demands of the surgery, which even the most rigorous of preoperative investigation cannot fully prepare the surgeon for.

There is an enormous trust needed between the patient, their relatives and the surgeon into whose hands they place their very lives. To undertake this surgery on a regular basis, there is the demand for a confidence which may occasionally be seen as arrogance in the surgeon. As I mentioned earlier, the well-known television and radio agony aunt Claire Rayner, herself and ex-nurse, said to me that she would hate to be operated upon by a surgeon without a degree of confidence that could be interpreted as arrogance. An experienced surgeon needs to exude an air of confidence to reassure the patient, but overt arrogance can be dangerous. All of us know that disaster lurks around the corner for the unsuspecting, and a heightened awareness is necessary at all times. Decisiveness based upon experience and a deep and broad knowledge is also a pre-requisite. Many surgeons play music whilst operating but I do not as it inevitably disturbs my concentration to some degree. It is interesting to observe that whenever I have been in an operating room with another surgeon playing music, on the occasions of an unsuspected serious problem the first thing one hears is 'Turn the damned music off.' That tells me all that I need to know about the distraction that it can cause. Secondly of course, the team needed for open heart surgery comprises eight or more people, and to think that even one of them, not to mention all of the others, would have the same taste in music as the surgeon is to stretch credibility. Enforcing one's own choice is likely to jar the ears of several of the others in the team.

However, no matter how challenging and tiring the case may be, the satisfaction that its completion can bring, as close to perfection as one can get, is immense. Conversely, disaster brings with it sadness and often, a sense of lonely exposedness. Rarely is there anyone to support the surgeon following the death of a patient. Yes, we have deep feelings too and having got to know a patient and their family we also feel a deep sense of loss and of having let someone down badly. We have failed. Addressing the family following such a disaster is painful and difficult. It demands a great deal of courage to speak the truth in all its details to help the family to understand what and why things have happened as they have. I have absolutely no doubt that telling the truth from the beginning is absolutely essential no matter how hard, and if a mistake has occurred that must be addressed immediately. These interactions have to be carried out with the utmost empathy and take as much time as the family need.

I have found that being completely honest is often repaid by the wonderfully comforting remarks by relatives who are so appreciative of what you, just another human being, have striven to achieve for their loved one. Any omission of the truth or certainly any attempt to cover something up is to be avoided at all costs. Sadly, I have also encountered hospital managers attempting to fabricate a story to remove the burden of guilt from themselves and their institution. This along with ridiculously long intervals between the death or unexplained injury of a patient and a full explanation to the family are the greatest cause of quite reasonable discontent felt by the families and along with inadequate communication, are the most common causes of litigation. The families and friends of people are wonderfully supportive if properly informed and dealt with in an empathic way. I am perplexed by the action of some of my colleagues and in particular of some management in these demanding situations. The proffered care of a family must continue even after the death of a loved one. The saying that 'time is a great healer' can be subtly changed in these contexts to 'the allowance of as much time as is truly needed to explain and listen to the family at such important meetings, can allow a better healing process for all concerned, than the possibly destructive, short sharp passing of basic and incomplete information.' This can be a difficult thing to teach the surgeon in training, but it is among the most important of lessons to be learnt in this most caring of all professions.

There is a relative truism that was told to me by Dr John Kirklin at the end of my time in Alabama. He said that if you carry out the correct procedure, in the right way and at the right time in the appropriate patient, with the appropriate experience and awareness, none should die. This is sometimes a difficult ideal philosophy to follow but on reflection they are very wise words. The reality of confronting patients in real need will often distort rationality. It is very difficult to say no to someone near the end of their life, but occasionally it is the correct decision to make. However, if this is done with great care and empathy and not in a rushed environment with the proper support around the patient and taking great care to carry the family with you, a full understanding can be achieved. But then one always has to consider that you may be wrong and we have all had patients that have pulled through the most harrowing of circumstances against the odds. There is rarely a clearly correct decision. All that one can do is to use the information gained from experience and published data to guide you. To be asked for a second opinion should also be embraced as part of the patient journey if they felt it would help them. It should not be seen as a slight on the surgeon first consulted, but a process of the fullest attempt to do the right thing for the patient. Despite all of this and the introduction of risk score analysis it is impossible to get it right all of the time.

This can also be a source of conflict between surgeons/physicians, lawyers and management. The popular deployment of multidisciplinary teams also does not solve all of the problems. Decisions can be carried by the intervention of a heavy handed loud individual intimidating others into silence. Also a senior and perceived more experienced participant can quieten others who otherwise would have important contributions to make. In some settings inexperience can dominate the process, driving forwards inappropriate decisions. In addition, uncertainty can draw out the management of a patient by the insistence of unnecessary investigations wasting time and adding extra cost. In truth, medicine and surgery has a degree of uncertainty that can never be completely irradicated.

Above all it has been a privilege to have been able to spend the last forty years tending to unwell people from all walks of life at the most vulnerable time in their lives. Receiving their trust to operate on their vital organs when an error can result in the death of the patient is humbling. Thankfully, the vast majority of patients are helped back to a normal life and the emotions that they express are very moving. Every patient had a different story to tell from, the most humble to the most senior figures in society. All are rendered low and vulnerable by life threatening illness. The advances in modern medicine and surgery allow for the correction of all but the most advanced disease states. To have been able to be a part of both the treatment of a fellow human being but also to make small advances in knowledge, moving the specialty forwards has been very special.

Finally it is important for me to acknowledge the support and companionship of my surgical and medical colleagues during these last forty years. At difficult times the only person who can really understand the predicament that we face is a colleague who has experienced similar circumstances. Also, the willingness of colleagues to offer help at any time of the day or night has been fundamental in delivering the best possible care for our patients. Indeed all of us regard it as a privilege to be asked for support and help by a colleague, knowing that each would do the same for the other without any hesitation. It has been a wonderful professional environment. Modern medical professionalism demands a reflective frame of mind. It is time for managers to exhibit the same degree of reflection on their own actions.

Working in the NHS in the Twenty-first Century

During my fifty years working within the National Health Service, I have witnessed huge changes. There have been several reorganisations by successive governments, but the overarching issues have been the inadequacy of funding, enormous wastage and latterly more aggressive and controlling management. The separation of government, who control the purse strings, and those providing care for the nation's people is vast and growing decade on decade. Nationalised health care has significant problems that have never been properly resolved. The basic question is 'To whom should the providers of health care be answerable?' And the only response has to be 'Those using the service.' In the current set up, the distance is too great between those providing the funds, those distributing them, and the consumer.

The modern NHS throws up challenges that we did not experience two decades and more ago. Consultant surgeons have been significantly emasculated. Often surgical instruments are poor and need replacing but budgets are claimed to be too tight to allow for that to occur on a regular basis. Discipline is often poor and attempts to retain control are met with complaints by theatre staff. In some institutions there is an atmosphere of low-grade fear amongst surgical colleagues which is very unhealthy. The working environment that I witness in other developed countries is quite unlike the situation here and more like the environment that we used to work in. Cardiac surgery demands people of character and emotional strength in all professional groups. The shortage of people wanting to work in the NHS is causing the appointment of many who are lacking in experience, who are then thrust into the front-line with little support. This causes fear within them and the likelihood that they will leave the specialty early. In addition the poor progression in terms and conditions allowed within the cardiac surgical unit is so poor that the staff leave for other areas of nursing that are less demanding, and which are often paid better. All of this is happening whilst senior managers claim success in saving money.

At the same time, money is wasted on consultancy companies, most of whom have little understanding of the real situation that we all face, when it ought to be spent on frontline services. Better advice could be obtained from experienced consultant and nursing staff, who, more often than is sensible are not listened to, or not consulted in the first place. In my role as thoracic services manager I had to contend with several management consultants brought in at various times under government reorganisations. More than one has said to me latterly that they had learnt more from us than they had been able to pass on. Indeed one group thanked me for the teaching that we have given them as they walked off with many tens of thousands of taxpayers' pounds.

There is a dissonance between the rate of growth of the population and those surviving longer and the provision of health care. In 1947 and 1948, at the inception of the health service, the population was approximately 42 million. It has increased to approximately 68 million. The number of diseases that could be treated and the cost of available treatments then was a fraction of the current situation. Thus costs have risen exponentially and way beyond progressive investment.

Successive generations of doctors have tried to bring about meaningful change, but most attempts have fallen on deaf ears. Probably the most effective change was brought about by the Blair government when waiting times for treatment fell with significant well-targeted investment. Subsequently the financial crash of 2008 wrought a new round of austerity under the Cameron/Osborne partnership which paved the way for the current disastrous situation, wherein the NHS has been described as 'broken' by the current health secretary. Doctors' and nurses' pay has been seriously eroded and the conditions of work deteriorated significantly. Through all of this senior management has been largely quiet and fostering their own situations. I have never witnessed morale as low as it is at the present time. Dilapidated hospitals, diminished nurse numbers and young doctors emigrating along with many of their established seniors to better conditions.

For much of the latter decades of the twentieth century, the UK PLC was spending approximately three percent of GDP on health whereas most developed Western countries such as Germany, France and the Scandinavian countries were spending between ten and twelve percent. Even the USA was spending around twelve and a half percent of GDP in addition to the huge private/insurance sector. If these differences are multiplied over decades the funding gap can be seen to be enormous. No wonder that making it up at all is a mammoth task. Tony Blair announced that he was going to increase UK spending from the current three percent at that time to the European average of seven percent. However, that only brought us to the level of Greece and other much poorer countries. We are still nowhere near the funding level of equivalent countries to our own, never mind catching up the deficit.

Senior hospital management and politicians seem reluctant to listen to criticism. Far too often their default position is to throw criticism back to the medical staff with the demand for increasing productivity. If the attitude towards doctors does not change, no end of substitution of the profession with enhanced non-medically trained staff will substitute for a well-trained and highly motivated medical profession. More recently a significant battle has developed between the medical profession and a new group of physician's assistants [PAs]. It makes no sense that the government and indeed the Royal Colleges can think that six years at medical school and a further decade of training can be replaced by a few years of protocol driven, 'on the job training' in the absence of a deep knowledge of the medical sciences. It is the patients that will pay dearly in the end. The public's deep dissatisfaction with general practice has translated into a flood of patients going straight to A & E departments, instead of their GP, overwhelming the capacity of the emergency departments to cope with the true emergencies which ought to be their bread and butter.

The renegotiated GP contract has a lot to do with the current situation. The old-style cradle to grave practice with community visits, cottage hospitals and night and weekend call has gone, removing the GP from the true family setting which was once their calling, and has removed many from being the patients' friend. It is almost impossible to see the same doctor twice, a situation that was endorsed by recent rule changes. The developed relationship and knowledge of a patient and their family that contact with the same doctor gives cannot be overestimated. The trust of the patient and the enhanced care through previous knowledge and the satisfaction gained by the doctor is immeasurable. A significant uplift in GP numbers, commensurate with the significant population rise accompanied by a small charge for a GP visit would begin to rectify the appalling situations that now prevail.

The fall in the standard of education of trainee doctors needs to be addressed. The profession is in dire need of protection from the educationalists, who invoke a style of approach to medical school training that deviates more and more from the importance of the basic sciences towards one more akin to the soft social sciences. A deep understanding of the structure and function of the body is the bedrock of medical practice, recognised as far back as Hippocrates and Aristotle.

It seems to have been completely forgotten that health provision is not a business in any normal sense of the word. The management should be good quality civil servants acting as administrators ensuring that the taxpayer's money is delivered to frontline services in the most efficient fashion.

Bullying and harassment of medical staff is rife and many work in fear of the call or letter from the (in)human resources department for some trivial misdemeanour or other. In short, morale in the health service in twenty-first century England appears to be at an all-time low. Again, in the words of the new Labour government Secretary of State for Health Wes Streeting, 'The NHS is broken.'

The vast majority of doctors are highly motivated bright professionals who want to do the best for their patients, but are bloodied and bowed by uncaring, unkind, often bullying and all too frequently poor-quality management, so far removed from the frontline of care that the day-to-day needs are lost in mountains of paperwork.

Is there a possible solution to this? Well, it will need a complete rethink of the way hospitals are managed and the way that so much money is wasted. Is it likely to happen? The disbandment of NHS England could be seen as a start down this road, but the problem as I see it lies buried in the bowels of the individual trust management structures. Many of us on the frontline hope and long for this to happen as without it the NHS funding stream as we know it will be forced to be torn apart and some form of hybrid insurance and tax -based system introduced. We know that the American insurance companies and private hospitals are itching to get a larger foothold in the United Kingdom, with a significant base already present. Perhaps their much more efficient systems would be a good development.

Despite all of this doom and gloom, medicine remains the noblest of all the professions and the capacity to do good for one's fellow man on a daily basis is incalculable. With the appropriate reduction in trust in religious bodies, as a result of the appalling behaviour within their ranks, and the law in disrepair, the medical and allied professions are the only ones that the population can turn to for true meaningful and productive care. It is vital that all of us with a calling to this most demanding of jobs continue to give hope and encouragement to the next generation, as without the proper investment in training and encouragement in the next generation of doctors we are lost.

How many other professions is one able to go home at the end of each day or night knowing that you have helped not just one, but several fellow human beings, even in the reduced circumstances of the NHS in 2025.

14

Life in Cambridge

I have often felt that my career may have taken a more rewarding path if I had managed to be a consultant on the London scene, specifically at Brompton hospital, which in several ways felt like an Alma Mater for me. I loved the Arts world that surrounds everyone in that, the prince of world cities, and to have been able to live in the region of the Fulham or Brompton roads would have been idyllic. However, the move to Cambridge brought with it a range of different life options. Living in a small village, Great Gransden, felt more like the environment that I had grown up in and the drive to and from work through the countryside was restorative.

The city itself, dominated by the ancient colleges with their wonderful hidden spaces, has a flourishing arts scene, not least in the sphere of music. There is a concert almost every evening of one kind or another. The academic scene is vibrant and ever-changing. It certainly was a wonderful environment for the children to grow up and be educated in. There are more excellent schools of private or state style per square mile than almost anywhere else in the country.

Being a London graduate I was not immediately immersed in college life. A few early years spent as a surgical supervisor at St John's college, organised by David Dunn, the senior medical tutor there, was extremely rewarding, but I did not have a college affiliation. That all changed a few years ago, when quite out of the blue, an invitation to become a life fellow of Clare Hall dropped onto the mat. To this day I have no idea how it came about and to some extent I have a degree of imposter syndrome, being surrounded by academic luminaries from all around the world.

Under the excellent presidency of Professor Alan Short, wonderfully supported by his wife Slaine, the college is punching way above its natural weight and has a loud voice in University affairs. A distinguished Architecture Professor, Alan has raised the bar of expectations of the college, and practically all have been achieved.

Dinners in college present a smorgasbord of new and interesting personalities. One day you are sitting next to the Royal Astronomer and the next a concert pianist or expert in artificial intelligence. All are warm and kind towards you as one stumbles through trying to make intelligent conversation on subjects far removed from one's own field. From candlelit dinners at top table in Magdalene college through to the vaulted medieval halls of Trinity, King's and St John's, the experience is life-enhancing. One hopes that the privilege that the students enjoy is fully appreciated and absorbed by them all.

I have been able to contribute in my own small way by staging exhibitions on Leonardo and my own series of large-scale photographs, 'A week in the life of a cardiac surgeon'.

More recently life has come full circle with two of my children, Joanna and Nicholas, now grown and with families of their own, living back in Cambridge. My youngest, Olivia, is pursuing a Master's degree course in another hauntingly beautiful city, Durham.

Several of the colleges hold evensong services in the college chapels and when one has the time it is spiritually uplifting to sit quietly and be transported to another world in beautiful choral music, in medieval settings witnessing an ageless tradition.

With London relatively close by, regular trips to theatre, opera and ballet still play a large part in my life as do the major galleries and museums. We are blessed with the wonderful Fitzwilliam museum in Cambridge with a relatively small but world class collection of works from all periods.

The accidents in life often bring the greatest rewards, and so it has been with my unpredicted move to Cambridge and a hugely rewarding life in this great medieval city. I am grateful to the God of fate that led me here.

> Isn't it strange that princes and kings, and clowns that caper in sawdust rings, and common people like you and me are builders for eternity. Each is given a bag of tools, a shapeless mass, a book of rules; Each must make ere life has flown a stumbling block or a stepping stone.
>
> R. L. Sharpe, 'A Bag of Tools', c. 1890

Endnotes

Chapter 1: Life in a Sleepy English Village

1. A. E. Houseman. 'Canto L' in *A Shropshire Lad.* (Harrap Ltd., London, 1982).
2. William Barrie, Yaoling Yang et al. 'Elevated Genetic Risk for Multiple Sclerosis Emerged in Steppe Pastoralist Populations.' (*Nature* 625, 2024) p. 321-328.
3. Salman Rushdie. *Knife*. p. 38. (Jonathon Cape, London, 2024).

Chapter 2: A Family at War

1. Horace *Odes* (III.2.13)
2. *Hartford Courant*, (Hartford, Connecticut, Friday 9 January 1931) p. 24.
3. Alan Clark. *The Donkeys*. (Pimlico, London, 1961 edition), p. 119.
4. Charteris, Brigadier-General, Earl Haig. Report from 28th April 1915. (Cassell 1929; G.H.Q. (Cassell 1931).
5. Dante Alighieri. 'Canto 16', *The Divine Comedy*. (The London Folio Society, London, 1st edition, Translation by Robin Kirkpatrick, 2023) p. 291.
6. Col. A. Crookenden. *The History of the Cheshire Regiment in the Great War*. (Naval & Military Press, Uckfield, 2005), p. 173.

Chapter 3: School Days

1. Leonardo da Vinci. Codex Foster III. 14r.

Chapter 4: Medical School at Last

1. J. Croker. 'Exchange between Boswell and Dr. Johnson' from Boswell's *Life of Johnson* (John Murray, London, 1839).
2. N. Robinson & F. Wells. 'Distribution and Localisation of Sites of Gamma Aminobutyric Acid Metabolism in the Adult Rat Brain.' (*Journal of* Anatomy, 114,3, 1973) pp. 365–378.
3. Obituaries. (*The Lancet*. 114. 25 July 1863), p. 114–115.
4. William Hunter MD FRCP. From, *Historical Account of Charing Cross Hospital and Medical School*. (John Murray, London, 1914), p. 31.
5. Dava Sobel. *Longitude*. (Fourth Estate, London. 1996).

Chapter 5: Now the Real Pain Begins – Pre-registration House Jobs

1. Leonardo da Vinci. Codex Atlanticus 289v.
2. Oliver Shah. 'Tony Blair, World King. In an interview with Oliver Shah.' (*Sunday Times Magazine*. 21 April 2024).

Chapter 8: Winchester, Cambridge and London Again

1. Canalis R., Ciavolella M and Finucci V. (eds), *Rethinking Medical Humanities. Perspectives From the Arts and the Social Sciences* (de Gruyter, Berlin, Leiden, 2023).
2. F. C. Wells. *The Role of Architecture and the Decorative Arts in Renaissance Medicine. In Disease and Disability in Medieval and Early Modern Art and* Literature, (Brepols, Turnhout, 2021), p. 204–228.
3. James Scott, Richard Cork, Zoe Penn, Andrew Hall, Anouk Mercier, David Ferry, Grace Saull, Lewis Khan, *The Healing Arts: The Arts Project at Chelsea and Westminster Hospital*. (Unicorn, Lewes, 2019).
4. F C Wells. 'The Iliac Streak: A New Radiological Sign of a Perforated Appendix in Peritonitis.' (*The British Journal of Clinical Practice*. April 1983 Vol. 37, No.4), p. 153–5.

5. Denton Cooley. *100,000 Hearts. A Surgeon's Memoir.* (Briscoe Center for American History, Austin, 2012), p. 82.
6. Ibid., p. 82.
7. T. Higenbottam, D. Wheeldon, F. Wells and J. Wallwork. 'Long-term Treatment of Primary Pulmonary Hypertension with Continuous Intravenous Epoprostenol (prostacyclin).' (*Lancet.* 1984 May 12;1(8385)), p. 1046–7.
8. Personal communication with the author and John Webster Kirklin, MD; 'A Conversation with the Editor', (*American Journal of Cardiology*,1998; 81) p. 1027–1044.
9. Alain Carpentier. 'Cardiac Valve Surgery – The "French Correction"', (*Journal of Thoracic and Cardiovascular Surgery*, September 1983 Number 3) p. 323–337.

Chapter 9: Fun with the Arts

1. K. D. Keele, *Leonardo da Vinci on Movement of the Heart and Blood.* (Harvey and Blythe Ltd. London, 1952).
2. B.J. Bellhouse and F.H. Bellhouse, 'Mechanism of Closure of the Aortic Valve.' (*Nature* 217 (5123), 1968), p. 66–7.
3. Royal Collection. W 1970 v. K.P. 113r.
4. Leonardo da Vinci. Windsor Royal Collection. W 1970r. Quaderni IV. 167a.
5. Leonardo da Vinci. Windsor Royal Collection. W 19071r. Quaderni II 1 r/c. 1513g.
6. Leonardo da Vinci. Windsor 1908 4r.
7. Codex Atlanticus 119 verso.
8. Francis Robicsek. 'Leonardo da Vinci and the Sinuses of Valsalva.' (*The Annals of Thoracic Surgery*, Vol. 52, issue 2, 1991), p.328-335.
9. Leonardo da Vinci. Codice Atlantico, Foglio 70r.
10. Siobhan Davies Studios, London. 'In Plain Clothes', (*Independent* Sunday 7 May 2006).
11. James Peto (ed). *The Heart.* (Yale University Press, New Haven and Wellcome Collection. 2007).
12. Mariléne Oliver and Francis Wells. 'Resurrecting Leonardo's Great Lady: A Collaboration.' (*Leonardo.* The MIT press, Volume 41, No 5, October 2008), p. 500–505.
13. Rinaldo Canalis, Massimo Ciavolella and Valeria Finucci (eds.) *Rethinking Medical Humanities. Perspectives from the Arts and the Social Sciences.* (De Gruyter, Berlin, Leiden, 2023).

14. Rinaldo Canalis and Massimo Ciavolella (eds.) *Disease and Disability in Medieval and Early Modern Art and Literature.* (Bepols, Turnhout, 2021).
15. Morteza Gharib et al. 'Leonardo's Visualisation of Gravity as a Form of Acceleration.' (*Leonardo* (2023) 56 (1)) p. 21–2.
16. Cyrano de Bergerac. *Voyages to the Moon and the Sun.* (Folio Society Books, London, 2023).
17. Tom Wolfe. *The Right Stuff*, (Farrar, Straus and Giroux, USA, 1979, Jonathon Cape Ltd., UK, 1983).

Chapter 10: Motoring Adventures with Sir Stirling Moss and Friends

1. Norman Tebbit. 'I loved my Spitting Image puppet'. (*The Oldie*, September 2020).
2. David Mason. *Thalidomide. My Fight.* (Allen & Unwin, London, 1976).
3. BBC News. '94-year-old Peer Passes Driving Test.' (Monday 21 July 2003, 15:38 GMT).

Chapter 11: 'New' Home Alabama

1. With respect to Rossington, Van Zant and Ed King. The song's writers.
2. Kolessov VI. 'Mammary Artery-Coronary Artery Anastomosis as a Method of Treatment for Angina Pectoris.' (*Journal of Thoracic and Cardiovascular Surgery*, 1967; 54), p. 535–44.

Chapter 12: So, This is What It is all About

1. Denton A. Cooley. *100,000 Hearts. A Surgeon's Memoir.* Chapter 13. (Dolph Briscoe Center for American History, Austin, 2012).
2. Terence English. *Follow Your Star. From Mining to Heart Transplants. A Surgeon's Story.* Pp. 130–1. (AuthorHouse©. UK Ltd, 2011).
3. M. Migliore, C. Choong, E. Lim, A. Goldsmith, A. Ritchie, F. Wells. 'A Surgeon's Case Volume of Oesophagectomy for Cancer Strongly Influences the Operative Mortality Rate.' (*European Journal of Cardio-thoracic Surgery* Vol 32, Issue 2, August 2007), p. 375–380.
4. H. M. Harrison. *Voyager in Time and Space. The Life of John Couch Adams Cambridge Astronomer.* (The Book Guild Limited, Market Harborough, 1994).

5. G. Baer, P. Talonen and F. Wells. 'Diaphragm Pacing.' (*Correspondence, Thorax*. 1988; 43), p. 743.
6. M. Jackson, M. King, Hockley, F. Wells and J. Shneerson. 'Early Experience with an Implantable Intratracheal Oxygen Catheter.' (*British Medical Journal*, 7 April 1990, Vol. 300.), p. 909–910.
7. D. Lindblom, L. Rodriguez and V. Bjork. 'Mechanical Failure of the Björk-Shiley Valve.' (*Journal of Thoracic and Cardiovascular Surgery*. 1986; 92), p. 894–907.
8. T. Treasure, A. Hollman. 'The Surgery of Mitral Stenosis 1898–1948. Why Did it Take 50 Years to Establish Mitral Valvotomy.' (*The Annals of The Royal College of Surgeons of England*, 1995; 77), p. 145–151.
9. R Langworth. *Churchill by Himself. The Definitive Collection of Quotations*. (Ebury Press, London, 2011), p. 574.